Tyldesley & Grieve's Muscles, Nerves and Movement in Human Occupation

Fourth edition

Ian R. McMillan

MEd, PgDip Ed Res, Dip COT, Cert Ed
Senior Lecturer in Occupational Therapy
School of Health Sciences
Queen Margaret University
Edinburgh, UK

Gail Carin-Levy

BSc (Hons) OT, COT
Lecturer in Occupational Therapy
School of Health Sciences
Queen Margaret University
Edinburgh, UK

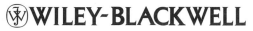
WILEY-BLACKWELL
A John Wiley & Sons, Ltd., Publication

This edition first published 2012 © 2012 by Ian R. McMillan, Gail Carin-Levy, Barbara Tyldesley and June I. Grieve

Blackwell Publishing was acquired by John Wiley & Sons in February 2007. Blackwell's publishing program has been merged with Wiley's global Scientific, Technical and Medical business to form Wiley-Blackwell.

Registered office: John Wiley & Sons, Ltd, The Atrium, Southern Gate, Chichester, West Sussex, PO19 8SQ, UK

Editorial offices: 9600 Garsington Road, Oxford, OX4 2DQ, UK
The Atrium, Southern Gate, Chichester, West Sussex, PO19 8SQ, UK
111 River Street, Hoboken, NJ 07030-5774, USA

For details of our global editorial offices, for customer services and for information about how to apply for permission to reuse the copyright material in this book please see our website at www.wiley.com/wiley-blackwell.

Library of Congress Cataloging-in-Publication Data
Tyldesley & Grieve's muscles, nerves and movement in human occupation. / Ian R. McMillan & Gail Carin-Levy – 4th ed. / Ian R. McMillan ... [et al.].
    p. ; cm.
Muscles, nerves, and movement in human occupation
Rev. ed. of: Muscles, nerves and movement / Barbara Tyldesley and June I. Grieve. 3rd ed. 2002.
Includes bibliographical references and index.
ISBN 978-1-4051-8929-3 (pbk. : alk. paper)
I. McMillan, Ian R.   II. Tyldesley, Barbara. Muscles, nerves and movement.   III. Title: Muscles, nerves and movement in human occupation.
[DNLM: 1. Movement–physiology. 2. Motor Skills. 3. Muscles–physiology. 4. Nervous System–anatomy & histology. 5. Nervous System Physiological Phenomena. 6. Occupational Therapy–methods. WE 103]
LC classification not assigned
612.7'6–dc23
                                                                        2011030349

A catalogue record for this book is available from the British Library.

Set in 10/12pt Calibri by Toppan Best-set Premedia Limited
Printed and bound in Singapore by Markono Print Media Pte Ltd

4   2015

Tyldesley &
Muscles, Nerves and
Movement in Human
Occupation

0

Contents

Preface to the fourth edition

The first edition of this book was published by Barbara Tyldesley and June Grieve in 1989 with the intention of studying anatomy combined with undertanding movement in daily living. Since then, subsequent editions have added chapters and further detail in numerous ways to promote and meet the original aim.

This new fourth edition enhances that original aim by revising the text, revising the practice note-pads which highlight some of the common conditions seen in clients/patients that students and therapists will encounter, adding key terms and a conceptual overview at the beginning of each chapter and providing a summary at the end of each chapter. There has also been a comprehensive revision of the figures and overall addition of colour throughout.

Section I introduces you to the idea of movement by looking at the basic units of structure and function, movement terminology and the structure and function of the central and peripheral nervous system that are involved in the control of movement.

Section II continues with the anatomy of movement in everyday living by examining the positioning movements of the shoulder and elbow, the manipulative movements produced by the forearm, wrist and hand, the nerve supply to the upper limb, the role of the lower limb in support and propulsion, the nerve supply to the lower limb and the role of the trunk in posture and breathing.

Section III looks at the sensorimotor control of movement that includes the sensory background to movement and motor control.

Section IV turns your attention to Human Occupation by firstly looking at occupational performance skills and capacities. The remaining part of this section examines different case scenarios where understanding anatomy, movement, the effects of conditions and how this influences human occupations are considered.

We trust this book will be useful not only to you as a student embarking on your career as an allied health professional, but also to practitioners in a variety of settings.

Ian R. McMillan, Gail Carin-Levy

Acknowledgements

We would like to extend our sincere thanks to all of the team associated with the production of this book at various stages: Cathryn Gates, Ruth Swan, Sarah Crawley-Vigneau and Joanna Brocklesby. We would also like to extend our thanks to Jane Fallows who completely revised and redrew all the figures for this new edition.

We very much appreciate the time and energy given by Linda Gnanasekaran who originally produced Chapter 13 in this edition.

We are also grateful to occupational therapists Ronnie Bentley, Linda Gwilliam and Louise Hogan who originally contributed to the case scenario exercises in Chapter 14 of this edition.

Finally and most importantly, we would like to take this opportunity to recognise the immense achivements of Barbara Tyldesley and June Grieve. They both pioneered the idea for this book to facilitate the education of health care students, with the first edition being published in 1989. Since then, countless numbers of students and qualified staff have utilised Tyldesley and Grieve's seminal textbook to deepen their understanding of the human body, the integration required for movement and its use in daily occupations.

'If we have seen further it is by standing on the shoulders of giants'
Isaac Newton 1676

Ian R. McMillan, Gail Carin-Levy

Section I
Introduction to movement

Components of the musculoskeletal and nervous system, movement terminology

- Basic units, structure and function: supporting tissues, muscle and nerves
- Movement terminology
- The central nervous system: the brain and spinal cord
- The peripheral nervous system: cranial and spinal nerves

1

Basic units, structure and function: supporting tissues, muscle and nerve

Key terms

connective tissues, articulations, skeletal muscle, neurone, muscle tone

Conceptual overview

This chapter addresses the basic components of structure that are organised to allow movement at joint level. Nerves, muscles and connective tissues work together to produce movement: connective tissues which provide stability and support; skeletal muscle which changes in length and pulls on bones to produce movements at joints; and neurones and nerves which conduct information between the environmental sensors, the control centres for movement and the muscles.

Tyldesley & Grieve's Muscles, Nerves and Movement in Human Occupation, Fourth Edition. Ian R. McMillan, Gail Carin-Levy.
© 2012 Ian R. McMillan, Gail Carin-Levy, Barbara Tyldesley and June I. Grieve. Published 2012 by Blackwell Publishing Ltd.

Framework and support: the connective tissues

The overall function of connective tissue is to unite or connect structures in the body, and to give support. Bone is a connective tissue which provides the rigid framework for support. Where bones articulate with each other dense fibrous connective tissue, rich in collagen fibres, surrounds the ends of the bones, allowing movement to occur while maintaining stability. Cartilage, another connective tissue, is also found associated with joints, where it forms a compressible link between two bones, or provides a low-friction surface for smooth movement of one bone on another. Connective tissue attaches muscles to bone, in the form of either a cord (tendon) or a flat sheet (fascia). The connective tissues may be divided into:

- **dense fibrous tissue**;
- **cartilage**;
- **bone**.

Dense fibrous tissue

Dense fibrous connective tissue unites structures in the body while still allowing movement to occur. It has high tensile strength to resist stretching forces. This connective tissue has few cells and is largely made up of fibres of collagen and elastin that give the tissue great strength. The fibres are produced by fibroblast cells that lie in between the fibres (Figure 1.1). The toughness

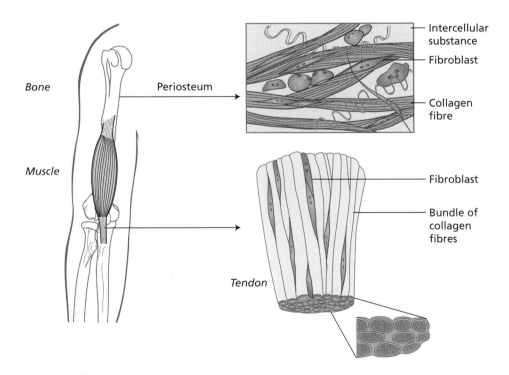

Figure 1.1 Dense fibrous connective tissue seen covering bone as periosteum, and forming the tendon of a skeletal muscle.

of this tissue can be felt when cutting through stewing steak with a blunt knife. The muscle fibres are easily sliced, but the covering of white connective tissue is very tough. Examples of this tissue are as follows:

- The **capsule** surrounding the movable (synovial) joints which binds the bones together (see Figure 1.7).
- **Ligaments** form strong bands that join bone to bone. Ligaments strengthen the joint capsules in particular directions and limit movement.
- **Tendons** unite the contractile fibres of muscle to bone.

In tendons and ligaments, the collagenous fibres lie in parallel in the direction of greatest stress.

- An **aponeurosis** is a strong flat membrane, with collagen fibres that lie in different directions to form sheets of connective tissue. An aponeurosis can form the attachment of a muscle, such as the oblique abdominal muscles, which meet in the midline of the abdomen (see Chapter 10, Figure 10.6). In the palm of the hand and the sole of the foot an aponeurosis lies deep to the skin and forms a protective layer for the tendons underneath (see Chapter 8, Figure 8.21).
- A **retinaculum** is a band of dense fibrous tissue that binds tendons of muscles and prevents bowstring during movement. An example is the flexor retinaculum of the wrist, which holds the tendons of muscles passing into the hand in position (see Chapter 6, Figure 6.15).
- **Fascia** is a term used for the large areas of dense fibrous tissue that surround the musculature of all the body segments. Fascia is particularly developed in the limbs, where it dips down between the large groups of muscles and attaches to the bone. In some areas, fascia provides a base for the attachment of muscles, for example the thoracolumbar fascia gives attachment to the long muscles of the back (see Chapter 10, Figure 10.6).
- **Periosteum** is the protective covering of bones. Tendons and ligaments blend with the periosteum around bone (see Figure 1.3).
- **Dura** is thick fibrous connective tissue protecting the brain and spinal cord (see Chapter 3, Figure 3.21).

Cartilage

Cartilage is a tissue that can be compressed and has resilience. The cells (chondrocytes) are oval and lie in a ground substance that is not rigid like bone. There is no blood supply to cartilage, so there is a limit to its thickness. The tissue has great resistance to wear, but cannot be repaired when damaged.

Hyaline cartilage is commonly called gristle. It is smooth and glass-like, forming a low-friction covering to the articular surfaces of joints. In the elderly, the articular cartilage tends to become eroded or calcifies, so that joints become stiff. Hyaline cartilage forms the costal cartilages which join the anterior ends of the ribs to the sternum (Figure 1.2). In the developing foetus, most of the bones are formed in hyaline cartilage. When the cartilaginous model of each bone reaches a critical size for the survival of the cartilage cells, ossification begins.

Reflective task

Look at some large animal bones from the butcher to see the cartilage covering the joint surfaces at the end. Note that it is bluish and looks like glass.

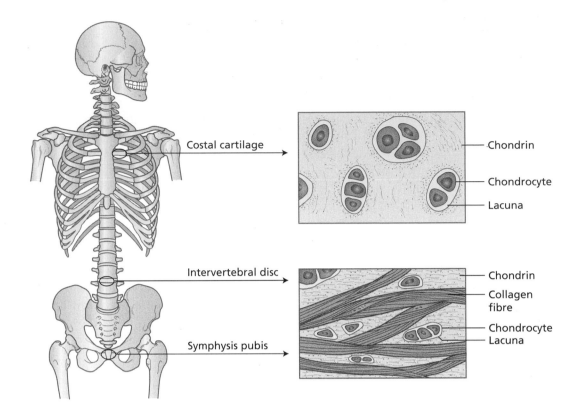

Figure 1.2   Microscopic structure of hyaline and fibrocartilage, location in the skeleton of the trunk.

Fibrocartilage consists of cartilage cells lying in between densely packed collagen fibres (Figure 1.2). The fibres give extra strength to the tissue while retaining its resilience. Examples of where fibrocartilage is found are the discs between the bones of the vertebral column, the pubic symphysis joining the two halves of the pelvis anteriorly, and the menisci in the knee joint.

Bone

Bone is the tissue that forms the rigid supports for the body by containing a large proportion of calcium salts (calcium phosphate and carbonate). It must be remembered that bone is a living tissue composed of cells and an abundant blood supply. It has a greater capacity for repair after damage than any other tissue in the body, except for blood. The strength of bone lies in the thin plates (lamellae), composed of collagen fibres with calcium salts deposited in between. The lamellae lie in parallel, held together by fibres, and the bone cells or **osteocytes** are found in between. Each bone cell lies in a small space or lacuna, and connects with other cells and to blood capillaries by fine channels called canaliculi (Figure 1.3).

In **compact bone**, the lamellae are laid down in concentric rings around a central canal containing blood vessels. Each system of concentric lamellae (known as a Haversian system or an osteon)

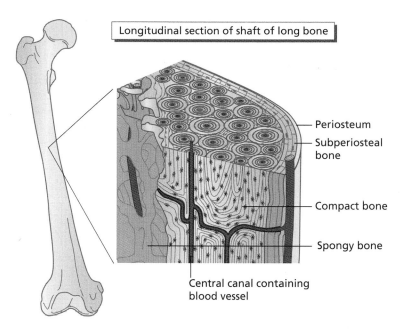

Longitudinal section of shaft of long bone

- Periosteum
- Subperiosteal bone
- Compact bone
- Spongy bone

Central canal containing blood vessel

Figure 1.3   A section of the shaft of a long bone.

lies in a longitudinal direction. Many of these systems are closely packed to form the dense compact bone found in the shaft of long bones (Figure 1.3).

Practice note-pad 1A: osteoporosis

Osteoporosis is literally a condition of porous bones, largely due to a depletion of calcium from the body. For a number of reasons, calcium loss exceeds calcium absorption from the diet, causing bone mass to decrease excessively. This leads to fractures occurring as a result of normal mechanical stresses upon the skeleton which it would normally withstand. Spontaneous fractures may also occur.

In **cancellous** or trabeculate bone, the lamellae form plates arranged in different directions to form a mesh. The plates are known as trabeculae and the spaces in between contain blood capillaries. The bone cells lying in the trabeculae communicate with each other and with the spaces by canaliculi. The expanded ends of long bones are filled with cancellous bone covered with a thin layer of compact bone. The central cavity of the shaft of long bones contains bone marrow. This organisation of the two types of bone produces a structure with great rigidity without excessive weight (Figure 1.4). Bone has the capacity to remodel in shape in response to the stresses on it, so that the structure lines of the trabeculae at the ends of the bone follow the lines of force on the bone. For example, the lines of trabeculae at the ends of weight-bearing bones, such as

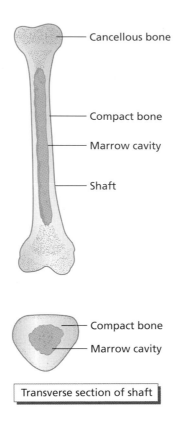

Cancellous bone

Compact bone

Marrow cavity

Shaft

Compact bone

Marrow cavity

Transverse section of shaft

Figure 1.4   Gross structure of long bone: longitudinal and transverse sections.

the femur, provide maximum strength to support the body weight against gravity. Remodelling of bone is achieved by the activity of bone-forming cells known as osteoblasts, and bone-destroying cells known as osteoclasts; both types of cell are found in bone tissue. The calcium salts of bone are constantly interchanging with calcium ions in the blood, under the influence of hormones (parathormone and thyrocalcitonin). Bone is a living, constantly changing connective tissue that provides a rigid framework on which muscles can exert forces to produce movement.

Reflective task

Look at any of the following examples of connective tissue that are available to you:

(1)   Microscopic slides of dense fibrous tissue, cartilage and bone, noting the arrangement of the cellular and fibre content.
(2)   Dissected material of joints and muscles which include tendons, ligaments, aponeurosis and retinaculum.
(3)   Fresh butcher's bone: note the pink colour (blood supply), and the central cavity in the shaft of long bones.
(4)   Fresh red meat to see fibrous connective tissue around muscle.

Articulations

Where the rigid bones of the skeleton meet, connective tissues are organised to bind the bones together and to form joints. It is the joints that allow movement of the segments of the body relative to each other. The joints or articulations between bones can be divided into three types based on the particular connective tissues involved. The three main classes of joint are **fibrous**, **cartilaginous** and **synovial**.

Fibrous joints

Here, the bones are united by dense fibrous connective tissue.

The **sutures** of the skull are fibrous joints that allow no movement between the bones. The edge of each bone is irregular and interlocks with the adjacent bone, a layer of fibrous tissue linking them (Figure 1.5a).

A **syndesmosis** is a joint where the bones are joined by a ligament that allows some movement between the bones. A syndesmosis is found between the radius and the ulna (Figure 1.5b). The interosseous membrane allows movement of the forearm.

A **gomphosis** is a specialised fibrous joint that fixes the teeth in the sockets of the jaw (Figure 1.5c).

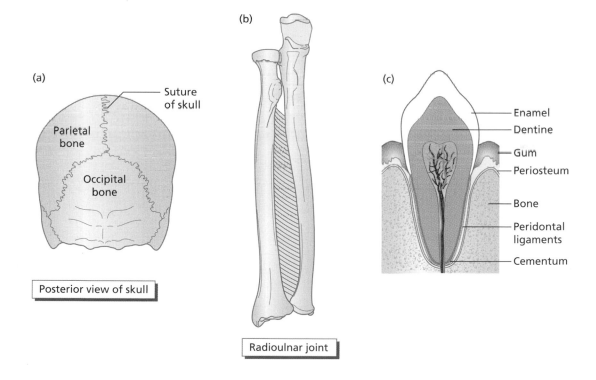

Figure 1.5   Fibrous joints: (a) suture between bones of the skull; (b) syndesmosis between the radius and ulna; (c) gomphosis: tooth in socket.

Cartilaginous joints

In these joints the bones are united by cartilage.

A **synchondrosis** or primary cartilaginous joint is a joint where the union is composed of hyaline cartilage. This type of joint is also called primary cartilaginous. The articulation of the first rib with the sternum is by a synchondrosis. During growth of the long bones of the skeleton, there is a synchondrosis between the ends and the shaft of the bone, where temporary cartilage forms the epiphyseal plate. These plates disappear when growth stops and the bone becomes ossified (Figure 1.6a).

A **symphysis** or secondary cartilaginous joint is a joint where the joint surfaces are covered by a thin layer of hyaline cartilage and united by a disc of fibrocartilage. This type of joint (sometimes called secondary cartilaginous) allows a limited amount of movement between the bones by compression of the cartilage. The bodies of the vertebrae articulate by a disc of fibrocartilage (Figure 1.6b). Movement between two vertebrae is small, but when all of the intervertebral discs are compressed in a particular direction, considerable movement of the vertebral column occurs. Little movement occurs at the pubic symphysis, the joint where the right and left halves of the pelvis meet. Movement is probably increased at the pubic symphysis in the late stage of pregnancy and during childbirth, to increase the size of the birth canal.

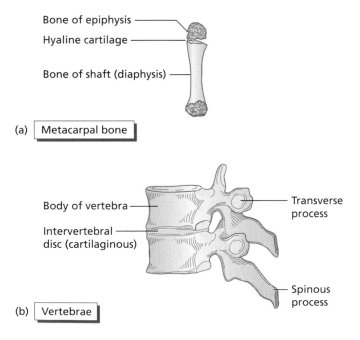

Figure 1.6 Cartilaginous joints: (a) synchondrosis in a child's metacarpal bone, as seen on X-ray; (b) symphysis between the bodies of two vertebrae.

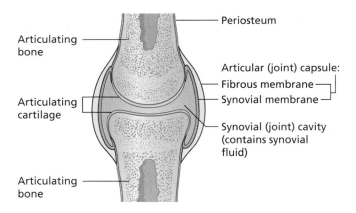

Figure 1.7   Typical synovial joint.

Synovial joints

Synovial joints are the mobile joints of the body. There is a large number of these joints, which show a variety of form and range of movement. The common features of all of them are shown in the section of a typical synovial joint (Figure 1.7) and listed as follows:

- **Hyaline cartilage** covers the ends of the two articulating bones, providing a low-friction surface for movement between them.
- A **capsule** of dense fibrous tissue is attached to the articular margins, or some distance away, on each bone. The capsule surrounds the joint like a sleeve.
- There is a **joint cavity** inside the capsule which allows free movement between the bones.
- **Ligaments**, bands or cords of dense fibrous tissue, join the bones. The ligaments may blend with the capsule or they are attached to the bones close to the joint.
- A **synovial membrane** lines the joint capsule and all non-articular surfaces inside the joint, i.e. any structure within the joint not covered by hyaline cartilage.

One or more bursae are found associated with some of the synovial joints at a point of friction where a muscle, a tendon or the skin rubs against any bony structures. A bursa is a closed sac of fibrous tissue lined by a synovial membrane and containing synovial fluid. The cavity of the bursa sometimes communicates with the joint cavity. Pads of fat, liquid at body temperature, are also present in some joints. Both structures have a protective function.

> **Practice note-pad 1B: osteoarthritis**
>
> Osteoarthritis is a degenerative disease occurring in middle-aged and older people. There is a progressive loss of the articular cartilage in the weight-bearing joints, usually the hip and the knees. Bony outgrowths occur at the margins of the joint and the capsule may become fibrosed. The joints become stiff and painful.

> **Practice note-pad 1C: rheumatoid arthritis**
>
> Rheumatoid arthritis is a systemic disease that can occur at any age (average 40 years) and it is more common in women. The peripheral joints (hands and feet) are affected first, followed by the involvement of other joints. Inflammation of the synovial membrane, bursae and tendon sheaths leads to swelling and pain which may be relieved by drugs. Deformity is the result of erosion of articular cartilage, stretching of the capsule and the rupture of tendons.

All of the large movable joints of the body, for example the shoulder, elbow, wrist, hip, knee and ankle, are synovial joints. The direction and the range of their movements depend on the shape of the articular surfaces and the presence of ligaments and muscles close to the joint. The different types of synovial joint are described in Chapter 2 where the directions of movement at joints are considered.

Skeletal muscle

Skeletal muscle is attached to the bones of the skeleton and produces movement at joints. The basic unit of skeletal muscles is the **muscle fibre**. Muscle fibres are bound together in bundles to form a whole muscle, which is attached to bones by fibrous connective tissue. When **tension** develops in the muscle, the ends are drawn towards the centre of the muscle. In this case, the muscle is contracting in length and a body part moves. Alternatively, a body part may be moved by gravity and/or by an added weight, for example an object held in the hand. Now the tension developed in the muscle may be used to resist movement and hold the object in one position.

In summary, the tension developed allows a muscle:

- to shorten to produce movement;
- to resist movement in response to the force of gravity or an added load.

Furthermore, muscles may develop tension when they are increasing in length. This will be considered in Chapter 2, in the section on types of muscle work.

Both muscle and fibrous connective tissue have elasticity. They can be stretched and return to the original length. The unique function of muscle is the capacity to shorten actively.

> **Reflective task**
>
> - Hold a glass of water in the hand. Feel the activity in the muscles above the elbow by palpating them with the other hand. The tension in the muscles is resisting the weight of the forearm and the water.
> - Lift the glass to the mouth. Feel the muscle activity in the same muscles as they shorten to lift the glass.

Structure and form

The structure of a whole muscle is the combination of muscle and connective tissues, which both contribute to the function of the active muscle. In a whole muscle, groups of contractile muscle fibres are bound together by fibrous connective tissue. Each bundle is called a fasciculus. Further coverings of connective tissue bind the fasciculi together and an outer layer surrounds the whole muscle (Figure 1.8).

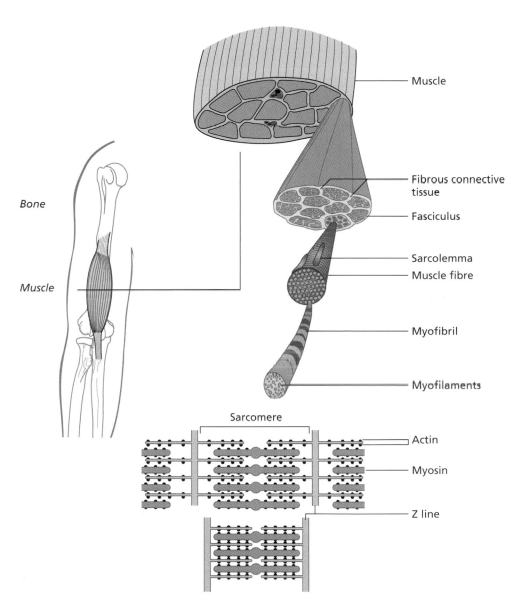

Figure 1.8   Skeletal muscle: the organisation of muscle fibres into a whole muscle, and a sarcomere in the relaxed and the shortened state (as seen by an electron microscope).

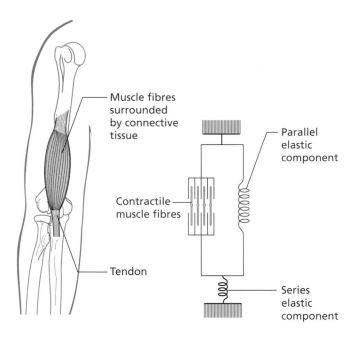

Figure 1.9   Elastic components of muscle.

The total connective tissue element lying in between the contractile muscle fibres is known as the parallel elastic component. The tension that is built up in muscle when it is activated depends on the tension in the muscle fibres and in the parallel elastic component. The fibrous connective tissue, for example a tendon, which links a whole muscle to bone is known as the series elastic component. The initial tension that builds up in an active muscle tightens the series elastic component and then the muscle can shorten. A model of the elastic and contractile parts of a muscle is shown in Figure 1.9. If the connective tissue components lose their elasticity, through lack of use in injury or disease, a muscle may go into contracture. Lively splints are used to maintain elasticity and prevent contracture while the muscle recovers.

The individual muscle fibres lie within a muscle in one of the following two ways:

- Parallel fibres are seen in strap and fusiform muscles (Figure 1.10a, b). These muscles have long fibres which are capable of shortening over the entire length of the muscle, but the result is a less powerful muscle.
- Oblique fibres are seen in pennate muscles. The muscle fibres in these muscles cannot shorten to the same extent as parallel fibres. The advantage of this arrangement, however, is that more muscle fibres can be packed into the whole muscle, so that greater power can be achieved.

The muscles with oblique fibres are known as unipennate, bipennate or multipennate, depending on the particular way in which the muscle fibres are arranged (Figure 1.10c, d). Some of the large muscles of the body combine parallel and oblique arrangements. The deltoid muscle of the shoulder (see Chapter 5, Figure 5.9) has one group of fibres that are multipennate and two groups

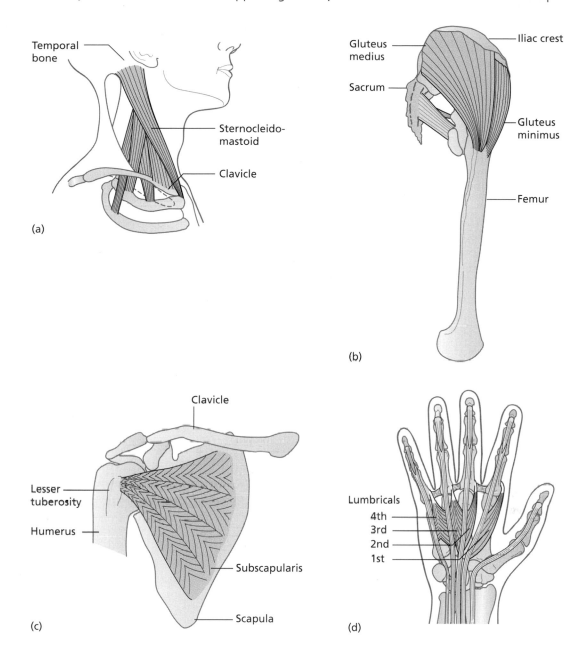

Figure 1.10   Form of whole muscle: parallel fibres (a) strap and (b) fusiform; oblique fibres (c) multipennate and (d) unipennate and bipennate.

that are fusiform, which combines strength to lift the weight of the arm with a wide range of movement. The form of a particular muscle reflects the space available and the demands of range and strength of movement.

Muscles have a limited capacity for repair, although a small area of damage to muscle fibres may regenerate. In more extensive damage, the connective tissue responds by producing more collagen fibres and a scar is formed. An intact nerve and adequate blood supply are essential for muscle function. If these are interrupted the muscle may never recover. Movement can then only be restored by other muscles taking over the functions of the damaged muscles.

Microscopic structure

A muscle fibre can just be seen with the naked eye. Each muscle fibre is an elongated cell with many nuclei surrounded by a strong outer membrane, the sarcolemma. If one fibre is viewed under a light microscope, the nuclei can be seen close to the membrane around the fibre. The chief constituent of the fibre is several hundreds of myofibrils, strands of protein extending from one end of the fibre to the other (Figure 1.8). The arrangement of the two main proteins, actin and myosin, that form each myofibril presents a banded appearance. The light and dark bands in adjacent myofibrils coincide, so that the whole muscle fibre is striated.

The electron microscope reveals the detail of the cross-striations in each myofibril. A repeating unit, known as the sarcomere, is revealed along the length of the myofibril. Each sarcomere links to the next one at a disc called the Z-line. The thin filaments of actin are attached to the Z-line and project towards the centre of the sarcomere. The thicker myosin filaments lie in between the actin strands. The darkest bands of the myofibril are where the actin and myosin overlap in the sarcomere.

The arrangement of the myosin molecules in the thick myosin filaments forms cross-bridges that link with special sites on the active filaments when the muscle fibre is activated. The result of this linking is to allow the filaments to slide past one another, so that each sarcomere becomes shorter. This, in turn, means that the myofibril is shorter, and since all the myofibrils respond together, the muscle fibre shortens.

Reflective task

Look at Figure 1.8, starting at the bottom, to identify the details of the structure of a muscle: (1) sarcomeres lie end to end to form a myofibril; (2) myofibrils are packed tightly together inside a muscle fibre; (3) muscle fibres are bound together in a fasciculus; and (4) fasciculi are bound to form a whole muscle.

In active muscles, the energy required to develop tension is released by chemical reactions. Most of these reactions occur in structures called **mitochondria** (Figure 1.11). All cells have mitochondria, but they are more abundant in muscle fibres where they lie adjacent to the myofibrils. The breakdown of adenosine triphosphate (ATP) and a 'back-up' phosphocreatine provide a high level of energy output in the muscle. The store of ATP is replenished in the mitochondria using oxygen and glucose brought by the blood in the network of capillaries surrounding muscle fibres (Figure 1.11). In this way, the muscle fibres have a continuous supply of energy, as long as the supply of oxygen is maintained (aerobic metabolism). Glycogen is another source of energy that

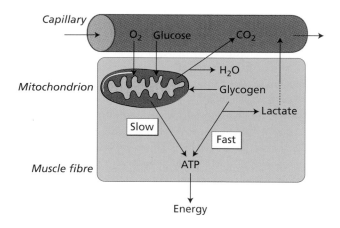

Figure 1.11   Energy for muscle contraction (simplified). The 'slow' pathway predominates in type I fibres, where ATP is replenished by aerobic reactions to provide the energy for long periods of low-level activity. The 'fast' pathway predominates in type II fibres, where glycogen provides energy without oxygen for short bursts of high-level activity.

is stored in muscle fibres. When there is insufficient oxygen to replenish ATP by oxidative reactions, energy is released from breakdown of glycogen to maintain the ATP levels. This occurs during a short burst of high-level muscle activity.

Adaptation of muscles to functional use

Not all muscle fibres in one muscle are the same. Two main types have been distinguished:

- **Slow** fibres, known as type I fibres, are red because they contain myoglobin which stores oxygen, like the haemoglobin in the blood, and they are surrounded by many capillaries. Energy supply for the slow fibres (called SO) is mainly from oxidative reactions. The slow fibres respond to stimulation with a slow twitch and they are resistant to fatigue.
- **Fast** fibres, known as type II fibres, are white with no myoglobin and have fewer capillaries per fibre. Energy is derived mainly from the breakdown of glucose and stored glycogen without oxygen. The fast fibres (called FG) respond with a fast twitch, but they are easily fatigued when the glycogen stores are used up.

Slow fibres are adapted for sustained postural activity, while the fast fibres are recruited for rapid intense bursts of activity, for example running, cycling and kitchen tasks such as cutting bread and chopping vegetables.

Skeletal muscle shows a remarkable capacity to adapt its structure to functional use. Both the relative proportion of slow and fast fibres and the number of sarcomeres in the myofibrils can change over time.

Muscle strength and bulk is increased by progressive resistance training programmes using weights or strength-training machines. The added strength is due to an increase in the number and size of the myofibrils, particularly in the fast muscle fibres which hypertrophy most readily.

Less increase occurs in the slow fibre type. There is little evidence that similar training programmes can strengthen the muscles of patients with chronic degenerative disorders of the neuromuscular system. Any change may depend on the number of remaining intact fibres. For these patients, improvement in stamina rather than strength will be more useful for daily living in any case. Training for endurance in healthy young adults has the effect of changes in some fast fibres, which become more like slow fibres. The presence of these type IIA or FGO fibres increases the length of time that the muscle can perform movement without fatigue.

Studies of the effects of ageing have shown a progressive decrease in the size of fast fibres with fewer changes in slow fibres. These changes are most likely to be the response to a less active life. Fast fibres can increase in size in elderly people, so that exercise programmes are beneficial when there are no pathological changes present.

Muscles also change the number of sarcomeres in the myofibrils if a muscle is held in a shortened or lengthened position, for example by a plaster cast. Sarcomeres are lost in the shortened position and added in the lengthened position. This is an adaptation to changes in the functional length of the muscle. Any benefit, however, may be overridden by the changes in the muscle which lead to muscle contracture.

Practice note-pad 1D: myopathies

Neuromuscular disorders that are myopathic originate in the muscle, and may be inherited or acquired. There is muscle weakness in the proximal muscles, which is slowly progressive with muscle wasting.

Duchenne muscular dystrophy is an inherited myopathy that affects boys only. There is a rapid progression of muscle weakness that begins in childhood.

Acquired myopathy can result from infections, or endocrine disorders, or as a complication of steroid drug treatment.

Basic units of the nervous system

The functions of the nervous system in movement are: to conduct motor commands from the brain to the muscles; to regulate the activity in the cardiovascular and respiratory systems which supply the muscles with essential nutrients and oxygen; and to monitor changes in the environment that affect movement.

The properties of **neurones** are:

- excitation: neurones generate impulses in response to stimulation;
- conduction of impulses between neurones (in one direction only).

Neurones are organised in networks or centres in the brain and the spinal cord. Activity in one centre is directed to a particular end, for example the location of a specific sensation. The output from one processing centre is then conducted to one or many other centres in a series of operations, for example from motor centres in the brain to the spinal cord. Information can also be conducted in parallel between processing centres.

The properties of neural networks are:

- processing of activity directed to a particular end;
- relay of the output of processing to other centres in the nervous system.

This section is primarily concerned with the structure and the activity in the basic units of the nervous system, the neurones. Neural processing in specific centres in the central nervous system will be considered in Section III.

The neurone: excitation and conduction

Each neurone has a **cell body** and numerous processes extending outwards from the cell. The processes are living structures and their membrane is continuous with that of the cell body (Figure 1.12). (Think of the cell body like a conker with spines projecting out in all directions.) The

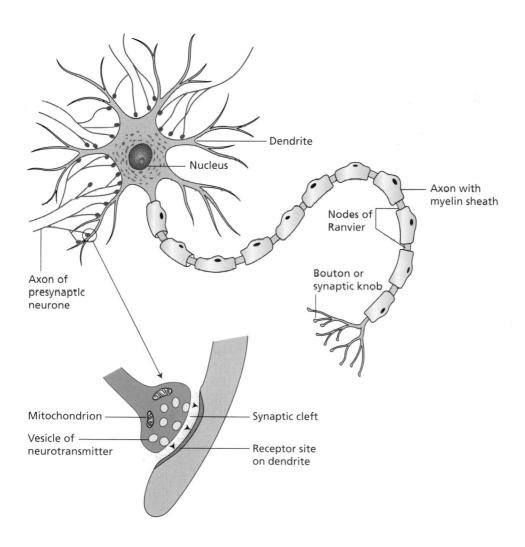

Figure 1.12   Neurone and synapse; synaptic cleft enlarged.

projections vary in length: short processes are called **dendrites**, and each neurone has one long process, the **axon**. The dendrites are adapted to receive signals or impulses and pass them on to the cell body. Some neurones, particularly in the brain, have thousands of complex branching dendrites, so that signals from a large number of other neurones can be received.

The axon is the output end of every neurone. The length of an axon varies from a few millimetres to 1 m. Cell bodies of motor neurones in the spinal cord in the lower back have long axons that extend down the leg to supply the muscles of the foot. The axon may be surrounded by a sheath of **myelin**, a fatty material, which increases the rate at which impulses are conducted down the axon. The myelin is laid down between layers of membrane of Schwann cells that wrap around the axon. Gaps in the myelin occur between successive Schwann cells forming nodes of Ranvier (Figure 1.12).

At the end of the neurone the axon branches, and each branch is swollen to form a bouton or synaptic knob. The boutons lie near a dendrite or cell body of another neurone. A typical motor neurone may have as many as 10 000 boutons on its surface which originate from other neurones. Axons also terminate on muscle fibres at a neuromuscular junction, on some blood vessels and in glands.

Practice note-pad 1E: multiple sclerosis (MS)

In multiple sclerosis, changes in the myelin sheath around axons result in the formation of plaques, which affects the rate of conduction of nerve impulses. Axons in the central nervous system (brain and spinal cord) are affected, while those in the peripheral nervous system are not. The visual system seems to be most sensitive to plaque formation. Disturbance of both movement and sensation occurs. Fatigue and cognitive impairment are other common features that affect function. The number of plaques and their sites vary between individuals and with time in the same individual, so that the disease sometimes follows a course of relapse and remission. In some individuals there is progressive deterioration.

An impulse is a localised change in the membrane of a neurone. When a neurone is excited, the membrane over a small area allows charged particles (ions) to pass across the membrane, a process known as depolarisation, and an impulse is generated. The area of depolarisation then moves to the adjacent area and the impulse travels down the membrane in one direction only. Each impulse is the same size, like a morse code of dots only, but the signals carried can be varied by the rate and pattern of the impulses conducted along the neurone.

A **synapse** is the junction where impulses pass from one neurone to the next. Impulses always travel in one direction at a synapse, i.e. from the axon of one neurone to the dendrites and cell body of the next neurone. This ensures the one-way traffic in the nervous system.

When an impulse arrives at the end of the axon, a chemical is released from the boutons into the gaps between them and the next neurone. The chemical is known as a neurotransmitter and the gap is the synaptic cleft (Figure 1.12). Each molecule of the neurotransmitter has to match special protein molecules, known as receptor sites, on the next neurone. When the transmitter locks on to the receptor site, the combination triggers the depolarisation of the membrane of the second neurone and impulses are conducted down it. Next, the transmitter substance is broken down by enzymes, taken up again by the boutons, re-formed and stored.

Each neurone has a threshold level of stimulation. The level of excitation reaching a neurone must be sufficient to depolarise the membrane, so that impulses are generated. Some impulses reaching a neurone affect the membrane in such a way that no impulses are propagated, this is known as **inhibition**. The source of inhibitory effects may be the presence of small neurones, the activity of which always produces inhibition, or the release of different transmitter substance from the boutons of the axon. The mechanism of inhibition will be discussed in more detail in Chapter 12.

Various transmitter substances have been identified in the nervous system. These include acetylcholine, adrenaline, dopamine and serotonin. Acetylcholine is the neurotransmitter released at most of the synapses in the pathways involved in movement, and also at the neuromuscular junctions. Drugs that prevent the release of acetylcholine at synapses are used as relaxants for muscles, for example in abdominal surgery.

Neuroplasticity

Neuroplasticity infers the human brain is capable of change as a result of our experiences and environment and that the brain is plastic in nature. The total number of neurones in the brain decreases after early adult life. Despite this loss, the brain retains its capacity to learn new skills and to use knowledge in different ways. For example, traumatic brain injury destroys neurones, either by direct damage to the neurones or as a result of reduced blood flow to the affected area of the brain. Recovery and rehabilitation may produce a, sometimes remarkable, return of function. It would appear that activity associated with a specific function can move to a different anatomical location within the brain. This suggests that the nervous system has the capacity to be modified and new connections can be made, although the reasons are not entirely understood.

Biochemical changes have been explored as a possible explanation for the plasticity of neurones. During the early development of the basic networks of the brain, protein substances called nerve growth factors (NGFs) are present, but these are absent in the adult brain. Attempts to reintroduce NGFs in patients with degenerative diseases of the nervous system have been largely unsuccessful.

Evidence from animal experiments has demonstrated that structural changes in neurones can occur in a damaged area in some parts of the brain. These changes include new synaptic connections made by undamaged neurones and the sprouting of the axons to form synapses at sites that were previously activated by injured axons. The time when the fibres make new connections coincides with the return of function.

Current knowledge supports some plasticity of neurones in response to learning new skills and after injury. The cell body of each neurone is relatively fixed, but the synaptic connections that it makes with other neurones can be modified.

Motor and sensory neurones

So far, the structure and properties of a typical neurone have been described. Electrochemical changes in the dendrites and cell body result in impulses that are propagated in one direction only, down the axon. In the organisation of the nervous system, the cell bodies of neurones lie in the central nervous system (brain and spinal cord) and the axons lie in the peripheral nerves that leave it to be distributed to all parts of the body.

Motor (efferent) neurones carry impulses away from the central nervous system to all parts of the body, or from the brain down to the spinal cord.

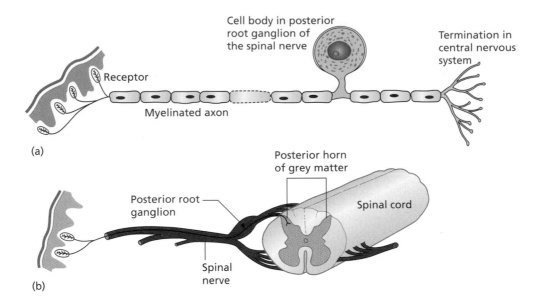

Cell body in posterior
root ganglion of
the spinal nerve

Termination in
central nervous
system

Receptor

Myelinated axon

(a)

Posterior horn
of grey matter

Posterior root
ganglion

Spinal cord

Spinal
nerve

(b)

Figure 1.13   Sensory neurones: (a) typical sensory neurone; (b) the position of a sensory neurone in a spinal nerve and the spinal cord.

Sensory (afferent) neurones develop in a different way. The cell bodies of the sensory neurones are found in ganglia just outside the spinal cord. There are no synaptic junctions on the cell bodies, and the axon divides into two almost immediately after it leaves the cell. The two branches formed by this division are a long process in a peripheral nerve that ends in a specialised sensory receptor, for example in the skin or a muscle, and a short process that enters the spinal cord and terminates in the central nervous system.

Figure 1.13a shows the arrangement of a typical sensory neurone. It is sometimes called 'pseudounipolar', since it has one axon but appears to be bipolar. Compare this with the multipolar motor neurone shown in Figure 1.12. Figure 1.13b shows the position of a sensory neurone in relation to the spinal cord, a spinal nerve and its branches. Note the cell body lying in a ganglion (swelling) and the axon entering the spinal cord. Sensory neurones carry impulses from the body towards the central nervous system, or from the spinal cord up to the brain.

Interneurones are those which lie only in the central nervous system and their axons do not extend into the nerves leaving it.

The motor unit

The motor neurones in the spinal cord, which activate the skeletal muscles, lie in a central H-shaped core of grey matter. These lower motor neurones are found in the anterior (ventral) limb of the grey matter. Neurones that activate a particular group of muscles lie together and form a motor neurone pool (Figure 1.14). The axons of these neurones lie in spinal nerves that branch to form the nerve supplying the muscle. There are fewer motor neurones in the pool than muscle fibres in the muscle, and therefore each neurone must supply a number of muscle fibres.

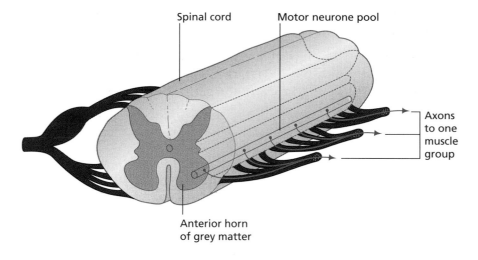

Figure 1.14   Motor neurone pool in the spinal cord.

Practice note-pad 1F: peripheral neuropathies

Neuromuscular disorders that are neurogenic originate in the nerve supply to the muscles, either in the spinal cord, in the nerve roots or in the peripheral nerves (see Chapter 4). Neuropathies of peripheral nerves affect sensory and motor axons, usually commencing distally, and are known as 'glove and stocking'. Muscle weakness and sensory loss occur. Peripheral neuropathy can occur as a complication of diabetes that Is not under control.

   Guillain–Barré syndrome is an acute peripheral neuropathy that affects motor axons. It usually follows a viral infection, and the resulting motor weakness involves the trunk and proximal limb muscles, mainly in the lower limbs. Recovery is nearly always complete unless there is severe involvement of the respiratory muscles or axonal damage.

A **motor unit** consists of one motor neurone in the anterior horn of the spinal cord, its axon and all the muscle fibres innervated by the branches of the axon (Figure 1.15). The number of muscle fibres in one motor unit depends on the function of the muscle rather than its size. Muscles performing large, strong movements have motor units with a large number of muscle fibres. For example, the large muscle of the calf has approximately 1900 muscle fibres in each motor unit. In muscles that perform fine precision movements, the motor units have a small number of muscle fibres (e.g. up to 100 in the muscles of the hand). The muscle fibres of one motor unit do not necessarily lie together in the muscle, but may be scattered in different fasciculi. The number of motor units that are active in a muscle at any one time determines the level of performance of the muscle.

There are two types of motor unit:

* **Low-threshold** motor units supplying slow type I muscle fibres are involved in the sustained muscle activity that holds the posture of the body. The number of active motor units remains

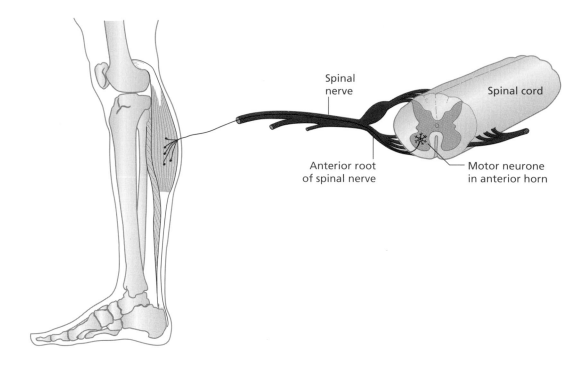

Figure 1.15 Motor unit.

constant, but activity changes between all the low-threshold neurones. The slow type I muscle fibres do not fatigue easily and the activity is maintained over long periods.

- **High-threshold** motor units with large-diameter axons supplying fast type II muscle fibres are involved in fast, active movements, which move the parts of the body from one position to another. These motor units soon fatigue, but they are adapted for fast, strong movements such as running and jumping.

In a strong purposeful movement, such as pushing forwards on a door, the motor units are activated or recruited in a particular order. The slow units are active at the start of the movement and then the fast units become active as the movement reaches its peak.

All muscle activity includes a combination of slow and fast motor units. The slow units contribute more to the background postural activity, while the fast units play a greater part in rapid phasic movements. In manipulative activities the shoulder muscles have sustained postural activity to hold the limb steady, while the hand performs rapid precision movements, such as writing, sewing or using a tool.

> **Practice note-pad 1G: motor neurone diseases**
>
> These are progressive disorders of the motor neurones in the spinal cord. Muscle weakness and fatigue of the muscles of the limbs and the trunk occur, which become generalised to affect swallowing and speech. There is no sensory loss. Depending on the sub-type, onset is usually around the age of 40 years, with rapid deterioration over 3–5 years.

Receptors

Receptors are specialised structures that respond to a stimulus and generate nerve impulses in sensory neurones. They are collectively the source of the sensory information that is transmitted into the central nervous system. While there is awareness of some receptor stimulation, a large amount of sensory processing and the resulting response occurs below consciousness. I can feel the pressure of the fingertips on the computer keys as I write and hear my mobile phone when it rings. At the same time, I am unaware of the receptors in the muscles in the neck and the balance part of the ear responding to changes in the position of the head so that my posture is adjusted to keep my eyes on the keyboard.

A system of receptors that respond to a specific stimulus is known as the **modality** of sensation, for example tactile modality. Several receptors of the same type may give input into one sensory neurone. The area covered by all the receptors activating one sensory axon is called a **receptive field**. There may be overlap in receptive fields, so that stimulation of one point may excite more than one sensory neurone (Figure 1.16). In the fingertips, for example, where the receptive fields are small and there is great overlap, a stimulus such as a pin prick can be very precisely interpreted.

When a receptor is stimulated, the membrane of the receptor ending is depolarised and impulses are generated. If the same stimulus continues for some time, the rate of firing of impulses falls and may stop, even though the stimulus is still present. This is known as **adaptation** of receptors. Different receptors adapt at different rates.

Slow-adapting receptors continue to produce impulses at the same rate all the time the stimulus is applied. The function of these receptors is to give continuous monitoring of background sensory information. Receptors found in muscles and joints are slow adapting. People are unaware of most of the activity of slow-adapting receptors.

Fast-adapting receptors generate a short burst of impulses in response to the stimulus, but activity ceases if the stimulus continues at the same level. Sensation from these receptors usually reaches consciousness. Touch receptors in the skin are fast adapting. When a person puts clothes on, he or she feels the clothes at first, and then is no longer aware of them. If the strength of stimulus changes, e.g. a belt becomes tighter, another burst of impulses is generated and the change is sensed.

Adaptation of receptors allows the nervous system to process the changing features of the environment inside and outside the body, while information of unchanging features is reduced.

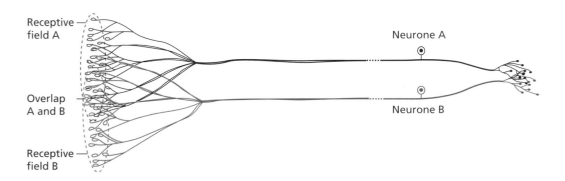

Figure 1.16   Receptors in the receptive fields of two neurones.

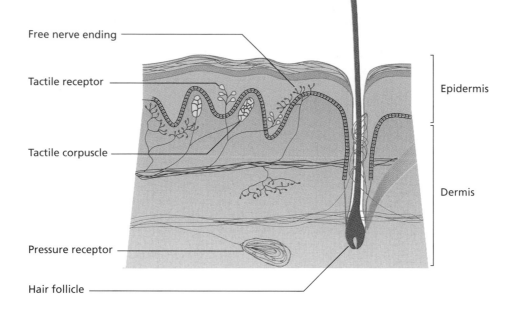

Free nerve ending

Tactile receptor

Tactile corpuscle

Pressure receptor

Hair follicle

Epidermis

Dermis

Figure 1.17   Section of the skin showing receptors.

Cutaneous receptors

Three types of receptor are found in the skin: thermoreceptors responding to temperature; nociceptors activated by noxious stimuli, which result in the perception of pain; and mechanoreceptors sensing touch and pressure (Figure 1.17).

Mechanoreceptors in the skin play a role in the regulation of movement. The sole of the foot has a high density of mechanoreceptors. These pressure sensors provide information about foot contact with the base of support, which is an important component of the maintenance of balance, both in standing and during movement. The jogger or athlete running along rough terrain in poor visibility relies on information from the soles of the feet to prevent tripping and falling. The palm of the hand and the fingertips also have a large number of mechanoreceptors. Writing with a pen, dressing and handling coins are all activites heavily dependent on information from the skin of the hand. The importance of these receptors is even greater when we cannot see the object, for example when doing up a back fastening on a skirt.

Nociceptors detect tissue damage that we perceive as pain. The noxious stimulus may be mechanical, thermal or the chemical products from damaged tissues. They should not be called pain receptors because pain is a perception, not a stimulus (see Chapter 11).

Proprioceptors

Proprioceptors lie in skeletal muscles, tendons and joints. They collectively signal the relative positions of the body parts. There are three types of proprioceptor: muscle spindles lying in parallel in between skeletal muscles fibres; Golgi tendon organs found at the junction between a muscle and its tendon; and joint receptors associated with the synovial joints.

A **muscle spindle** has a capsule of connective tissue enclosing 5–14 specialised small muscle fibres known as intrafusal fibres. The central part of these intrafusal fibres of the spindle contains the nuclei and is non-contractile. Wound round this central area is the primary sensory ending, called the annulospiral ending. The main stimulus for the activation of muscle spindles is a change in length of the muscle.

A **Golgi tendon organ** is found at the junction between the muscle fibres and the tendon in a skeletal muscle. A spindle-shaped capsule of connective tissue containing collagen strands encloses the nerve ending. Increase in tension in the muscle pulls on the collagen fibres in the tendon organ and stimulates the nerve ending. In a muscle there are fewer tendon organs than muscle spindles.

Joint receptors are found in all the synovial joints lying in the capsule and ligaments. Some of the receptors are free nerve endings and others are encapsulated In a similar way to those found in the skin. These receptors are activated by the changing angulation of a joint during movement.

The cutaneous, muscle and joint receptors are collectively known as somatosensory receptors. They contribute to the sense of limb position (body scheme) and the sense of movement of body parts. The function of proprioceptors in the regulation of movement will be considered in Chapter 12.

Muscle tone

The functional activity of the muscles of the body depends on nervous stimulation and the conduction of impulses to and from the muscles. A muscle cannot function without its nerve supply. Even when we are at rest, there is low level nervous activity in the muscles. If a person feels their own muscles or those of a partner, the muscles are not limp but 'lively'. This is known as **muscle tone**. A low level of muscle tone is present in a relaxed conscious person. Even when the body Is asleep some muscle tone is present, except in periods of deep sleep. Muscle tone has also been described as the state of readIness of the body musculature for the performance of movement. Postural tone allows people to hold static postures. For example, in many self-care activities, the muscles around the shoulder hold the hand close to the head while the hand combs the hair or cleans the teeth. In this position, it is important to resist any tendency for the shoulder muscles to lengthen and allow the limb to fall down.

Postural tone originates in the proprioceptors (muscle spindles) lying in parallel with the skeletal muscle fibres. When there is a change in length of a muscle, the spindles are stimulated. Impulses pass in sensory neurones to the spinal cord where they synapse with the lower motor neurones of the same muscle. These are large-diameter motor neurones, known as skeletomotor neurones. There are two types of skeletomotor neurone corresponding to the fast type II muscle fibres and the slow type I muscle fibres. The response in these muscle fibres restores the muscle to its original length. The pathway of this muscle stretch reflex is shown in Figure 1.18. Note that it is a monosynaptic reflex with no interneurones involved in the spinal cord.

Reflective task

Feel the muscles around the shoulder of another person while the arm is hanging by his or her side. The muscles are not limp, but they are 'lively'. Now ask the person to lift his or her arm sideways to the horizontal and hold the position. Feel the muscles again, and notice that they are more lively, the tone of the muscles has increased.

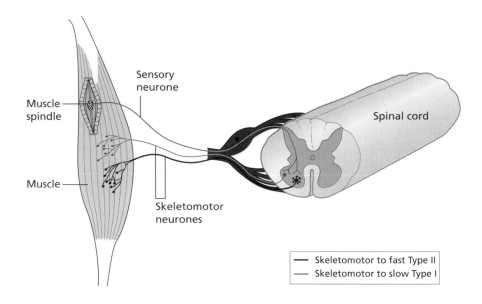

Figure 1.18   Pathway of the muscle stretch reflex showing skeletomotor neurones.

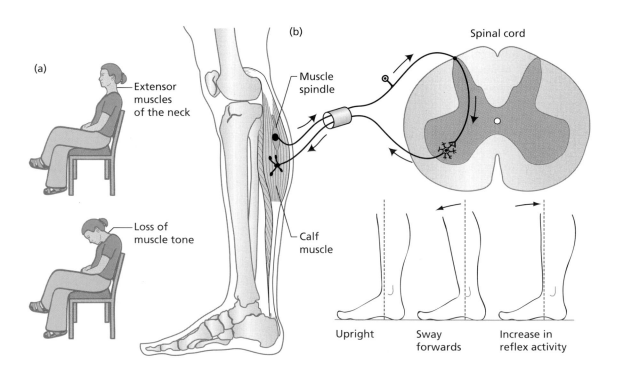

Figure 1.19   Examples of postural tone: (a) the head in sitting; (b) calf muscles in standing.

When a person stands upright, the background level of stretch reflex activity increases in the antigravity muscles of the neck, trunk and lower limbs, which prevents the body from collapsing in response to the pull of gravity. In sitting upright the head is held up by the activity in the muscles at the back of the neck to prevent the head from falling forwards (Figure 1.19a). In standing, the tendency for the body to sway forwards is counteracted by activity in the muscles of the calf (Figure 1.19b). When postural tone is too high or too low, for example in many neurological conditions, movement is affected. A person with low tone has difficulty in maintaining balance while performing fast and accurate movement. In the presence of high tone, movements overshoot and the performance of fine motor skills is impaired.

Summary

This chapter has addressed the structure and properties of the basic units of the musculoskeletal and nervous systems:

- The connective tissues provide support for the whole body.
- Bone forms the rigid framework and has a remarkable capacity for repair after injury.
- Fibrous connective tissue binds and attaches bones to each other as well as joining muscle to bone. Fibrous tissue contains collagen strands which have both tensile strength and elasticity.
- Cartilage also joins some bones and forms the low-friction surface for the articulating surfaces of bones at the movable joints of the body.
- Bones articulate at joints which allow varying degrees of movement. Fibrous and cartilaginous joints show limited movement together with a high level of stability. The greatest movement occurs in the synovial joints.
- The stability of these joints depends on the shape of the articulating surfaces, the number and the strength of the ligaments that join the bones, and the presence of short muscles close to the joint. The joints with a structure that provides poor stability usually have a wide range of movement.
- Skeletal muscle changes in length in response to nervous stimulation to produce movement of bones at their articulations.
- Active muscle also resists change in length in response to the force of gravity or an added load. The strength of a muscle depends on the number and size of the individual muscle fibres.
- Two main types of muscle fibre are found in all muscles. Slow fibres are adapted for sustained activity and are resistant to fatigue. Fast fibres have rapid response times, but they are easily fatigued. The relative proportion of slow and fast fibres in a muscle depends on its functional use and can change over time.
- The neurones of the nervous system are specialised to: respond to stimulation; conduct information to and from the muscles and the organs of the body; and integrate information from different sources in neural networks found in the central nervous system.
- Receptors are specialised endings of neurones which respond to specific stimuli.
- Cutaneous receptors respond to changes in the external environment. Those in the hand and the foot are important for sensory information about the surfaces in contact with them, for example objects held in the hand and the texture of the supporting surface in the foot.
- Proprioceptors, lying in the muscles, tendons and joints, collectively respond to changes in the length and tension in muscles, and the angulation of joints. The nervous system processes

the information from the proprioceptors to provide knowledge of the position and movement of the parts of the body.

- Muscle tone is the force with which skeletal muscles resist changes in length and hold a position.
- The neural background to muscle tone is the muscle stretch reflex, a monosynaptic pathway from and to the same muscle via the spinal cord. Postural tone is important to counteract the force of gravity in upright standing.

2

Movement terminology

Key terms

the anatomical position, movement terms, biomechanical principles

Conceptual overview

This chapter outlines the anatomical terminology used to describe direction of movement and three planes of movement: sagittal, coronal and transverse (or horizontal). The different terms used to describe movement at joint level will be described in relation to the various types of joints in addition to a brief overview of biomechanical principles that affect muscle work – and, ultimately, produce movement that enables activity.

Tyldesley & Grieve's Muscles, Nerves and Movement in Human Occupation, Fourth Edition. Ian R. McMillan, Gail Carin-Levy.
© 2012 Ian R. McMillan, Gail Carin-Levy, Barbara Tyldesley and June I. Grieve. Published 2012 by Blackwell Publishing Ltd.

The anatomical position

All movement starts from a posture or position, which must be first defined before proceeding to the changes that follow. A common reference must be used to describe the positions, relationships and directions of movement. This reference is the anatomical position, standing upright with the palms of the hands facing forwards, the feet parallel and facing forwards (Figure 2.1). Note that the natural standing position, with the palms of the hands facing the sides, is not used.

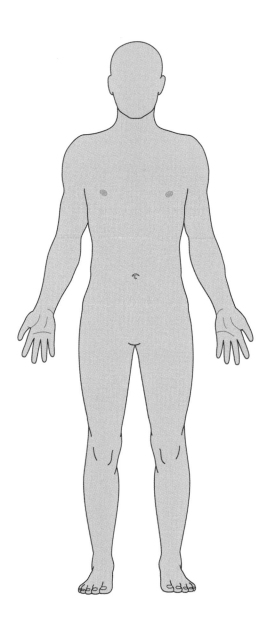

Figure 2.1   The anatomical position.

Reflective task

- Look at the articulated skeleton to see the difference between the anatomical position and the natural standing position. In the anatomical position, the bones of the forearm are parallel, and the whole of the palm of the hand can be seen from the front.
- Stand in a natural position, and then change to the anatomical position. Note the change in position of the forearm and hand. Check that the feet are slightly apart and facing forwards.

Planes and axes of movement

The reference anatomical position can now be divided into three planes which lie at right angles to each other. The planes are the fixed lines of reference for movement (Figure 2.2).

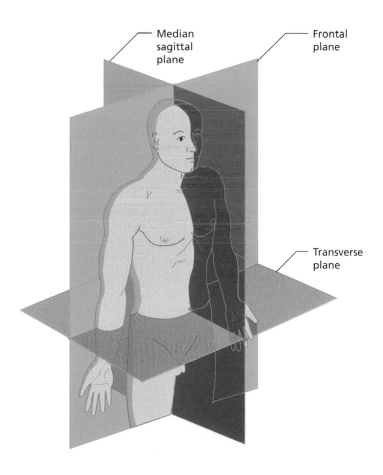

Median sagittal plane

Frontal plane

Transverse plane

Figure 2.2   Planes of movement.

Sagittal (median) plane

The sagittal or median plane is a vertical plane passing through the body from front to back which divides the body into right and left halves. Any parallel plane dividing the body into unequal right and left halves is also said to be a sagittal plane. It is parallel to the sagittal suture in the midline of the skull. The terms medial and lateral relate to this plane. A structure nearer to the median plane is medial, and one further away from it is lateral. For example, the medial ligament of the knee is on the inside of the joint, while the lateral ligament is on the outside.

Coronal (frontal) plane

This plane passes through the body from top to bottom and divides the body into front and back halves. It is at right angles to the sagittal plane. Frontal planes are parallel to the frontal suture of the skull across the crown of the head. The terms anterior and posterior relate to this plane. The anterior shaft of the femur is the front of the bone in the anatomical position, while the posterior shaft is the back of the bone.

Transverse (horizontal) plane

This is parallel to the flat surface of the ground. Planes in this direction divide the body into upper (cranial) and lower (caudal) parts. Crossing the body in this direction, planes are at right angles to the sagittal and frontal planes. The terms superior and inferior relate to this plane. The superior radioulnar joint is near to the elbow (above or towards the head), while the inferior radioulnar joint is adjacent to the wrist (below or towards the ground). When the limbs move to different positions, the terms superior and inferior can become confusing, for example if the arm is above the head. Another way of identifying structures may then be used. The terms proximal and distal mean nearer to the centre of the body or further away from the centre, respectively. The superior radioulnar joint can therefore also be named the proximal joint, and likewise the inferior as distal.

The axis of movement at a joint is at right angles to the plane. Bending the elbow is a movement in the sagittal plane about an axis passing through the frontal plane at the joint. Turning the head from side to side is a movement in the horizontal plane about a vertical axis through the joint between the first and second vertebrae of the neck. It may help to understand plane and axis by thinking of the plane of movement of the wheels of a car, around the axle (axis) at the hub of the wheels. Movements can be classified in terms of the three planes and axes described. Many functional activities, however, occur in diagonal planes. The leg swing in walking does not occur exactly in the sagittal plane at the hip, but in a diagonal plane between the sagittal and frontal planes, so that the foot comes to the ground near to the midline of the body. Movement at the shoulder which carries the arm forwards and slightly across the body is in a diagonal plane.

Structure and movements at synovial joints

Most of the movements of the body occur at the synovial joints. See Chapter 1 for the structure of a typical synovial joint. The synovial joints are classified by the axes of movement (uniaxial, biaxial and multiaxial) and by structure, as follows.

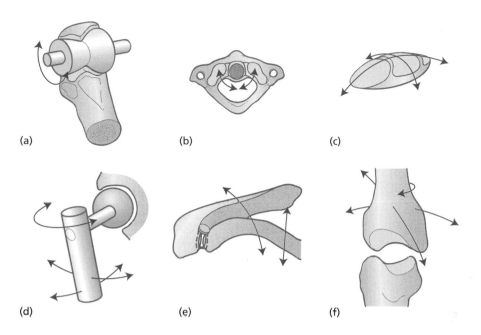

Figure 2.3   Types of synovial joint: (a) hinge; (b) pivot; (c) ellipsoid; (d) ball and socket; (e) plane; (f) saddle.

- A **hinge joint** allows movement in one direction only, in the sagittal plane. It is a uniaxial joint. Examples of a hinge joint are the elbow (Figure 2.3a) and the ankle.
- A **pivot joint** is restricted to rotational movement around a vertical axis in the horizontal plane. It is a uniaxial joint. Examples are the atlantoaxial joint in the neck, which turns the head to look sideways (Figure 2.3b), and the joints in the forearm that allow the hand to turn so that the palm faces backwards.
- An **ellipsoid joint** has oval joint surfaces that allow movement in the sagittal and frontal planes, but no rotation. It is a biaxial joint. Examples are the radiocarpal (wrist) joint (Figure 2.3c), and the joints at the base of the fingers (metacarpophalangeal joints).
- A **ball and socket joint** allows movement in three planes (Figure 2.3d). It is a triaxial or multi-axial joint. Examples are the shoulder and hip joints.
- A **plane joint** has flat articular surfaces that allow limited gliding or twisting movement between the bones. An example is the joint between the acromion of the scapula and the clavicle (Figure 2.3e). Plane joints may be arranged in series, so that the cumulative effect of the limited action at each joint gives considerable movement overall. The synovial joints between the bony arches of adjacent vertebrae are examples of plane joints, which together give the overall movements of the trunk (see Chapter 10, Joints of the vertebral column).
- A **saddle joint** has a surface that resembles a saddle (a concave convexity) with a reciprocally curved surface sitting on it. The movements are in two planes with a limited range of rotation as well. The first carpometacarpal joint at the base of the thumb is a saddle joint (Figure 2.3f).

The range of movement possible at each synovial joint depends on three main factors.

- The shape of the bony articulating surfaces determines both the direction and extent of the movement. For example, the shallow socket of the shoulder joint allows a wide range of movement.
- The position, strength and tautness of the surrounding ligaments affects range. By regular stretching exercises from an early age, gymnasts and ballet dancers can stretch certain joint ligaments to achieve a greater range of movement.
- The strength and size of the muscles surrounding the joint affects range. Bulging muscles around a joint halt movement when the two moving segments come into contact. For example, bending the elbow is limited by contact of the forearm with the upper arm. Other muscles may restrict movement by their position in relation to a joint. Tight hamstring muscles at the back of the thigh limit bending of the hips in touching the toes.

Movement terms

Starting from the anatomical position, paired terms are used to distinguish the direction of movement of body segments in the three planes described (Figure 2.4).

Flexion and **extension** are movements in the sagittal plane. Flexion movements bend the body part away from the anatomical position. Extension is movement in the opposite direction back to the anatomical position and beyond into a reversed position (Figure 2.4a). In flexion, the angle between the bones is usually decreased, e.g. flexion of the elbow bends the forearm forwards

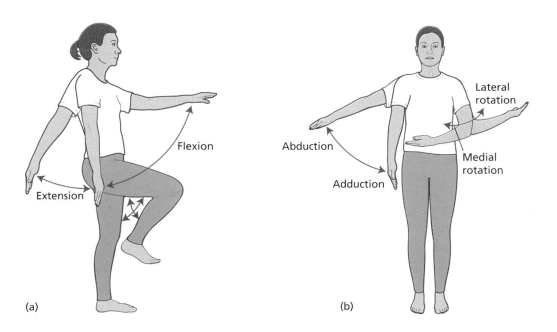

(a)   (b)

Figure 2.4   Movements at joints: (a) flexion and extension; (b) abduction and adduction; medial and lateral rotation.

and upwards towards the arm, and flexion of the knee takes the leg backwards towards the thigh. Flexion movements curl the body into a ball, while extension stretches the body out.

Abduction and **adduction** are movements in the frontal plane. Abduction movements carry a body part away from the midline. Adduction is movement in the opposite direction towards the midline (Figure 2.4b). In the hands and feet, the movements are related to the central axis of the segment. The fingers move away from the middle finger, and the toes move away from the second toe.

Reflective task

Do not confuse aBduction and aDduction: the letter b comes earlier in the alphabet, and is followed by d, the return movement being adduction. The prefixes come from latin and you will recognise that 'ab' means 'away from', as in abscond – to escape; and 'ad' means 'towards', as in addition.

When the return movement continues beyond the anatomical position, the terms 'hyperextension' and 'hyperadduction' may be used (hyper means 'more than').

Rotation is movement in the horizontal plane about a vertical axis. When the bone is rotating away from the midline, or towards the posterior surface, the movement is known as lateral rotation (or external rotation). In the reverse movement, the bone turns in towards the midline of the body and the movement is known as medial rotation (or internal rotation) (Figure 2.4b).

Circumduction is a term used to describe a sequence of movements of flexion, abduction, extension and adduction. The bone moves round in a conical shape, with the apex of the cone at the moving joint and the base at the distal end of the bone. True circumduction does not include rotation.

The paired movement terms are also used to name the groups of muscles producing them. Muscles that bend the fingers are known as flexors of the fingers, while the extensors straighten the fingers. The abductors of the hip carry the leg sideways.

Reflective task

- Stand in the anatomical position. Move each of the large joints in turn, e.g. shoulder, elbow, wrist, hip, knee, ankle.
- Record the movements possible at each of the joints.

Most body movements do not start at the anatomical position, but they are described with reference to that position. To analyse a movement, the starting position must first be defined. For example, lifting a glass from a table to the mouth starts with the shoulder in a neutral position, the elbow flexed, the wrist extended and the fingers flexed around the glass. The changes at each joint are then described as the movement proceeds. To drink, the shoulder must be flexed and the elbow flexed further to bring the glass to the lips.

Group action and types of muscle work

Muscles produce movements at joints by pulling on the bones to which they are attached. To describe a muscle, its attachments are named. One end of the muscle is usually fixed and the bony attachment at the other end moves. The attachment that is usually held steady is known as the **origin** of the muscle and is usually more proximal. The moving end is called the **insertion** and is often more distal. Some muscles can work from either end. For example, the muscle that extends the hip (gluteus maximus) pulls the thigh backwards as in climbing stairs (Figure 2.5a). If

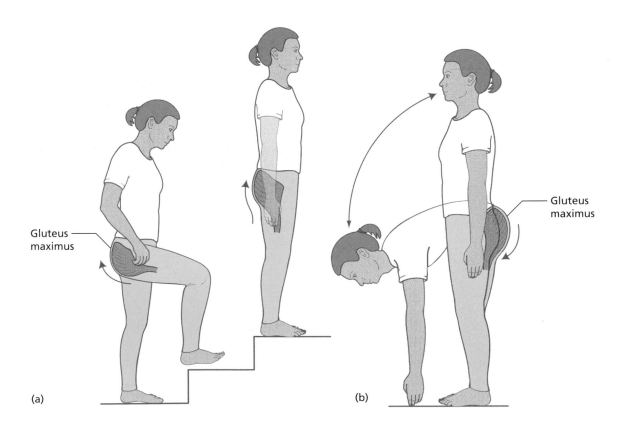

Gluteus maximus

Gluteus maximus

(a)   (b)

Figure 2.5   Muscle attachments. Action of the gluteus maximus in extension of the hip: (a) distal attachment moves; (b) proximal attachment moves.

the trunk is flexed forwards, this hip extensor acts in reverse to pull the pelvis upwards and straighten the trunk on the leg (Figure 2.5b).

Group action in muscles

No muscle acts alone. All of the muscles arranged round a joint are involved in the movement at that joint (Figure 2.6). In the case of the elbow joint, there are four muscles crossing the front of the joint and two that lie posteriorly. The anterior group is the flexors and the posterior group the extensors. When the elbow is actively flexed, the flexors are the **prime movers** (or agonists) and the extensors become the **antagonists**. The extensors are reciprocally relaxed during elbow flexion, but will act as controllers of the extent and speed of the movement. Other muscles are active to support the proximal joints, and are known as **fixators**. They are able to fix the origin of the prime movers. When the biceps is active as a prime mover, the muscles attached to the trunk, scapula and humerus are active as fixators to fix the origin of biceps. If the muscles acting as prime movers pass over more than one joint, other muscles known as **synergists** are active to prevent undesirable movements occurring at the other joints. For example, the flexors of the fingers cross the wrist and other joints in the hand. When gripping the handle of a tool or a racquet, the wrist extensors act as synergists to prevent wrist flexion and allow the finger flexors to exert maximum holding power on the handle.

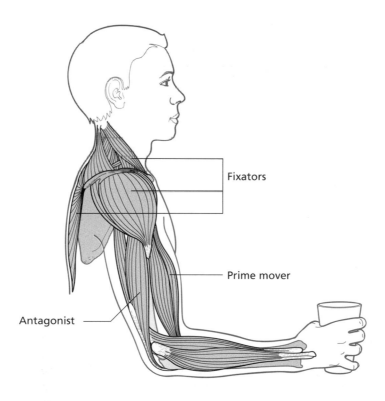

Figure 2.6 Group action of muscles in lifting a glass: prime mover, antagonist and fixators.

Types of muscle work

Muscle action is not only used to make a body part move, it may also be necessary to hold the position of a body part, such as the forearm supporting a book in the hand. Muscles are also used to control the effect of an external force acting on a body part. When moving from standing to sitting down on to a chair, the extensors of the leg work to control the effect of gravity, which is pulling the body down on to the seat. The term 'muscle contraction' may be a misleading one, because muscle action may involve the shortening of the muscle, or the muscle staying the same length or a controlled lengthening of the muscle. For this reason, muscle action (muscle work) is categorised into concentric, eccentric and static work.

- **Concentric work** (sometimes called isotonic shortening) applies to muscles that are shortening to produce a movement. When a saucepan is lifted off a stove, the elbow flexors are working concentrically: they shorten to lift the pan (Figure 2.7a).
- **Eccentric work** (sometimes called isotonic lengthening) applies to an active muscle that is lengthening. The muscle activity is controlling the rate and extent of movement as the attachments are drawn apart by external forces, such as gravity. When a saucepan is put down on to a stove, gravity is assisting the movement, so the elbow flexors must work eccentrically to control the movement, allowing the pan to be placed carefully on the hotplate (Figure 2.7b).
- **Static work** (also called isometric work) applies to the active muscles that remain the same length to hold a position. 'Isometric' means same length. If the saucepan is held still over the stove, the elbow flexors are working isometrically to prevent it from dropping down.

Static work is the most tiring form of muscle work and should not be performed for long periods without rest. Fatigue is largely due to poor blood flow and accumulation of waste products in the muscle, partly because the static state reduces the pumping action of contracting muscles on the circulation of the blood. The terms isometric and isotonic were first used by physiologists to distinguish two types of muscle response in isolated frog muscle. Isotonic means the same tension, and applies to a muscle that changes in length without a change in the tension within the muscle. In the human body, true isotonic muscle activity rarely occurs, because over the whole range of movement changes in muscle tension occur in response to the changing effects of gravity and leverage (see later for discussion of leverage). Isometric work occurs in the body when muscles

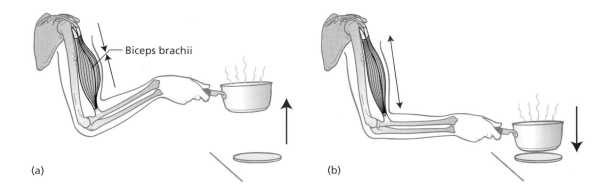

(a)

Biceps brachii

(b)

Figure 2.7   Types of muscle work: (a) concentric; (b) eccentric.

are not changing length but they are active to hold the position of a body segment and any added load. The term is also used in exercise programmes, when the muscles are working against the resistance of springs or weights.

Reflective task

- Ask a person to lift the forearms to a horizontal position and feel the tension in the elbow flexors by palpating the muscles above the elbow.
- Place a tray in the hands with the forearms in the same position. Note the change in the tension (hardness) of the elbow flexors even though there has been no change in length of the muscles. This is because the elbow flexors are having to develop tension to support the added load of the tray.

Biomechanical principles

Mechanical principles that apply to buildings and machines, such as bridges, cranes and trucks, are equally appropriate when applied to the human body and its segments. Therapists commonly use terms such as muscle tension, strength and power in the rehabilitation of weak muscles. In this section, the terms used in biomechanics to describe the mechanical components of muscle action will be defined. Their application to both body movement and the adaptation of the environment will also be considered.

Active muscle becomes tense and this **tension** developed inside a muscle generates a **force** at its point of attachment to a bone. This force produces movement at the joint over which the muscle is acting. The work done by the active muscle is the product of the force generated by its action and the distance moved by the body part.

Forces outside the body also produce movement. One external force is **gravity**, which is a constant downward force acting at the centre of a body segment, for example the thigh or the trunk. The whole weight of an object or of a body segment, for example the forearm, acts vertically downwards through the centre of gravity of the part. The position of the centre of gravity of any symmetrical object of uniform density can be found in the following way:

Reflective task

- Take a piece of card of symmetrical shape: square, oblong or circular. Draw diagonals across it. The point where the diagonals meet is the centre of gravity.
- Thread a string through the centre of gravity and note how the card is balanced at this point.

The force of gravity acting on each body segment produces movement at joints. Other external forces acting on a body segment include the weight of an object, for example a book held in the hand and the resistance offered by an object, for example a heavy lid on a box.

What happens to a joint at any instant depends on the net effect of all the **moments of force** acting around it. A moment of force is the product of its magnitude and its distance from the joint to which it is being applied (force × distance). In the body, moments of force act in different

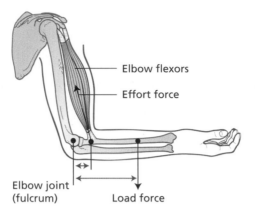

Elbow flexors

Effort force

Elbow joint
(fulcrum)

Load force

Figure 2.8 Moments of force at the elbow: force × distance from the fulcrum for effort and load.

directions around a joint. If they cancel out, the position of the joint remains constant. If they do not cancel out, movement will occur. The balance between the opposing moments may be very fine, leading to slow, precise movements, for example in finger dexterity. A large difference in the balance of moments of force leads to rapid and accelerative movement, which may be seen at the shoulder in sweeping a floor or cutting a hedge.

In bending the elbow (Figure 2.8), the flexors exert a moment of force which depends on: (i) the force exerted by the muscles and (ii) the distance between the insertion of the muscles on the bones and the centre of the elbow joint. Gravity also exerts a moment of force in the opposite direction which is the product of: (i) the weight of the forearm and hand and (ii) the distance between the centre of gravity of this body segment and the centre of the joint. If the moment of force of the elbow flexors is greater than the moment of force due to the weight of the forearm, movement occurs.

The **power** output of a muscle is a combination of strength and speed of action. High levels of muscle power are needed when the speed of action is crucial to lift heavy loads in a few seconds.

In the process of rehabilitation of weak muscles, the upper limb may be supported by a sling, which will allow movement but will reduce the force due to gravity. This encourages weak muscles to perform tasks that may be impossible when the full effect of gravity must be overcome. As the muscles of the upper limb become stronger, movements can be achieved without the support.

Adaptation of the environment can reduce the need for using strong muscle forces against gravity. Reaching above the head demands strong muscles around the shoulder. In the kitchen, frequently used items can be placed in cupboards at the level of the elbow when standing or when sitting in a wheelchair. Chairs with seats at an adequate height reduce the muscle work in the lower limbs in standing up from sitting, compared with low seats.

Stability

An essential feature of all movement is the need to keep the body in stable equilibrium, so that we do not fall over while the body is changing position. There are obvious stability problems for a gymnast balancing on a beam or a ballet dancer poised on the toes, but the balance requirements of everyday activities are taken for granted. People do not have to think about balance at each step as they walk, but become aware of the problem when standing on a jolting train or bus.

The mechanical properties of the bones, connective tissues and muscles contribute to body stability. Some joints form locking mechanisms, for example the knee and the joints of the vertebral column. The tensile strength of ligaments and tendons is important to anchor bones at joints. This is most effective at joints with limited movement, for example the sacroiliac joint of the pelvis. The muscles of the neck act as guy-ropes to support the head, while the abdominal and long back muscles stabilise the trunk. Head control relies on stability in the upper trunk and the shoulder girdle.

The mechanical principle that determines stability is:

An object is in stable equilibrium when the line from its centre of gravity lies within its base of support.

The following task illustrates this principle.

Reflective task

Return to the piece of card used to find the centre of gravity. Place the card flat on a table and move it towards the edge of the table. Note when the card falls off the table.

You will observe that the card falls as soon as the point of the centre of gravity is no longer over the table. In the same way, the upright body is only stable when the vertical line from the centre of gravity lies within the base of support, which is usually the feet. If the line of gravity moves outside the foot base when moving around, a person will fall over. If the body was rigid like a plaster figure, the addition of a weight on one side would move the centre of gravity to that side and the figure would topple over. In the body, the postural mechanisms of the nervous system ensure that this does not happen. Figure 2.9a shows how the added weight of a bucket held in the hand moves the line of gravity to the right and beyond the foot base, so that the body will fall to that side. Figure 2.9b shows how the body segments alter their position to move the line of weight back over the base of support (the feet) and the body becomes stable again. This realignment of body segments occurs automatically (see Chapter 11 for more detail).

Position of the centre of gravity

In upright standing, the centre of gravity of the body is located just anterior to the upper border of the sacrum (see Chapter 10, Figure 10.2). This position, low in the trunk and over the feet, offers stability. The centre of gravity changes position during movement, for example lifting the arms raises the centre of gravity, whereas bending the knees lowers it.

The important principle to remember is that the stability is greater when the centre of gravity is lower, so it follows that all efforts to help the balance of the body should be directed to positions where the centre of gravity is lowest. When bending to pick up a child or a box, the knees should be bent and the trunk flexed to move the centre of gravity down and over the feet. A hoist used to move a patient will be most stable if it is adjusted to the lowest position.

Base of support

The upright body is least stable when the feet are parallel and close together, because in this position the base support is small (Figure 2.10a). As the feet are moved further apart the base support is increased and a more stable position is achieved (Figure 2.10b).

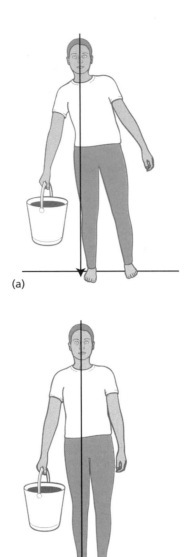

(a)

(b)

Figure 2.9   Stability in carrying a weight at the side of the body: (a) unstable; (b) stable.

In standing, the centre of gravity moves horizontally in reaching forwards or to the side. The body remains in balance as long as the new position of the vertical line of gravity lies within the base of support provided by the feet. In preparation for standing up from the sitting position, stability can be increased by moving the feet back and leaning the trunk forwards (see Chapter 8, Figure 8.9c). In this way, the foot base is aligned with the centre of gravity in the trunk before standing up.

Walking aids such as a stick, crutches or pulpit frame all increase the size of the base support and therefore allow more swaying of the body above without falling (Figure 2.10c). Standing with

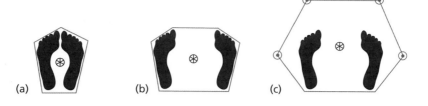

Figure 2.10   Base support: (a) feet together; (b) feet apart; (c) feet with walking frame.

the feet apart and knees bent is a stable position for a therapist to adopt when assisting a transfer by a patient.

When the centre of gravity falls outside the postural base, **rescue reactions** occur automatically to attempt to restore balance. These are: (a) stepping; (b) sweeping; and (c) protective reactions.

- **Stepping reactions.** When a force is applied to the body which pushes or pulls the body off balance, for example bumping into someone in a crowd, the response is to take a step forwards or sideways. The step increases the area of the base of support and balance is restored.
- **Sweeping reactions.** When stepping is inappropriate, for example when standing on a wall, the arms swing backwards if the body were falling forwards. Sweeping reactions also enable people to grab stable objects as they fall.
- **Protective reactions.** If balance is lost and a person does fall, powerful protective reactions occur to protect the head and the body. The arms are thrown out and the trunk is rotated to break the fall. These reactions are not easily suppressed, for example a hand may be pushed through a pane of glass as a result of a protective reaction.

> **Reflective task**
>
> Stand behind a partner who is also standing upright. Push him/her from behind. Repeat a few times with the same (and not too great!) force. Push once from the side unexpectedly. Observe the responses to the pushing. Did it change after a few repetitions in the same direction?

These responses are also known as **equilibrium reactions**. The initiation of equilibrium reactions by the sensory systems will be considered in Chapter 11, Regulation of posture.

Principles of levers

In the body, the bones form rigid levers and each joint is a pivot or fulcrum. The principles of levers therefore apply to all posture and movement in the body.

'Moment of force' has already been defined. It is the product of the force and its distance from the fulcrum. A moment of force is always tending to produce movement, and a lever is only balanced when the moments of force acting around the fulcrum are equal and opposite.

This principle may be illustrated by the example of an adult sitting on a see-saw with a small child. By putting the child at the far end on one side of the see-saw, the adult can balance the

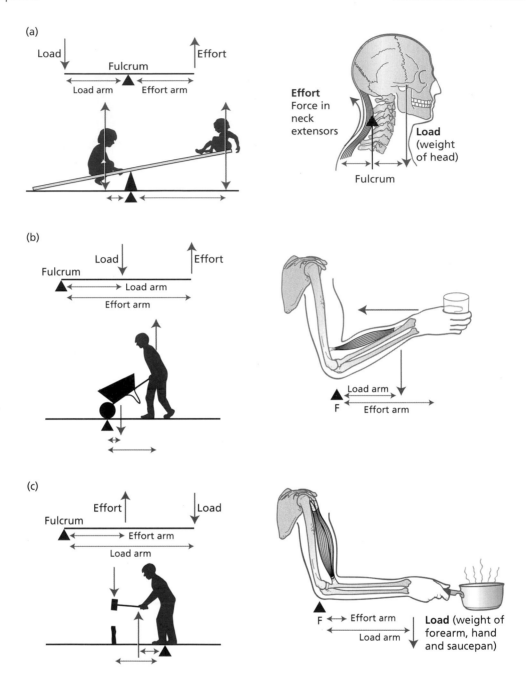

Figure 2.11   Levers: (a) first order; (b) second order; (c) third order.

see-saw by sitting near to the central pivot or fulcrum. This shows how a large force at a short distance can balance a small force at a larger distance (Figure 2.11a). Levers do not always have the fulcrum in the middle, the forces may both be acting on the same side of the fulcrum. A wheelbarrow is an example of this type of lever (Figure 2.11b). The wheel in contact with the ground forms the fulcrum. The load in the barrow is near to the fulcrum, and the effort is applied by the hands to the handles at a greater distance from the fulcrum on the same side.

The muscles acting on the joints exert effort forces on the bony levers. The part of a lever between the fulcrum and the point of application of effort can be called the effort arm.

The total force of the weight of any body segment and any added weight is the load force. The part of a lever between the fulcrum and the point of application of the load can be called the load arm.

For movement to occur against gravity, the muscle moment (effort force × effort arm) must be greater than the gravity moment (load force × load arm). If either the force or its point of application is changed, the leverage changes.

Levers are classified into first, second and third class. Figure 2.11 shows the arrangement of effort, fulcrum and load in each of the three orders of levers, with examples of each. Most of the muscles of the body act as third-order levers since the muscles are attached near to the joint that they move. The advantage of this arrangement is that it gives a greater range and speed of movement, which is important in throwing and swinging actions of the upper limb, as well as in walking and running actions in the lower limb. A few muscles, for example the brachioradialis in the forearm, act as second-class levers (Figure 2.11b). The tension in this muscle is important to relieve the stress on the bones of the forearm when weights are held in the hand.

The principles of levers can be used to increase the strength of muscles by exercise against gradually increasing loads. For example, activities for weak shoulder muscles should first involve gravity-assisted movement and then movements with the elbow flexed so that the load arm is short (Figure 2.12a). As the muscles become stronger, the shoulder can be used to reach with the extended upper limb (load arm longer) (Figure 2.12b). Eventually, reaching with an object held in the hand (load force larger) can be achieved (Figure 2.12c).

In weight-training programmes, the muscles are exercised against increasing resistance placed at increasing distances from the joint which forms the centre of the movement. In order to increase the strength of abdominal muscles, sit-ups are performed first without weights, next with a weight

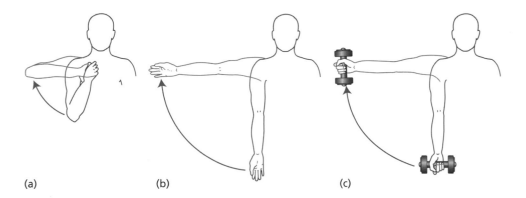

(a)   (b)   (c)

Figure 2.12   Principles of levers. Increase in effort required to lift the arm sideways: (a) short load arm; (b) long load arm; (c) long load arm plus added weight.

held in front of the chest, and finally with the weight held in the outstretched arms. In **lifting** and **carrying loads**, the effort is reduced if the moment of force of the trunk plus the added load is reduced. Figure 2.13 shows how the length of the load arm (the distance between the line of gravity of the body and the fulcrum in the lower back) changes in different starting positions for lifting a child. Position (c) requires least effort for the back muscles as the load arm is shortest.

Leverage is also applied in adapting tools used in daily living for people with weak muscles or painful joints. If the lid of a jar is opened by a tool with a long handle then less effort will be required than when grasping the lid itself. Scissors and shears with long handles will be easier to use than those with short handles (Figure 2.14). In the adaptation of tools and equipment for use by people with weak muscles it is important to remember two rules:

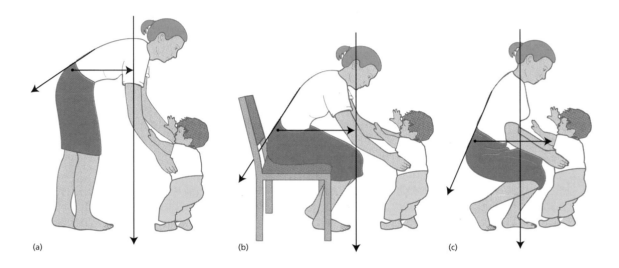

(a)   (b)   (c)

Figure 2.13   Changes in moment of load force in lifting with different starting positions: (a) standing with straight legs; (b) sitting; (c) bent knees. 1 = line of gravity; 2 = load arm; 3 = effort force.

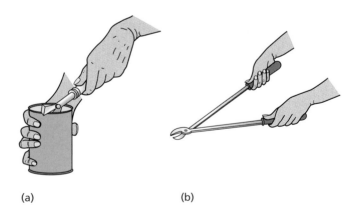

(a)   (b)

Figure 2.14   Adaptation of tools to reduce effort: (a) tin opener with extended handle; (b) long-handled shears.

- Put the load as near to the pivot as possible.
- Apply the effort as far away from the pivot as possible.

Summary

- The anatomical position, from which movement is defined, is the upright human standing with the feet parallel and the palms of the hands facing forwards.
- Three hypothetical planes of reference, at right angles to each other, divide the body and define the axes of movement of the body segments.
- Movements at the individual joints are described as:
  - flexion and extension in the sagittal plane;
  - abduction and adduction in the frontal plane;
  - medial (internal) and lateral (external) rotation in the horizontal plane.
- Most of the movement of the body occurs at synovial joints. These are classified by the shape of their articulating surfaces, which determines the number of axes of movement.
- Muscle action occurs in groups of muscles arranged around the joints. The prime movers or agonists produce the required movement and the opposing group of antagonist muscles relaxes.
- In some movements, muscles are required to fixate the origin of the prime movers. Other muscles, known as synergists, may be active to prevent unwanted movements at other joints.
- Muscle action involves the shortening of the muscle fibres to move bones; this is known as concentric muscle work.
- Muscles are often active when they are lengthening to control an external force, for example gravity acting on a body segment. This is known as eccentric work.
- A third type of muscle work involves active muscles remaining at the same length to hold a position and/or a load. This is static work, which is the most tiring owing to poor blood flow to the active muscles.
- The need to maintain the stability of the body is a major factor in movement.
- Stability depends on the line from the centre of gravity of the body falling within its base of support, usually the feet. If the body becomes unstable, rescue or equilibrium reactions occur to restore balance.
- Stepping reactions increase the base of support and sweeping reactions allow a stable object to be grabbed. If balance is lost, protective reactions occur to protect the head and body.
- The weight of a body segment forms the load force which acts at a joint or fulcrum. The muscles provide the effort force to counteract this load force and produce movement. The principle of levers states that loads placed near to joints require less effort force to move them. Similarly, the use of tools with long handles reduces the effort which must be applied to operate them.
- The movement terminology defined in this chapter is used in Section II to describe the actions of particular groups of muscles and in Chapter 13 in the descriptions of occupational performance skills.

3

The central nervous system: the brain and spinal cord

Key terms

major structures within the brain, spinal anatomy, spinal neurones, spinal reflex pathways

Conceptual overview

This chapter deals with the central nervous system, from the development of the nervous system in the foetus to the organisation of the adult brain and spinal cord. The anatomy of the brain will be examined, looking at key anatomical areas and relating them to function and dysfunction. Finally, the spinal cord will be discussed, highlighting briefly the key structures and neural pathways which enable movement.

Tyldesley & Grieve's Muscles, Nerves and Movement in Human Occupation, Fourth Edition. Ian R. McMillan, Gail Carin-Levy.
© 2012 Ian R. McMillan, Gail Carin-Levy, Barbara Tyldesley and June I. Grieve. Published 2012 by Blackwell Publishing Ltd.

PART I: THE BRAIN

Introduction to the form and structure

At first glance the brain seems to be composed only of the two cerebral hemispheres (Figure 3.1). Although they are the largest feature of the brain, they conceal many other important areas. The two symmetrical hemispheres have a folded surface with their inner aspects lying close together in the midline. Underneath the posterior end of each cerebral hemisphere is the cerebellum, which also has two hemispheres that are joined together in the midline. Part of the pons is visible anterior to the cerebellum, and below the pons is the cone-shaped medulla oblongata. The medulla leads down into the spinal cord at the foramen magnum ('large hole') in the base of the skull.

Development of the brain

A look at the development of the brain shown in Figure 3.2a will help in the understanding of the position and form of the adult brain areas.

The **forebrain** first grows laterally and backwards. It then folds forwards on itself and takes on the appearance of a hand wearing a boxing glove with the thumb touching the palm when viewed from the side. Hidden by the extensive growth of the cerebral hemispheres, the forebrain also develops less rapidly to form the basal ganglia. The wall of the remaining part of the forebrain thickens to form the thalamus and hypothalamus, collectively known as the diencephalon or 'between brain'. The structures in the diencephalon provide important links between the cerebral hemispheres and other parts of the central nervous system for both sensory and motor activity.

The **midbrain** continues in the same position during development, increasing in total size, but obscured in the external view of the brain by the lower temporal lobes of the cerebral hemispheres. In the adult, the midbrain looks like the 'waist', area with the expanded forebrain above and hindbrain below. Find the midbrain in the sagittal section of the brain (Figure 3.3). The midbrain provides routes for pathways carrying impulses up or down to various levels of the central nervous system and is also important for integration of information from the eyes and ears.

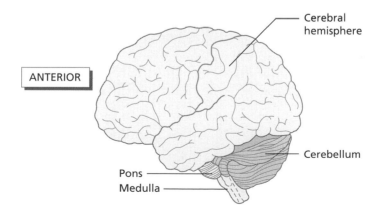

Figure 3.1 External appearance of the brain, lateral view of the left side.

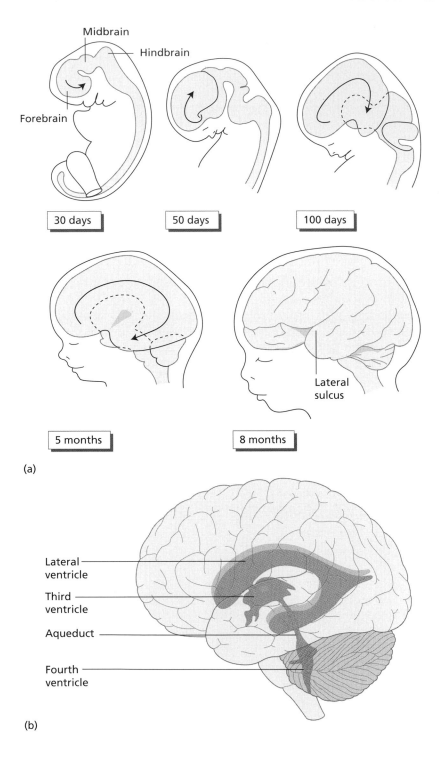

Figure 3.2 (a) Development of the brain showing folding of the forebrain; (b) adult brain viewed from the left showing the position of the cavities.

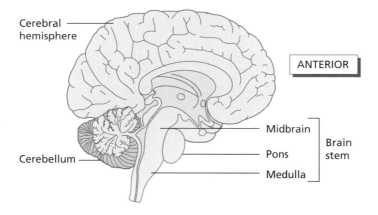

Figure 3.3   Median sagittal section of the brain.

The **hindbrain** develops into the pons and medulla oblongata. The cerebellum, also part of the hindbrain, grows out from the pons to lie under the posterior lobes of the cerebral hemisphere in the adult brain. Three fibre tracts link the cerebellum to the midbrain, pons and medulla.

The **brain stem** is the term used to describe the long cylindrical base of the brain which links the diencephalon to the spinal cord below. The brain stem is composed of the midbrain, pons and medulla (Figure 3.3). If the outgrowths of the cerebral hemispheres and cerebellum are removed from the brain, the complete brain stem can be seen with the diencephalon above.

The developing brain retains an internal cavity which forms the ventricular system containing cerebrospinal fluid. The cavity within each cerebral hemisphere follows the shape of the clenched hand and is known as the lateral ventricle. The cavity in the centre of the diencephalon is a thin slit between the two thalami, called the third ventricle. The central cavity of the midbrain is a narrow canal called the cerebral aqueduct which leads down into the fourth ventricle, the cavity of the hindbrain. The fourth ventricle lies behind the pons and upper part of the medulla, with the cerebellum forming the roof of the cavity. Figure 3.2b shows the cavities of the brain in position in the adult brain.

> **Reflective task**
>
> Look at a model of the brain and diagrams of sections through the brain in other anatomy textbooks to identify the position and relationships of the following brain areas: cerebral hemispheres, thalamus, basal ganglia, midbrain, pons, cerebellum and medulla oblongata.

Cerebrospinal fluid

The central nervous system is surrounded and protected by the bones of the skull and the vertebral column. Further protection is provided by the cerebrospinal fluid, which is found in all the cavities of the brain and in the central canal of the spinal cord. The same fluid is also found surrounding the brain and spinal cord, in between two of the three layers of protective connective

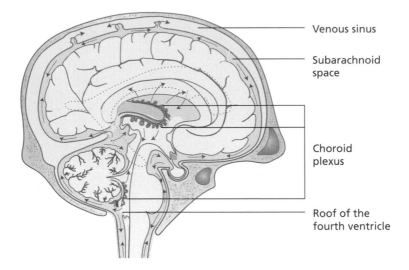

Figure 3.4   Circulation of cerebrospinal fluid seen in a sagittal section of the brain.

tissue known as the meninges; these will be described later. The main function of the fluid is to act as a shock absorber. It also carries nutrients and other essential substances to the nerve tissue. Figure 3.4 shows a sagittal section of the brain and part of the spinal cord to illustrate the way in which the cerebrospinal fluid circulates through the central cavities and around the outside of the central nervous system. The fluid is secreted from special patches of blood capillaries called choroid plexuses situated in each of the ventricles of the brain. The ventricles are found in the areas of greatest growth and expansion during development. Cerebrospinal fluid is formed by a process of filtration from the capillaries of each choroid plexus at the rate of 500 ml/day. Follow the arrows in Figure 3.4 to see how the fluid flows downwards in the brain and then through openings in the roof of the fourth ventricle into the space between the coverings of the brain. The absorption of cerebrospinal fluid into the blood takes place mainly in the venous sinus between the two cerebral hemispheres, known as the superior sagittal sinus.

Organisation of neurones into grey and white matter

The brain is composed of neurones (see Chapter 1) and their supporting cells, the neuroglia. Surprisingly, half the volume of the central nervous system is made up of neuroglia, which are special support cells found in between the neurones, and of capillaries which supply the high oxygen demands of nerve tissue. The neuroglia act as transporting and insulating cells, and also co-operate in the function of the neurones. Sections through the brain reveal areas of light and darker shade, the white and the grey matter, respectively. The overall pink colour of living brain tissue reflects the abundant blood supply.

The **grey matter** is all the cell bodies and dendrites of the neurones which form the core of the central nervous system. In the brain the core is not continuous, but the cells are collected together to form many nuclei of grey matter. For example, the thalamus is a nucleus of grey matter where ascending pathways from the spinal cord synapse on the way to many areas of the cerebral hemisphere. Grey matter also forms the outer layer or cortex of the cerebral hemispheres and the cerebellum. The cell bodies of the cortical neurones are laid down in layers in an organised way. The cortical grey matter is folded and each raised part, seen on the surface, is known as a gyrus. Each depression in between the gyri is called a sulcus (Figure 3.5a). A very deep sulcus is some-times called a fissure.

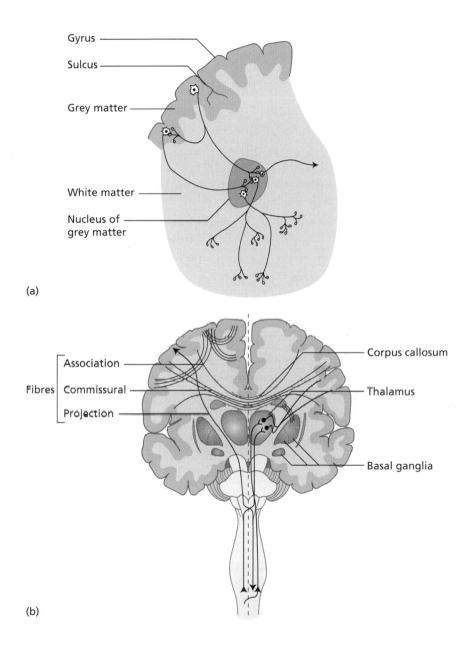

Gyrus

Sulcus

Grey matter

White matter

Nucleus of grey matter

(a)

Fibres
Association
Commissural
Projection

Corpus callosum

Thalamus

Basal ganglia

(b)

Figure 3.5   (a) Grey matter: cortex with gyrus, sulcus and deep nucleus; (b) white matter: projection, association and commissural fibres.

The **white matter** is the axons of neurones. It is found surrounding the nuclei in the brain stem and forming the core of the cerebellum and the cerebral hemispheres. The white matter is mainly organised into bundles of axons lying in particular directions (Figure 3.5b). Commissural fibres connect the right and left cerebral hemispheres. The main bridge between the two lies above the diencephalon and is known as the corpus callosum. It contains an estimated one million nerve fibres. Association fibres link one gyrus to another gyrus in the same hemisphere. Projection fibres convey information between the surface grey matter and both the lower centres of the brain stem and the spinal cord. Each of the projection fibres carries impulses in one direction only, either upwards or downwards.

Reflective task

Look at a brain model and diagrams of sections of the brain to identify

(1) the position and relations of the cerebral hemispheres, the cerebellum and the brain stem (midbrain, pons and medulla) (see Figure 3.3);
(2) the cortical layer of grey matter in the cerebral hemispheres and cerebellum which forms the outer surface like the skin of a fruit;
(3) the nuclei of grey matter in the brain stem and in the core of the cerebral hemispheres and cerebellum;
(4) the white matter found below the layers of cortex, and also surrounding the nuclei in the brain stem.

It is important to build up a three-dimensional picture of the shape, position and relations of the areas of the brain. Diagrams of sections taken through the brain at different levels can be compared with slices in various directions of a Swiss (jelly) roll or a piece of marble. Each slice shows one particular colour in a different way, but the shapes can be put together to determine the three-dimensional shape inside. This task is not easy, but can be achieved with practice.

The **location** and overall **functions** of each of the main brain areas will now be considered in the following order: cerebral hemispheres (frontal, parietal, temporal and occipital lobes), basal ganglia, thalamus, hypothalamus and limbic system, brain stem and cerebellum.

Cerebral hemispheres

The great expansion of the cerebral hemispheres (or cerebrum) to envelop nearly all other brain areas distinguishes the primates, especially humans, from other animals. It is, therefore, not surprising that the surface of the hemispheres (cerebral cortex) has been studied extensively for over two centuries. The microscopists of the mid-nineteenth century noted variations in the basic cellular architecture in different regions of the cerebral cortex. The result of these studies was a detailed mapping into 52 areas numbered by Brodman (1909) and used in practice to this day for purposes of description. Meanwhile, evidence from brain damage was accumulating to suggest that different areas of the cerebral cortex have particular functions. In 1861 Broca had identified a particular area in the left hemisphere concerned with speech, from the post-mortem examination of a patient with a severe motor speech defect. Evidence from head injuries in soldiers in the trenches in World War I, and studies of the electrical activity of the surface of the brain during surgical intervention led to the identification of distinct motor and sensory areas related to particular parts of the body.

The **primary areas** identify and localise information from the sense organs, skin and muscles (sensory), or send out motor commands to the muscles for the correct force, timing and speed of movement (motor). Other areas, called **association areas**, process information from the primary areas at a higher level for recognition and meaning. For example, there is a primary sensory area receiving information from receptors in the skin, muscles and joints. An adjacent association area has links with the primary area and with other areas involved in perception and memory. The integration of all this information leads to the ability to recognise objects held in the hand without vision, known as stereognosis.

In recent years, **neuroimaging studies** using positron emission tomography (PET) have extended our knowledge of brain function by identifying the active brain areas during the performance of activities using the upper limbs. Studies have shown that the number and the location of active areas vary in different individuals performing the same task, and activity may occur in both the right and left hemispheres during the performance of a single-handed task. Similarly, functional magnetic resonance imaging (fMRI) scans can measure the changes in blood flow as a result of neuronal activity linked to different functions. This technology can assist in mapping different areas of the cortex in response to undertaking different activities. More recently, TMS (transcranial magnetic stimulation) studies involve placing a magnetic coil near a specific area of the person's head to extrinsically stimulate functional movements, i.e. make someone perform a specific movement. If this is combined with fMRI, the specific location of that function can be very accurately mapped on the cortex.

PET scan studies have shown that the function of one brain area can shift to another area with related function after brain damage. A group of people who had been blinded in early life showed activity in the areas of the brain normally concerned with vision when they performed tactile tasks. Normal subjects doing the same tactile tasks showed no activity in the visual areas. These results confirm the **plasticity** of neurones in the brain, particularly in early life.

The lobes of the cerebral hemispheres

Each cerebral hemisphere is divided into four lobes, named after the skull bones that cover them. In each hemisphere, the lobes are separated by two deep sulci: the central sulcus and the lateral sulcus (Figure 3.6a).

- The **frontal lobe** lies anterior to the central sulcus, and above the lateral sulcus.
- The **parietal lobe** lies behind the central sulcus.
- The **occipital lobe** is at the posterior end of the hemisphere, above the cerebellum at the base of the skull.
- The **temporal lobe** lies below the lateral sulcus.

Each lobe continues on to the medial surface of the hemisphere (Figure 3.6b). The median sagittal sulcus separates the right and left frontal, parietal and occipital lobes (Figure 3.6c).

It is important to realise that the surface of the cerebral hemispheres extends from the level of the eyebrows in front, to the base of the skull at the back of the head, and down to the level of the ears at the side. This becomes obvious when a life-sized model of the brain is placed inside the cranial cavity of the skull.

The overall functions of each lobe of the cerebral hemispheres will be described in turn. It is important to stress that the numerous interconnections among the four lobes means that no individual lobe functions alone.

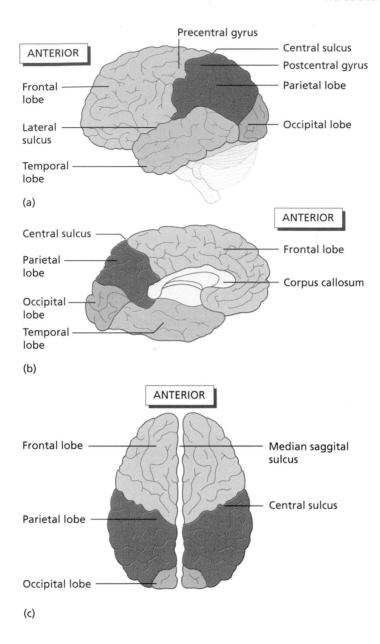

Figure 3.6 Lobes of the cerebral hemispheres seen in: (a) lateral view; (b) medial view; (c) view from above.

Frontal lobe

The frontal lobe is a large part of the cerebral hemisphere found underneath the frontal bone of the skull. The part of the frontal lobe particularly concerned with the performance of movement lies more posteriorly in the lobe, leading up to the central sulcus. The larger anterior part of the lobe, which lies above the orbit of the eyes (supraorbital area), is involved in planning and problem-solving aspects of both movement and behaviour. This part of the frontal lobe is also called the prefrontal lobe.

Practice note-pad 3A: stroke

Stroke is brain tissue damage that results from disruption of the blood supply to a localised area of the brain. It may be caused by haemorrhage from a blood vessel, but is more commonly due to arterial occlusion by a thrombus or an embolism.

The disruption of the blood supply results in infarct (tissue death) of the affected area, giving rise to a lesion. The symptoms and prognosis for each patient will be determined primarily by the location, extent and causal mechanism. A stroke can occur in any area of the brain, but usually affects one cerebral hemisphere, giving rise to difficulties associated with the functions of that hemisphere. See practice note pads 3B to 3E.

The band of grey matter lying immediately in front of the central sulcus (precentral gyrus) is the **primary motor area**, which is concerned with the generation of movement in the whole of the opposite side of the body (Figure 3.7a). Adjacent to this area are the premotor area and the supplementary motor area which are discussed in more detail below.

The cell bodies of the neurones in the motor cortex project not to individual muscles, but to functional groups of muscles. Direct links to the small muscles of the hands, the feet and the face are particularly important, and damage to the primary motor area often results in loss of precision movements.

There is representation of half of the body in an 'upside-down' position in each primary motor cortex. The head is represented in the lower cortex on the lateral side, then the upper limb and trunk above, and finally the lower leg and feet in the cortex on the medial surface of the lobe. In Figure 3.8, a vertical section through the cerebral hemisphere at the level of the primary motor area is shown (frontal section). Note that the sizes of the body parts are not in normal proportions. The body parts that move with the greatest degree of precision have larger areas of representation, so that the face and hand are large, while the trunk and leg are small. A figure constructed with these dimensions has a head like a hippopotamus, the hands of a giant, and the trunk and legs of a dwarf, and is known as the 'motor homunculus'.

The **premotor area** lies anterior to the primary motor area on the lateral surface of the lobe (Figure 3.7a). Visual and auditory information from the occipital and temporal lobes, respectively, is integrated in the premotor area to guide movement, more specifically it helps guide body movement by integrating sensory information and controls muscle groups that are closest to the axis of the body (midline). Neurones project from this area to the primary motor area on the same and the opposite side. Projection fibres from the premotor area descend directly to the spinal cord, or indirectly via the primary motor cortex.

The **supplementary motor area** (SMA) also lies anterior to the primary motor area, but mainly on the medial side of the frontal lobe (Figure 3.7b). Neuroimaging studies have recorded an increase in cerebral blood flow in the supplementary motor area immediately before the

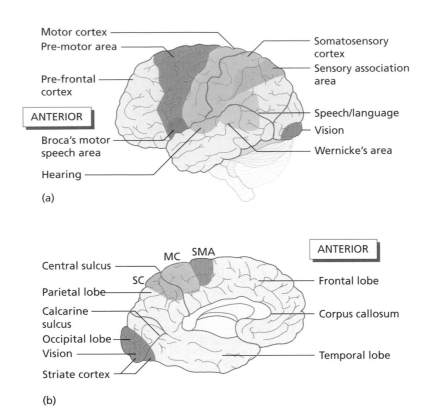

Figure 3.7   Main functional areas of the cerebral hemispheres: (a) lateral view; (b) medial view. MC = primary motor cortex; SMA = supplementary motor area; SC = somatosensory area.

execution of complex sequences of movements of the fingers, and when both hands are involved. These studies suggest a role in the planning of movement that is internally generated.

The **motor speech area** identified by Broca lies in the lower part of the frontal lobe in the lip of the lateral sulcus (see Figure 3.7a). The function of this area, usually only found in the dominant hemisphere, is in the production of fluent speech.

The **prefrontal area** (supraorbital area) occupies the large anterior area of the frontal lobe and connects with all the other lobes of the cerebral hemispheres, the thalamus, the limbic system and many other brain areas. Interaction with the limbic system is concerned with the emotional aspects of movement. The prefrontal area is also concerned with the planning of goal-directed movement and behaviour and in modifying the plan in response to changes in the environment. These are known as the executive functions.

Parietal lobe

The parietal lobe lies posterior to the frontal lobe and beneath the parietal bone of the skull. The overall function of the parietal lobe is the processing of sensory input from receptors in all parts of the body and also from the special sense organs (eyes and ears). This provides awareness of the position of the parts of the body during movement and spatial awareness of the environment.

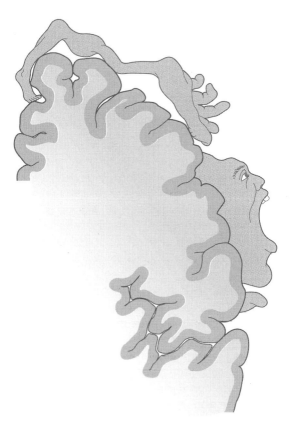

Figure 3.8   Primary motor cortex seen in frontal section to show the representation of body parts.

Practice note-pad 3B: frontal lobe lesion

- A lesion in the primary and premotor cortex on one side leads to muscle weakness in the muscles of the opposite side of the body, known as contralateral hemiplegia. Muscle tone may be low (flaccid) or high (spastic). Fine skilled movements of the extremities are particularly affected.
- Lesions in the prefrontal cortex area lead to problems in planning movement and the ongoing review of movement whilst it is being carried out. Loss of insight into movement performance may be a major factor in the rehabilitation process. Frontal lobe lesions are also associated with innapropriate social behaviour and lack of insight. The inability to plan and monitor movement and behaviour resulting from lesions in the prefrontal cortex is known as dysexecutive syndrome.

The **somatosensory area** is the primary area, lying immediately behind the central sulcus in the postcentral gyrus (Figure 3.7a). Pathways from receptors in the skin, muscles and joints of the opposite side of the body connect with the primary sensory cortex via the thalamus. The areas of the body are represented in an 'upside-down' position in the same way as in the primary motor cortex. The area of cortex representing the hand is large, particularly the palmar surface of the thumb and index finger. The lips also have a large area of representation for the complex sensory input required for speech and the mastication of food.

Practice note-pad 3C: parietal lobe lesion

This type of lesion infers a loss of somatic sensation on the opposite side of the body, particularly in the distal parts of the limbs. The main features are inability: to localize tactile information; to appreciate temperature; to judge the weight of objects; and to appreciate the position of the limbs (proprioception). The inability to recognise objects without vision is known as astereognosis. In right-sided parietal lesions there may be loss of body and spatial awareness on the contralateral side. Individuals may ignore one side of the body or objects in one side of space and this is known as unilateral neglect.

The **sensory association area**, lying posterior to the somatosensory area, is where processing of the sensory information occurs. An object, such as a key, held in the hand and moved about can be recognised even with the eyes closed. Information about the size, shape, weight, temperature and texture arriving at the cortex can be integrated with reference to memory, so that the exact nature of the object can be identified. This ability is known as stereognosis.

The parietal lobe, by receiving sensory information from the joints and muscles, synthesises a **body scheme**, which is the position of all body segments in relation to each other and to the environment. The parietal lobe also receives input from visual and auditory areas of the cortex. Objects and sounds in the environment are located and identified. All of this spatial information processed by the parietal lobe is essential for the ability to use objects and tools.

Temporal lobe

The temporal lobe, found beneath the temporal bone of the skull, processes auditory information from the ear and also plays an important role in memory.

Sound falling on the ear is transmitted by nerve impulses from the cochlea of the inner ear to the **primary auditory area** below the lateral sulcus in the temporal lobe (see Figure 3.7a). The pathway is mainly crossed to the opposite temporal lobe, but each auditory area receives some impulses from both ears. The primary area links with auditory association areas in the superior temporal gyrus, which interpret the sound frequencies. In the dominant hemisphere, the extension of the auditory association area around the tip of the lateral sulcus and into the parietal lobe is known as Wernicke's area (Figure 3.7a) and plays a role in receptive aspects of speech and language. Visual and auditory input from the written and spoken word are integrated in this area.

Practice note-pad 3D: temporal lobe lesion

When the primary auditory area is affected in one temporal lobe, slight loss of hearing occurs in both ears, but the loss is greater in the contralateral ear. Posterior lesions on the left temporal lobe may affect receptive aspects of language (Wernicke's area). Consequently, the individual is unable to understand spoken or written words (receptive dysphasia).

The temporal lobe is also involved in **memory**. Neuroimaging using PET scanning has shown the importance of a buried gyrus in the temporal lobe, called the hippocampus, in the ability to find the way around in the environment. This may be part of the spatial aspects of memory.

Occipital lobe

The occipital lobe lies beneath the occipital bone of the skull. All visual information transmitted from the eye is first processed by the occipital lobe.

The **primary visual area**, known as the striate cortex, lies at the posterior pole of the occipital lobe and extends mainly on to the inner or medial surface, on either side of the calcarine sulcus (Figure 3.7b). Sections of the primary visual area reveal a horizontal stripe of white matter, hence the name striate cortex. Information from the retina of both eyes arrives in each striate cortex. The left half of the visual field for both eyes is processed in the right striate cortex. Conversely, the right half of the visual field for each eye is relayed to the left striate cortex.

The **prestriate cortex** is an association area surrounding the primary area on the medial surface of the lobe (Figure 3.7b). Links to the parietal and temporal lobes are involved in the recognition of objects and faces, and in the understanding of the written word.

Practice note-pad 3E: occipital lobe lesion

- **Hemianopia.** Damage to the primary visual area in one occipital lobe may result in loss of sight in an area of the opposite half of the visual field of each eye. In small lesions, there may be apparent normal central vision known as macular sparing.
- **Visual agnosia.** Damage to the prestriate occipital cortex leads to loss of the ability to recognise objects on the contralateral side, even though the objects can be seen clearly. Bilateral damage results in severe recognition problems for objects and faces.

Sensory information from the eyes plays a major role in movement. Vision is important in placing the foot accurately on the ground in locomotion. Reaching and manipulating objects depends on knowledge from vision of their position and relations with all the features of the visual environment.

Summary

- **Frontal lobe:** planning and performance of movement; modifying goal-directed movement and behaviour in response to decision making or changes in the environment (executive function); motor speech.
- **Parietal lobe:** location of sensation in specific parts of the body; integration of sensation from the skin, the joints and the muscles during movement; stereognosis; body scheme; spatial relations of objects.
- **Temporal lobe:** hearing; receptive speech and language; topographical orientation; memory.
- **Occipital lobe:** reception of visual images from the retina of the eye; processing of visual information for recognition.

Lateralisation

The functional asymmetry of the right and left hemispheres, first recognised by Broca in the mid-nineteenth century gained new interest from 'split brain' studies by Sperry in the 1970s. Sperry

Practice note-pad 3F: traumatic brain injury

Trauma to the head can result in multiple lesions within the brain, both at the primary site of impact and as a result of secondary complications. This infers potential contusions and lacerations of brain tissue. The effects of shearing and rotational forces cause diffuse axonal damage throughout the brain.

The presenting features are complex, variable and related to diffuse cerebral damage. Individuals may have problems related to:

- movement: changes in muscle tone leading to abnormal patterns of movement;
- sensory processing: balance and walking;
- perception: visuospatial, object and face recognition, disordered movement;
- cognition: attention, memory and speech;
- social interaction: loss of engagement in social situations, loneliness, withdrawal, depression;
- personality changes;
- behaviour: anger, frustration, irritability, apathy, loss of insight.

devised an experiment using two screens placed in positions so that information could be presented to only one of the visual fields at a time. This, in turn, meant that only one hemisphere received the information. These experiments showed that each hemisphere processes particular types of information, verbal on the left and spatial on the right.

Both sides of the normal brain receive the same basic input, so that any differences between the two must lie in their capacity to process different types of information. The **dominant** hemisphere (usually the left) contains the areas for speech and language, and this side is particularly concerned with analytical functions. The **non-dominant** hemisphere plays a greater role in non-verbal, creative activity requiring spatial processing (Figure 3.9).

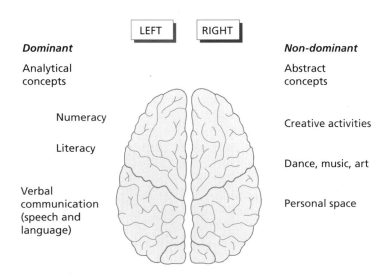

Figure 3.9   Lateralisation of function in the right and left hemispheres.

Basal ganglia

The basal ganglia (or basal nuclei) are found in the diencephalon at the base of the cerebral hemispheres and in the midbrain. In Figure 3.10 the lateral cerebral cortex has been made to appear transparent to reveal three of the basal ganglia: the caudate, putamen and globus pallidus. (The caudate and putamen are sometimes called the corpus striatum. The putamen and the globus pallidus are sometimes called the lentiform nucleus.) Two other basal nuclei are the sub-thalamic nucleus and the substantia nigra. The latter is in the midbrain.

The basal ganglia together form a complex interdependent system, which functions as a whole. It has been recognised that the basal ganglia are important in movements that rely heavily on sensory cues from the environment, for example walking across the threshold of a door. Information from all the sensory and motor areas of the cerebral cortex is processed in the basal ganglia and is projected back to the motor areas of the cortex via the thalamus (Figure 3.11). In this way, the

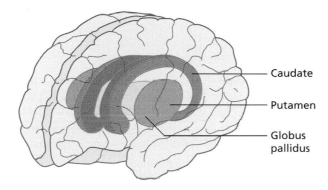

Figure 3.10   Basal ganglia in position at the base of the cerebral hemispheres.

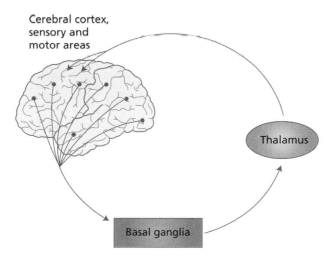

Figure 3.11   Motor control loop from the cerebral cortex to the basal ganglia and back to the cortical motor areas, via the thalamus.

basal ganglia act as a bridge between the cerebral cortex and the thalamus for the initiation and control of movement. The effect of the basal ganglia on the motor areas of the cerebral cortex appears to be in the form of a brake during the execution of movement.

The basal ganglia have no direct link with the muscles via the spinal cord. Their influence on movement is via the descending pathways from the cortical motor areas with which the basal ganglia interact.

Practice note-pad 3G: parkinson's disease

The progressive degeneration in the neurones of the substantia nigra in the brain stem, which project to other basal nuclei, leads to a reduction of dopamine (a neurotransmitter) in the basal ganglia. The resulting effects include: a resting tremor in distal joints that disappears during movement; cogwheel rigidity in muscles; and difficulty initiating and producing movement.

Thalamus

The thalamus lies in the diencephalon, at the base of the forebrain and enveloped by the cerebral hemispheres. The slit-like third ventricle lies in the midline, and each thalamus is an oval mass of grey matter on either side of it. Return to Figure 3.5 to find the thalamus on each side of the brain, close to the midline, as seen in a frontal section of the brain.

All sensory information, except for smell, passes through the thalamus before reaching the cerebral cortex. The output from the thalamus radiates out to the cerebral cortex of the same side (ipsilateral) like the spokes of an umbrella with the thalamus at its centre. The reticular formation (see later section, Brain stem), which acts as a sift to most of the sensory information originating at the level of the spinal cord, regulates the level of activity in the thalamus. The thalamus also has a function in the motor system via links with the basal ganglia and cerebellum (see Chapter 12).

Figure 3.12 is a sagittal section through one cerebral hemisphere showing the corona radiata of projection fibres (both motor and sensory) all converging at the base of the hemisphere. Figure

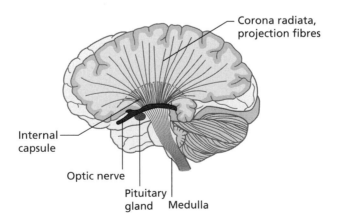

Figure 3.12   Cortical projection fibres converging to form the internal capsule.

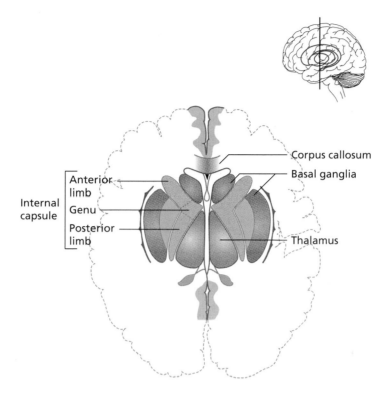

Figure 3.13 Horizontal section at the level of the internal capsule.

3.13 is a transverse section to show where these fibres lie between the thalamus and the basal ganglia. At this point the bundle of nerve fibres is known as the **internal capsule**. All of the ascending and descending information passing between the spinal cord and the cerebral cortex passes through the internal capsule. Because of the convergence of a large number of projection fibres into this narrow area, damage in the region of the internal capsule has widespread effects on both sensory and motor function.

Hypothalamus and limbic system

The **hypothalamus** is smaller than the thalamus and lies beneath it in the floor of the third ventricle (Figure 3.14a). Like the basement of a house with thermostats and stopcocks, the hypothalamus contains groups of neurones for the control of body temperature and body water. The output from the hypothalamus is to the autonomic division of the peripheral nervous system (see Chapter 4) which controls the diameter of blood vessels, the secretion of sweat glands and the release of hormones from the pituitary gland.

The hypothalamus is the control area for all the mechanisms that maintain homoeostasis (a constant internal environment) in the body. This area can be referred to as the 'visceral brain'.

The **limbic system** as a whole is a complex series of interconnected structures lying in the forebrain and midbrain, linked by a large cable of white matter known as the fornix. The limbic

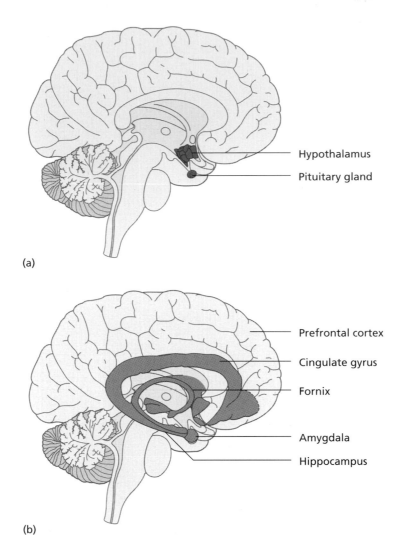

Figure 3.14   Position of: (a) hypothalamus; (b) limbic system seen in medial view of the left side of the brain.

forebrain includes an area of cerebral cortex (cingulate gyrus) lying medially above the corpus callosum, and the hippocampus lying buried in the temporal lobe (Figure 3.14b).

The functions of the limbic system structures are diverse and include:

● involvement in our emotions and motivations, especially those related to survival (fear, anger and apprehension);
● the retention of recent memory, particularly the hippocampus in the temporai lobe;
● receiving inputs from the basal ganglia and assisting learning, planning and coordination of movement;

- emotional aspects of movement. Feelings of pleasure and anger produce physiological responses via activity in the hypothalamus. The effects of emotional factors, for example motivation and insight, on movement are the outcome of interaction between the limbic system and the prefrontal area.

Brain stem

When the cerebral hemispheres and the cerebellum are removed from the brain, the whole of the brain stem is revealed (Figure 3.15). The brain stem is the region where most of the cranial nerves (see Chapter 4) enter the brain. These nerves carry sensory information from the eyes, the ears and the face, as well as motor commands to the muscles of the face and those moving the eyes.

From above downwards, the brain stem consists of **midbrain**, **pons** and **medulla oblongata**. The midbrain contains the substantia nigra, one of the basal ganglia (Figure 3.16a). The pons

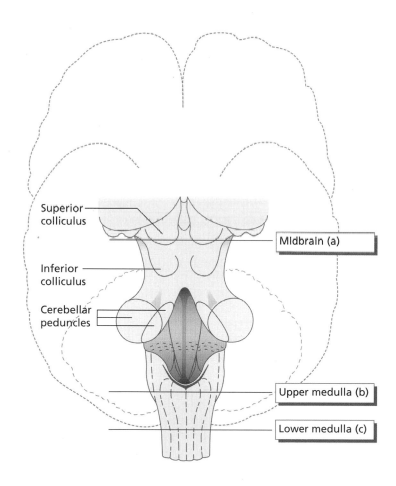

Figure 3.15   Brain stem, posterior. Sections at (a), (b) and (c) are shown in Figure 3.17.

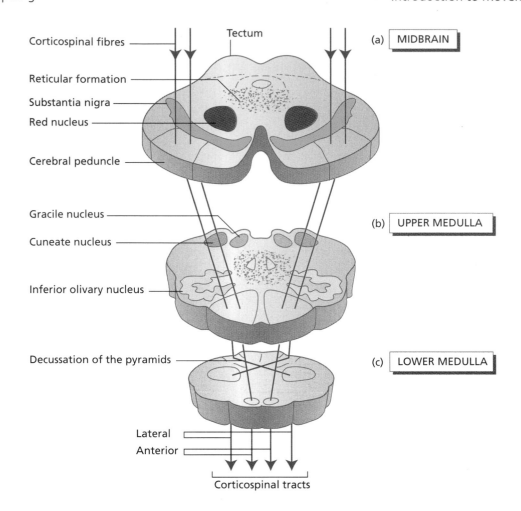

Corticospinal fibres
Tectum
(a) MIDBRAIN

Reticular formation
Substantia nigra
Red nucleus

Cerebral peduncle

Gracile nucleus
(b) UPPER MEDULLA

Cuneate nucleus

Inferior olivary nucleus

Decussation of the pyramids
(c) LOWER MEDULLA

Lateral
Anterior

Corticospinal tracts

Figure 3.16 Transverse sections through (a) midbrain; (b) upper medulla; (c) lower medulla. Note substantia nigra (basal ganglia); brain stem nuclei; descending pathway crossing in the medulla.

can be easily identified on the anterior side of the brain stem where a bulge is formed by the transverse fibres linking the two halves of the cerebellum. The medulla oblongata is the cone-shaped lower end of the brain stem that leads down into the spinal cord.

The white matter of the brain stem contains ascending and descending tracts. Some of these tracts form direct routes between the cerebral cortex and the spinal cord which cross to the opposite side in the brain stem (Figure 3.16). Other tracts, described in Chapter 12, originate in motor nuclei in the brain stem. The cerebellum lies posteriorly to the brain stem and exerts its influence on movement via output to descending tracts in the brain stem.

The brain stem motor centres play an important role in the control of posture during movement by activation of the extensor (antigravity) muscles supporting the head, trunk and lower limbs; and the proximal muscles which stabilise the upper limbs in manipulative movements.

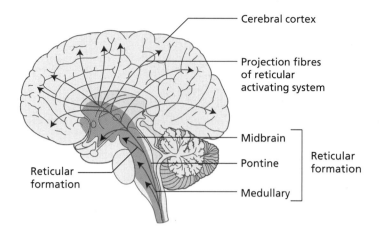

Figure 3.17   Brain stem reticular formation.

Reticular formation

The reticular formation is a diffuse network of neurones in the core of the brain stem extending from the midbrain to the medulla. Some groups of neurones are collected together in nuclei, but in general the reticular formation, unlike other brain areas, consists of scattered cell bodies with the fibres lying in between. The network receives branches from the ascending pathways through the brain stem. The neurones of the reticular formation in the midbrain project to all areas of the cerebral cortex and form the ascending reticular activating system (ARAS) (Figure 3.17). The activity in these neurones affects the level of arousal and attention. The ARAS controls the 'body clock', which alternates the cycle of sleeping and waking.

In the lower pons and medulla the reticular formation contains the vital centres, which control the heart from the cardiac centre, the blood pressure from the vasomotor centre and breathing from the respiratory centres. These vital centres respond to changes in blood composition and the activity in sensory nerves from receptors in blood vessels and the lungs. Continuous or intermittent activity in the centres results in stimulation of the muscle of the heart, the walls of blood vessels and muscles involved in breathing such as the diaphragm.

Cerebellum

The cerebellum lies behind the pons and below the occipital lobe of the cerebral hemispheres in the posterior cranial fossa of the skull. Three stalks of white matter, the superior, middle and inferior peduncles, connect the cerebellum to the brain stem like a three-pin plug (Figure 3.18).

The cerebellum has two halves which are connected by a central area known as the vermis. The outer layer of grey matter of the cerebellum is folded into uniform narrow gyri. The inner white matter forms a tree shape with the folded grey matter as the leaves. This was called the arboretum vitae (the tree of life) by the early neuroanatomists. The cerebellum also has a number of deep nuclei, the largest being the dentate nucleus.

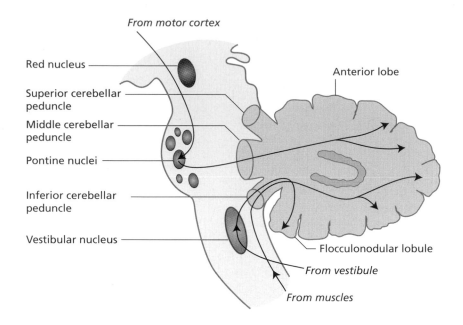

From motor cortex

Red nucleus

Superior cerebellar peduncle

Middle cerebellar peduncle

Pontine nuclei

Inferior cerebellar peduncle

Vestibular nucleus

Anterior lobe

Flocculonodular lobule

From vestibule

From muscles

Figure 3.18   Input to the cerebellum from: the motor cortex; the vestibule of the ear; the muscles.

The cerebellum does not generate movement, but it regulates both movement and posture indirectly by adjusting the output to the major descending motor system from the brain to the spinal cord. Figure 3.18 shows how information enters the cerebellum from:

- the vestibule of the ear (see Chapter 4) about the position of the head;
- the proprioceptors in the muscles and joints about the position of all the body segments;
- the motor cortex about the current motor commands to the descending motor system.

By comparing the intended movement (motor commands) with the sensory information that reflects the actual performance, the cerebellum compensates for errors in movement. The cerebellum has been compared with the control system of a guided missile which ensures that it lands on the target.

Practice note-pad 3H: cerebellar dysfunction – ataxia

The performance of movement (on the ipsilateral side) is uncoordinated, clumsy or jerky. This is known as ataxia. Movements often overshoot or undershoot the intended goal (dysmetria), for example in walking on a narrow base, turning suddenly or touching the nose with a finger. Muscle tone is usually decreased. Intention tremor occurs in proximal muscle groups during purposeful movement.

Another function of the cerebellum concerns its role in learning motor skills. Motor programmes, which are developed, stored and updated by the cerebellum, can be executed without reference to consciousness. More details of motor learning will be described in Chapter 12.

Summary of brain areas: function in movement

- **Motor areas of the cerebral cortex:** generate the motor commands to the muscles for the performance of movement:
  - **primary motor area:** generates the motor commands based on activity received from the somatosensory area, the basal ganglia and the cerebellum;
  - **premotor area:** integrates information from the visual and auditory cortical areas and links with the primary motor area in the planning of movement;
  - **supplementary motor area:** plans complex voluntary movement and integrates bilateral movement.
- **Sensory areas of the cerebral cortex:** identify and locate stimuli from the senses, the skin and the muscles; further processing leads to recognition and meaning:
  - **primary somatosensory area:** identifies and locates tactile and proprioceptive information;
  - **striate area:** processes visual images from the retina of the eyes; further processing in the prestriate area leads to visual recognition;
  - **primary auditory area:** processes sounds in the environment and in speech; further processing in the association areas lead to sound discrimination and receptive speech.
- **Thalamus:** transmission and some processing of: all sensory information except for smell to the cerebral cortex for integration and interpretation; motor command information from the basal ganglia and cerebellum to the cortical motor areas.
- **Basal ganglia:** planning, initiation and regulation of skilled movements that are mostly automatic, for example walking.
- **Limbic system and prefrontal cortex:** involved in the emotions, such as fear, anger and anxiety, which influence movement and behaviour.
- **Cerebellum:** regulates movement and posture by comparing the motor commands for intended movement with sensory feedback about the actual performance; stores motor programmes for learned motor skills.
- **Brain stem:** adjusts the activity in the descending motor system for the control of posture during movement.
- **Reticular formation:** adjusts arousal and attention level during movement; vital centres for breathing and circulation of the blood.

PART II: THE SPINAL CORD

The spinal cord appears to be a simple structure by comparison with the brain, but its role in the function of the central nervous system is nevertheless very important. Basic movement patterns of the limbs and trunk are processed in the spinal cord. A large part of the body's sensory information is received by the spinal cord and is passed on to higher levels in the brain.

Position and segmentation of the spinal cord

The embryonic neural tube grows in diameter and length with the bony vertebrae developing round it. The internal cavity of the tube remains as a small central spinal canal containing cerebrospinal fluid. A pair of spinal nerves grows out from the developing spinal cord between adjacent vertebrae. The segment of the cord that gives rise to each pair of spinal nerves is named in relation to the corresponding vertebra, for example the segment lying under the first thoracic vertebra is known as T1.

There are 31 **spinal segments**, named as follows: eight cervical (C1–C8), 12 thoracic (T1–T12), five lumbar (L1–L5), five sacral (S1–S5) and one coccygeal.

The first pair of cervical nerves lies between the skull and the first cervical vertebra, and C1–C7 all emerge *above* the corresponding vertebrae. The eighth pair of cervical nerves emerges between the seventh cervical and first thoracic vertebrae.

All of the thoracic and lumbar nerves emerge *below* the corresponding vertebra.

The sacral nerves descend in the vertebral canal of the sacrum and emerge through the anterior foraminae of the sacrum, which can be seen in the anterior view of the pelvis in Appendix I. The vertebral column grows in length more rapidly than the spinal cord, so that in the adult the lower end of the spinal cord lies at the level of the disc between the first and second lumbar vertebrae. The lower end tapers to a point and is attached by a strand of connective tissue (filum terminale) to the lower end of the sacrum and to the coccyx.

Reflective task

- Look at an articulated skeleton, or the individual vertebrae loosely strung together. Put a piece of plastic tubing 45 cm long into the vertebral canal and note where the lower end lies. The tubing should be thicker towards the upper and lower ends to represent the spinal cord accurately. Note that the vertebral canal is larger in the cervical and upper lumbar regions to accommodate the cervical and lumbar enlargements of the spinal cord.
- Identify the intervertebral foramina between adjacent vertebrae where the spinal nerves emerge. Starting at the skull, see how the spinal segment and pair of spinal nerves C8 appear.
- Look at Figure 3.19, a sagittal section through the spinal cord and vertebral column with the spinal nerves emerging from the cord. The cervical and lumbar enlargements accommodate the large number of neurones that supply the upper and lower limbs, respectively.
- Look at Figure 3.20 to see a transverse section of the spinal cord lying in position surrounded by the bony vertebra. The right and left sides of the spinal cord are symmetrical and are separated by two longitudinal sulci, one anteriorly and one posteriorly.

Spinal meninges

The spinal cord is protected externally by three membranes of connective tissue which are also continuous over the surface of the brain. The three layers (Figure 3.21), from superficial to deep, are the dura mater, the arachnoid mater and the pia mater.

The **dura mater** is a thick layer densely packed with collagen fibres and some elastin which lines the cranial vault of the skull and the vertebral canal of the spine as far down as the level of the second sacral vertebra. The epidural space lies between the dura mater and the periosteum and ligaments of the vertebral column. Anaesthetics injected into the epidural space of one spinal segment may spread upwards or downwards to affect the spinal nerves emerging from adjacent segments.

The **arachnoid mater** is a thin membrane lying in close contact with the dura mater, separated by a thin film of fluid. Deep to the arachnoid mater is the subarachnoid space containing cerebrospinal fluid. The arachnoid mater ends at the level of the second sacral vertebra. This means that between the third lumbar vertebra (where the spinal cord ends) and the second sacral vertebra, cerebrospinal fluid can be extracted for examination without risk of damaging the spinal cord. This procedure, a lumbar puncture, is usually done by inserting a blunt needle between the laminae of the third and fourth lumbar vertebrae.

The **pia mater** is a loose membrane of connective tissue which covers the whole surface of the brain and spinal cord, and dips down into all the sulci. There is a rich network of blood vessels associated with the pia mater providing a major part of the blood supply to the brain and spinal cord.

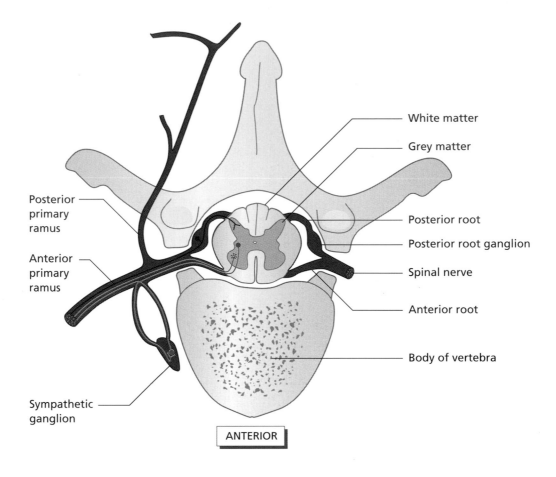

White matter

Grey matter

Posterior primary ramus

Anterior primary ramus

Posterior root

Posterior root ganglion

Spinal nerve

Anterior root

Body of vertebra

Sympathetic ganglion

ANTERIOR

Figure 3.20   Transverse section of the spinal cord surrounded by the corresponding vertebra.

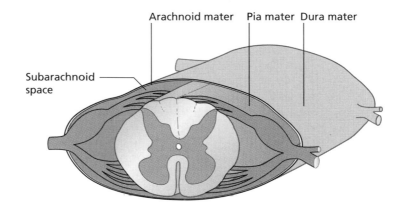

Arachnoid mater   Pia mater   Dura mater

Subarachnoid space

Figure 3.21   Meninges surrounding the spinal cord.

The meninges protect the spinal cord and brain from infection, and the cerebrospinal fluid acts as a shock absorber.

Organisation of neurones into grey and white matter

The internal structure of the spinal cord is organised into an H-shaped central core of grey matter with anterior and posterior horns, surrounded by white matter. Transverse sections of the spinal cord at different levels can be seen in Figure 3.22. The anterior horn is large in the cervical, lumbar and sacral regions where the lower motor neurones supplying muscles of the limbs are found. The grey matter in all thoracic segments, lumbar segments 1 and 2, and sacral segments 2, 3 and 4 have a lateral horn where the cell bodies of neurones which form part of the autonomic nervous system (see Chapter 4), supplying organs, glands and blood vessels, are found.

The **white matter** contains bundles of nerve fibres or tracts carrying impulses up or down the spinal cord. These are known as ascending and descending **tracts**, respectively (Figure 3.23b).

The white matter of the spinal cord is largest at the upper end and smallest at the lower end. Fibres leave the descending tracts at each segment to enter the grey matter. The ascending tracts are formed from sensory neurones in spinal nerves, the axons of which enter the white matter at all levels either directly or after synapsing in the posterior horn. Figure 3.23a shows how the posterior column of white matter increases in size as it receives fibres from successive spinal nerves.

The **grey matter** which forms the core of the spinal cord is organised as follows.

The **anterior horn** contains motor neurone pools, each supplying particular groups of muscles acting on one joint. Their axons lie in the anterior roots of spinal nerves to be distributed to all parts of the body. These motor neurones include the skeletomotor neurones described in Chapter 1.

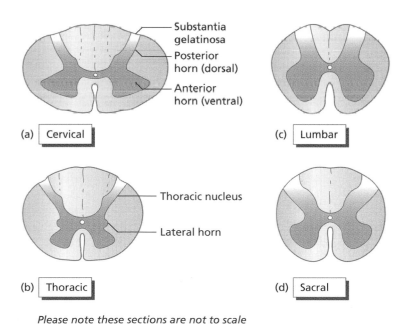

Please note these sections are not to scale

Figure 3.22   Transverse sections of the spinal cord: (a) cervical; (b) thoracic; (c) lumbar; (d) sacral.

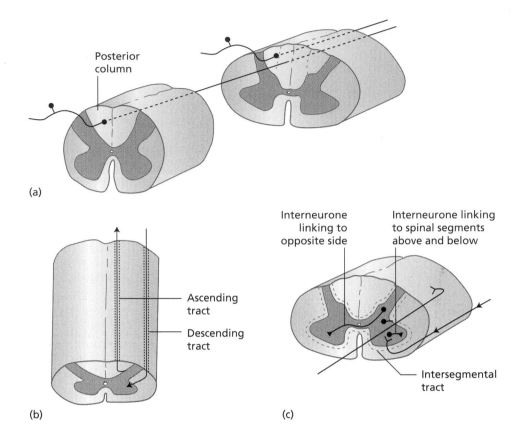

Figure 3.23   Spinal cord: (a) formation of ascending tract; (b) ascending and descending tracts; (c) interneurones.

The **posterior horn** contains second-order neurones which receive tactile, proprioceptive and nociceptive information from the sensory neurones entering the spinal cord. The axons of the second-order neurones of the posterior horn form the ascending tracts of the white matter.

Interneurones lie in the central core of grey matter. In the posterior horn, interneurones form the transmission cells between sensory neurones entering the spinal cord and the ascending tracts in the white matter. Inhibitory interneurones are found in the anterior horn which relax antagonist muscles when the agonist muscle contracts (see Reciprocal innervation in the next section). All segments of the spinal cord are connected by interneurones, the fibres of which lie in the inter-segmental tract, so that activity spreads to other spinal levels above and below. Activity is also spread across the spinal cord by interneurones in bilateral activities. Figure 3.23c shows the position of the different types of interneurone in the spinal cord.

Ascending and descending tracts

The white matter is divided for description into three columns or funiculi: posterior (dorsal), lateral and anterior (ventral). The ascending and descending tracts are named after the two areas that

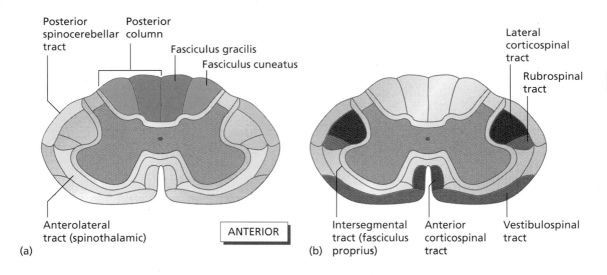

Figure 3.24 Spinal cord showing the position of the main (a) ascending and (b) descending tracts.

they link. For example, the spinothalamic tract is an ascending pathway that links the spinal cord with the thalamus, and the corticospinal tract is a descending route from the cerebral cortex to the spinal cord. Figure 3.24a shows the position of the main ascending tracts and Figure 3.24b shows the descending tracts. It must be remembered that all of the tracts are present on both sides of the spinal cord. Detail of the function of these tracts will be discussed in Chapters 11 and 12. At this stage the general way in which the white matter is organised should be appreciated. Each tract is rather like a cable of wires, but evidence indicates that there is some overlap of function. A narrow band of white matter surrounds the whole of the central core of grey matter. The fibres of this intersegmental tract connect different segments of the spinal cord. The fibres vary in length, some pass from one segment to another and others pass nearly the whole length of the cord, branching up, down and across the cord.

Spinal reflex pathways

The function of the spinal cord in movement is to regulate the activity in muscles via local pathways between the segments of the spinal cord and the nerves supplying the muscles. These pathways are known as **spinal reflexes**. Each spinal reflex has five components:

- sensory receptors which respond to a stimulus;
- a sensory (afferent) path to the spinal cord via a spinal nerve and its posterior root;
- one or more synapses in the spinal cord;
- a motor (efferent) path away from the spinal cord;
- an effector (usually a muscle) which produces the response.

Examples of spinal reflexes are the muscle stretch and the flexor reflex.

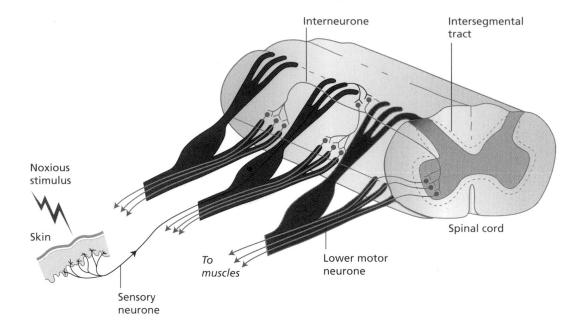

Figure 3.25 Flexor reflex: spread of activity to three spinal segments.

In the **muscle stretch reflex** (see Chapter 1) the stimulus is a change in length of the muscle that stimulates the receptors (muscle spindles) lying in parallel with the muscle fibres. This is a monosynaptic reflex and the effector is the same muscle which shortens. The function of this reflex is to maintain a posture of the body when external forces are tending to disturb it (see Figure 1.19).

The **flexor reflex** is a protective reflex that withdraws a limb away from a harmful stimulus. The receptors are nociceptors in the skin. The response is to activate all flexor muscles in the affected limb. We are aware of this when touching a hot saucepan with the hand or treading on a sharp obstacle on the floor. At the same time, activity spreads via interneurones to the opposite side of the spinal cord to activate extensor muscles of the opposite limb and maintain balance. The pattern of activity in the spinal cord in the flexor and crossed extensor reflex involves the spread of impulses to several spinal segments (Figure 3.25) and to both sides.

Spinal reflexes can be seen in the newborn baby when the influence from higher levels of the nervous system is not yet fully developed. The young child acquires head control, followed by the equilibrium reactions that allow the body segments to align over the feet and lead to standing and walking. The spinal reflexes remain as the basis of normal movement.

Reciprocal innervation

The performance of smooth movement requires the co-operation of opposing muscle groups acting around a joint, for example flexors and extensors, abductors and adductors. This is achieved by the reciprocal innervation of the lower motor neurones of antagonist muscle groups. Excitation of the lower motor neurones of one muscle group is accompanied by inhibition of the motor neurones of the antagonist group. In this way, the antagonist relaxes and allows the agonist to contract.

The input to the lower motor neurones may be from spinal reflex sensory stimulation or from descending pathways in the spinal cord carrying motor commands from the motor centres in the cerebral cortex or brain stem. In each case, the excitatory neurones in the spinal cord branch in the grey matter. One branch of each of these neurones excites the motor neurones of prime mover muscles. Another branch relays to interneurones that form inhibitory synapses with the motor neurones supplying the opposing muscle group. This is known as **reciprocal innervation** or reciprocal inhibition, whereby the activity in opposing muscles is balanced and graded during movement.

Figure 3.26 shows the reciprocal innervation of lower motor neurones in the flexor and crossed extensor reflex. In the lower limb responding to the stimulus, the flexors are excited and the opposing extensors are inhibited. In the opposite limb, the excitation and inhibition are reversed.

Reciprocal innervation is the basis of integrated muscle action in both the maintenance of the balance of the body and the execution of voluntary movement.

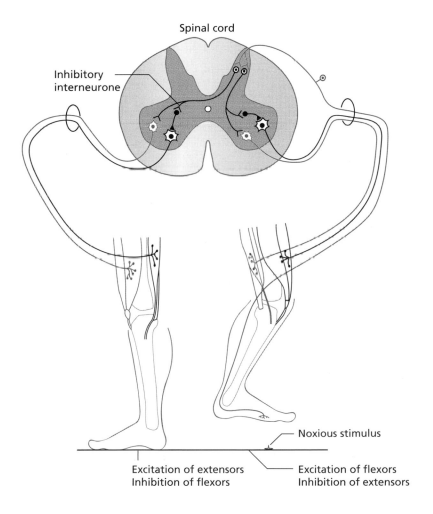

Figure 3.26   Reciprocal innervation in the flexor reflex.

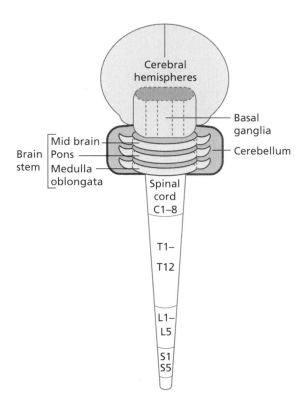

Figure 3.27 Hierarchical organisation of the central nervous system.

Summary of the functions of the spinal cord

- Conveys ascending sensory information from all areas of the body to higher levels of the central nervous system.
- Conveys descending information from all levels of the central nervous system to the muscles, organs and glands.
- Generates basic movement patterns, for example locomotion.
- Regulates muscle tone in response to changes in body position and movement.
- Co-ordinates the activity in opposing muscle groups by reciprocal innervation.
- Forms the final common pathway from the central nervous system to the muscles.

Summary

- This chapter described the location and structure of the parts of the central nervous system, the brain and the spinal cord, together with an outline of their function. This provides a first look at the components of the sensory and motor systems which is developed further in Chapters 11 and 12.

- The neurones of the central nervous system are organised into grey matter, formed by the cell bodies of neurones, and white matter, formed by the axons. The grey matter forms the core of the central nervous system and is also found in an outer cortical layer in the cerebral hemispheres and the cerebellum.
- The spinal cord retains the segmentation found in the early stages of development. The white matter of the spinal cord contains ascending and descending tracts carrying information towards and away from the brain, respectively.
- Reflex pathways within the spinal cord regulate muscle tone to the correct level required to hold a position and to allow movement. The reciprocal innervation of the motor neurones of opposing muscle groups in the spinal cord is the basis of movement that is balanced and graded.
- The components of the central nervous system are hierarchically organised, with each successive level functioning at a more complex level. This hierarchy can be compared to a commercial company/organisation with the muscles acting as the workers (Figure 3.27):
  - The **cerebral hemispheres** are the senior management group of the company responsible for executive decision making, planning for the future, quality control, ethical policies, reviewing of past performance and overall control of the company. Various departments exist at this level that specialise in particular functions and have efficient lines of communication between them.
  - The **basal ganglia** are the middle management group facilitating commands and instructions handed down from above to lower levels. This group is responsible for everyday actions of the company that do not require the attention of the senior management group. A control centre (hypothalamus) is situated in this level that maintains the status quo (homeostasis) of the services required by the company, for example water levels, heating and ventilation.
  - The **cerebellum** is the computerised guidance control system of the company which is in communication with all the other departments in the company. This is a highly specialised department that compares past performance with future intention. Files of past performance are stored in its computer memory.
  - The **brain stem**, consisting of the midbrain, pons and medulla, is the maintenance department which organises the support staff to maintain optimum background conditions for efficient production. This department includes the reticular formation, which deals with the vital functions of the company round the clock.
  - The **spinal cord** is a very large elevator to all different levels of the company. Information is constantly being transmitted up and down this area with multiple connections to the workers who perform the tasks for the company. Information is also passed through specific channels (peripheral nervous system, see Chapter 4) from the workers to the elevator and ultimately to the senior management group if required.

4

The peripheral nervous system: cranial and spinal nerves

Key terms

spinal nerves, dermatomes and myotomes, peripheral nerves, cranial nerves, autonomic nervous system, sympathetic and parasympathetic systems

Conceptual overview

This chapter discusses various components of the peripheral nervous system, looking specifically at spinal, peripheral and cranial nerves. The origin of spinal nerves will be discussed as the path from the spinal cord to the various plexuses is followed, highlighting the difference between the anterior (motor) and posterior (sensory) roots, and following on to the peripheral nerves and their function. The twelve pairs of cranial nerves will also be discussed with their vital functions illustrated. The chapter ends with a summary of the autonomic nervous system with its importance as a regulatory system highlighted as the sympathetic and parasympathetic divisions are discussed.

Tyldesley & Grieve's Muscles, Nerves and Movement in Human Occupation, Fourth Edition. Ian R. McMillan, Gail Carin-Levy.
© 2012 Ian R. McMillan, Gail Carin-Levy, Barbara Tyldesley and June I. Grieve. Published 2012 by Blackwell Publishing Ltd.

Introduction

The peripheral nervous system provides the link between the central nervous system and all parts of the body. The nerves of the peripheral nervous system transmit information to and from the brain and the spinal cord.

Sensory information, originating in a variety of receptors all over the body, is transmitted to the spinal cord and the brain by the peripheral nervous system. The receptors in the sense organs and the skin monitor changes in the external environment, while those in blood vessels, glands and organs of the body respond to the internal environment. During movement, the proprioceptors in the muscles and the joints are activated by the changing position of the body. All this information is carried to the central nervous system in the peripheral nerves.

Motor commands originating in the brain and spinal cord are transmitted by the peripheral nervous system to the skeletal muscles to execute or modify movement. By the same route, the activity in the organs and glands is regulated to maintain a constant internal environment.

All the nerves of this system contain axons of sensory and motor neurones bound together by connective tissue. There are two functional categories of axons found in the peripheral nerves. The **somatic** component consists of all the sensory and motor axons associated with activity in the muscles, the joints and the skin. The **visceral** component is all the axons carrying nerve impulses to the glands, organs and blood vessels. The visceral nerve fibres are part of the autonomic nervous system.

Damage to the nerves of the peripheral nervous system at any point from their origin in the central nervous system to their terminations inside the muscles will result in loss of both muscle function and sensation in the skin. Trophic changes, such as flushing and dryness of the skin, will also occur if the visceral fibres are damaged.

The nerves of the peripheral nervous system are arranged in a bilateral system of paired nerves. The cranial nerves leave the brain, and the spinal nerves leave the spinal cord.

Twelve pairs of cranial nerves, the cell bodies of which are located in the brain, can be seen most clearly in a ventral view of the brain (Figure 4.1). The pairs of cranial nerves appear at irregular intervals as a result of the folding of the embryonic neural tube in the development of the brain. The cranial nerves are summarised in Appendix II, Table A2.1.

The spinal nerves consist of the 31 pairs of nerves leaving the spinal cord. Each pair of spinal nerves emerges from the vertebral canal between adjacent vertebrae at the intervertebral foramina. The latter can be seen in the lateral view of a thoracic vertebra in Appendix I. The lower end of the spinal cord in adults lies at the level of the disc between the first and second lumbar vertebrae. The lower spinal nerves therefore lie in the spinal canal below this level before emerging at their corresponding level. This sheath of lumbar and sacral nerves is known as the cauda equina (horse's tail).

> **Reflective task**
>
> Look at an articulated skeleton and return to Figures 3.19 and 3.20 to revise the emergence of the 31 pairs of spinal nerves from the vertebral column.

85

86

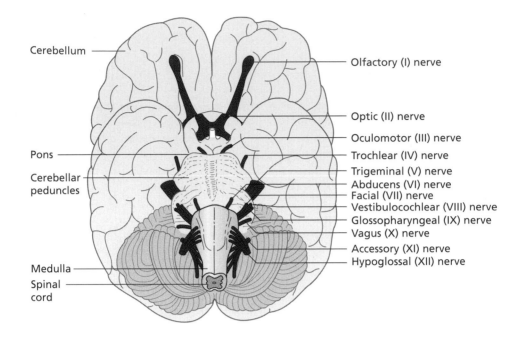

Figure 4.1   Cranial nerves seen in a ventral view of the brain.

Spinal nerves

Each spinal nerve begins at the spinal cord with two roots: the anterior (ventral) root, and the posterior (dorsal) root. Each root consists of a series of rootlets which eventually join. Diagrams of the formation of a spinal nerve represent each root as a single trunk for clarity.

The **anterior root** consists of axons that grow out from multipolar nerve cells in the spinal cord. These axons are all **motor (efferent)**, carrying impulses away from the cord. Those originating in the anterior horn are lower motor neurones supplying muscles. Visceral motor fibres of the autonomic nervous system are also found in the anterior roots. The cell bodies of these autonomic neurones lie in the lateral grey matter of certain segments of the spinal cord (described later).

The **posterior root** develops in a different way. A ridge of cells on each side of the neural tube in the embryo forms a pair of ganglia (cells) for each segment of the spinal cord. Fibres grow centrally from each ganglion into the spinal cord, and also laterally to lie alongside the fibres originating in the anterior root. The fibres of the posterior root are all **sensory (afferent)**, carrying information from the receptors in the skin, the muscles and the joints. The cell bodies lie in the posterior root ganglion, isolated from the hundreds of synaptic connections possible for the cell bodies of neurones in the grey matter of the spinal cord. Axons of the sensory neurones enter the spinal cord, branch to segments of the cord above or below, or turn into the posterior white matter to reach the brain stem before synapsing.

The **spinal nerve** is the common nerve trunk formed by the anterior (motor) root and the posterior (sensory) root joining, distal to the posterior root ganglion. Spinal nerves are mixed; each contains motor and sensory nerve fibres. Alternative terms are efferent and afferent respectively.

Each spinal nerve contains all the somatic and visceral nerve fibres that supply the corresponding body segment. The thoracic spinal nerves follow the basic plan described. The other spinal nerves show considerable mixing, branching and joining. This regrouping of nerve fibres forms a **plexus**.
There are four major plexuses formed by the anterior primary rami of the spinal nerves:

- cervical plexus (C1–C4) to the muscles of the neck;
- brachial plexus (C5–T1) to the muscles of the upper limb;
- lumbar plexus (L1–L4) to the muscles of the thigh;
- sacral plexus (L4–S4) to the muscles of the leg and foot.

Figure 4.2 shows the four plexuses formed by the spinal nerves. The lumbar and the sacral plexus can be considered together as the lumbosacral plexus supplying the whole of the lower limb.
As a result of the formation of a plexus, some nerve fibres from one spinal nerve may eventually lie alongside those from a different spinal nerve in one peripheral nerve.

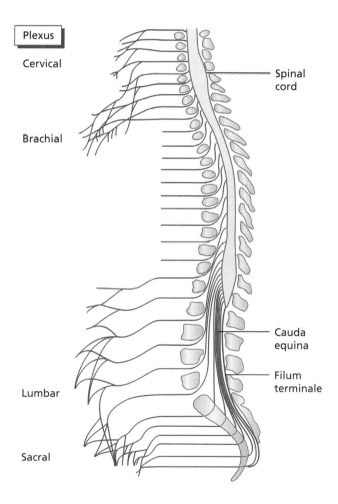

Figure 4.2 Spinal nerves emerging from the vertebral column and formation of the cervical, brachial, lumbar and sacral plexuses.

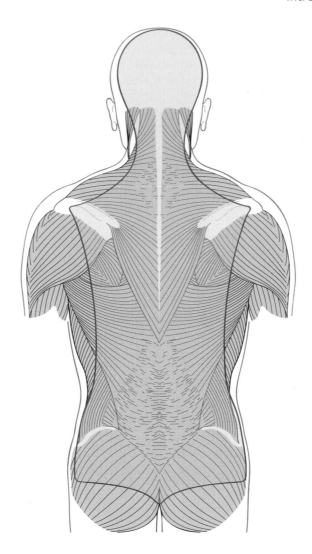

Figure 4.3   Area of skin supplied by the posterior branches of the spinal nerves.

The first branch of each spinal nerve after it emerges from the vertebral column supplies the deep muscles of the back and the skin covering them (Figure 4.3). This branch is known as the posterior primary ramus. Visceral nerve fibres of the autonomic nervous system lying in the spinal nerve connect with sympathetic ganglia, which lie on the sides of the bodies of the vertebrae, by grey and white rami. Look at Chapter 3, Figure 3.20 to see the position of the posterior primary ramus of a spinal nerve and the rami of the sympathetic ganglion. The autonomic fibres will be considered later in this chapter.

Dermatomes and myotomes

A **dermatome** is an area of skin supplied by all the sensory nerves fibres of one spinal nerve. An example of a dermatome is a band of skin around the trunk innervated by the sensory nerve fibres

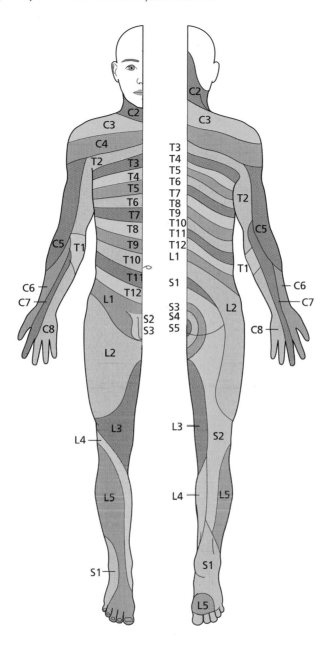

Figure 4.4   Dermatomes. The cutaneous distribution of the spinal nerves in (a) anterior and (b) posterior view.

of the second pair of thoracic nerves. A map of the dermatomes of all the spinal nerves is shown in Figure 4.4. In the trunk, the dermatomes form a series of bands, one for each spinal nerve from T2 to L1 in order. There is some overlap, and each dermatome may receive nerve fibres from three or four spinal nerves. In the limbs, the arrangement of dermatomes is more complicated. Each limb develops from a bud, which grows out in the embryo, and some dermatomes are carried to

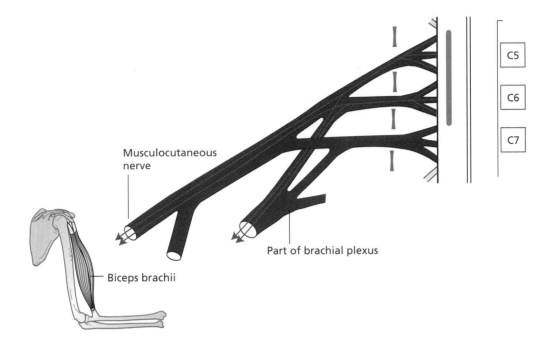

Musculocutaneous
nerve

C5

C6

C7

Part of brachial plexus

Biceps brachii

Figure 4.5 Formation of a peripheral nerve (musculocutaneous) from two spinal segments (C5 and C6).

the ends of the limb. C7 and C8 are carried in this way to the hand, while L4, L5 and S1 reach the skin of the foot. From the diagram, it can be seen that damage to the spinal nerves in the upper part of the neck (C4, C5) will give loss of sensation around the shoulder, while severance of lower roots (C7, C8) will affect sensation in the hand.

A **myotome** is all the muscles supplied by one spinal segment and its pair of spinal nerves. For example, nerve fibres from the first thoracic nerve (T1) are distributed to a long finger flexor muscle in the forearm and some of the intrinsic muscles of the hand. Each individual muscle, however, receives fibres from two or three spinal nerves (Figure 4.5), so that injury to one spinal segment may have only a limited effect on one particular muscle.

The segmental origin of the nerves supplying the muscle groups of the limbs is given in Appendix II, Table A2.2.

Peripheral nerves

Branches of the spinal nerves, and the plexuses formed from them, are distributed to all the parts of the body. These branches are known as peripheral nerves. The structure of a peripheral nerve is shown in Figure 4.6. Half of the total bulk of a nerve is connective tissue, surrounding both the nerve and also the bundles of axons within the nerve. Each nerve has its own blood supply, which branches along the length of the nerve in both directions.

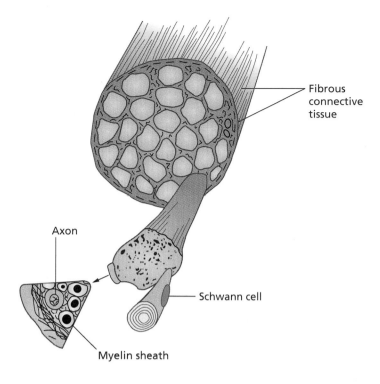

Figure 4.6 Transverse section of a peripheral nerve showing the axons and connective tissue.

Peripheral nerves are 'mixed'; they contain sensory (afferent) fibres and motor (efferent) fibres. Some branches of peripheral nerves enter muscles. Other branches pierce the deep fascia around the body to supply the skin.

Muscular branches contain:

- skeletomotor neurones supplying the skeletal muscle fibres;
- fusimotor neurones controlling the sensitivity of muscle spindles in the muscle;
- visceral motor neurones regulating the diameter of blood vessels in the muscle;
- sensory neurones from the proprioceptors in the muscle.

Cutaneous nerves contain:

- sensory neurones from thermal, mechanoreceptors and nociceptors in the skin;
- motor neurones supplying blood vessels, sweat glands and the small muscles at the base of hair follicles.

One nerve often connects with other cutaneous nerves in the same area, so that severing one cutaneous nerve may reduce sensation in the area, but does not abolish it. An example of a cutaneous nerve is the superficial terminal branch of the radial nerve (see Chapter 7). This nerve pierces the deep fascia above the wrist, and branches to supply an area of skin on the back of

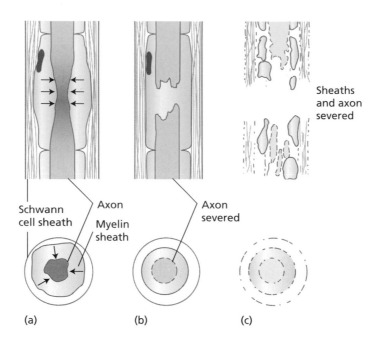

Figure 4.7   Injury to peripheral nerve: (a) axon and Schwann cell sheath intact, swelling of the myelin sheath; (b) axon severed, sheaths intact; (c) axon and sheaths severed.

the hand. Damage to this nerve usually results in a very small area of sensory loss owing to overlap from the other cutaneous nerves in the hand. Damage to the vasomotor fibres supplying the blood vessels leads to flushing and dryness of the skin.

> **Practice note-pad 4A: peripheral nerve injury**
>
> Peripheral nerve injuries can have a variety of causes. Fractures and lacerations may involve peripheral nerve damage, but the axons of peripheral nerves are also affected in diseases of the anterior horn of the spinal cord or peripheral neuropathies (see Practice note-pad 1F).
>
> In cases where a nerve is stretched or crushed, but no axons are actually severed, there may still be some conduction of nerve impulses, but conduction may be poor due to swelling or haemorrhage (Figure 4.7a). Some loss of movement and muscle tone occurs, but sensory information related to touch and pain remains intact.
>
> If the axons are severed (Figure 4.7b) there may be complete loss of movement and sensation. Recovery will depend upon the extent of involvement of the sheaths around the axon, Schwann cell sheath and endoneurium (Figure 4.7b, c).

Cranial nerves

Twelve pairs of cranial nerves emerge from the brain. Unlike the spinal nerves, the cranial nerves do not lie in a regular sequence because of the elaborate folding and the differential growth rates of the various areas in the developing brain. All the fibres of one cranial nerve emerge together from the brain either as a single bundle or as a row of filaments that join together at a short distance from the brain stem. (Remember, in each mixed spinal nerve, motor and sensory fibres are separated into two distinct roots leaving the spinal cord.)

The components of a cranial nerve are similar to the basic plan of spinal nerves, except that not all cranial nerves are 'mixed'. Some contain sensory fibres only, for example the optic nerve from the retina of the eye, and some are motor only, for example the nerves supplying the muscles at the back of the eye.

Each cranial nerve has one or more nuclei of grey matter in the brain stem, where motor fibres originate and sensory fibres terminate. The sensory fibres of some cranial nerves, particularly from the sense organs, synapse in other brain areas before relaying in the nucleus of the specific cranial nerve. The nuclei of the cranial nerves lie at all levels in the brain stem.

Collectively, the cranial nerves have many diverse functions:

- conduction of information from the primary sense organs: smell, taste, vision, hearing and balance;
- movement of the eyes, ocular reflexes (pupillary constriction and lens accommodation);
- detection of the position of the head in space to provide information for postural reflexes;
- production of facial expression;
- regulation of the heart and digestive organs;
- swallowing and speech.

A summary of the 12 pairs of cranial nerves is given in Appendix II, Table A2.1.

Movement of the head and eyes

The integration of head and eye movements allows the view of an object to be centred on the part of the retina where visual acuity is greatest, the fovea, while the head moves in space. For example in manipulative tasks, the head turns in various directions and the eyes track the objects as they are moved around. This is achieved by the brain stem reflex known as the **vestibulo-ocular reflex** (VOR). This reflex involves four of the cranial nerves: the vestibular nerve detecting the movements of the head and three cranial nerves that supply the muscles at the back of the eye. When the head remains static, the eyes can move to scan an area in the visual field ahead. This also requires the co-operation of the same cranial nerves.

The position of the head is sensed by receptors that lie in the utricle, saccule and semicircular canals of the inner ear (see Chapter 11). Information from these receptors is transmitted along the vestibular nerve, which is one division of the eighth cranial nerve, into the vestibular nucleus in the brain stem. A tract in the white matter of the brain stem links the vestibular nucleus with the nuclei of the three cranial nerves (III, IV and VI) that supply the muscles at the back of the eye (Figure 4.8).

As the head turns to one side, the eyes are turned in the opposite direction to keep a constant image on the fovea of the retina. If the head continues to turn, the eyes will move rapidly in the same direction of head movement to focus on a new fixed point. The combination of slow eye movement in the opposite direction followed by a rapid movement in the same direction is known as nystagmus. The same eye movements occur when the body remains still and the field of view is moving, for example looking out of a window while sitting in a moving train.

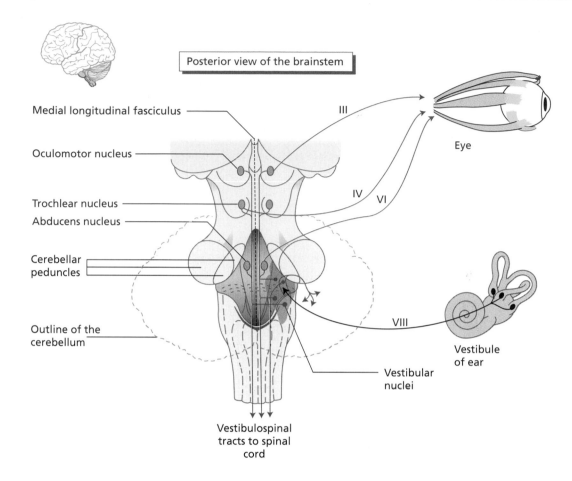

Figure 4.8   The vestibulo-ocular reflex, brain stem and cranial nerves.

Facial expression

The **facial** VII and **trigeminal** V **nerves** co-operate in movements of the face and the mouth. These movements are important for speaking and chewing, and for the expression of mood and emotion.

The **facial nerve**, containing motor fibres to the muscles of the face, emerges from the pons and leaves the skull through a foramen in the temporal bone close to the middle ear. The nerve then passes through the parotid salivary gland just in front of the ear and divides into five branches like the digits of a goose's foot (Figure 4.9a). Between them the branches supply all the muscles of the scalp and face, except for the muscles of mastication, which receive motor fibres of the trigeminal nerve. Movements of the lips and tongue, essential for speech, are made by co-ordination of activity in the facial nerve with the hypoglossal nerve to the muscles of the tongue.

Figure 4.9b shows the position of the main muscles of the face. Combining in different ways, they produce all of the movements involved in facial expression, speech and the mastication of food.

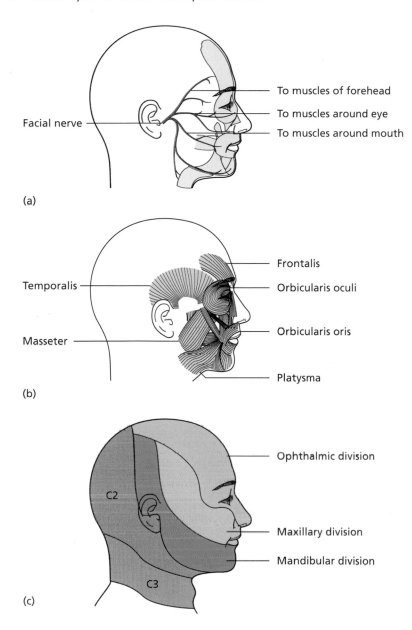

Figure 4.9   a) Facial nerve and branches to the muscles of the face; (b) distribution of the three divisions of the trigeminal nerve; (c) muscles of the face.

> **Practice note-pad 4B: Bell's palsy**
>
> Bell's palsy is a facial nerve disorder of unknown origin. It frequently follows exposure to cold on one side of the face or a mild viral respiratory infection. Facial paralysis occurs on one side, affecting the eyelid, forehead and the muscles moving the lips. Recovery from Bell's palsy is usually spontaneous.

The trigeminal nerve is important for sensation in the skin of the face. The three divisions of this nerve supply particular areas (Figure 4.9c). The ophthalmic branch enters the orbit and then branches to the skin of the forehead and the front of the scalp. The maxillary branch passes through the floor of the orbit and then turns downwards to the skin over the cheek and to the teeth of the upper jaw. The mandibular branch supplies the skin over the side of the head and the lower jaw. Loss of sensation in the face leads to difficulty in activities such as shaving and putting on make-up. Motor branches of the nerve supply the temporalis and masseter muscles used in the mastication of food.

Autonomic nervous system

The autonomic nervous system innervates smooth muscle, cardiac muscle and the glands of the body. It is largely a motor system, which regulates many important reflexes, for example the vaso-motor control of blood pressure and the motor control of the bladder. During movement, autonomic fibres in the peripheral nerves regulate the blood flow to the active muscles, by their effect on the smooth muscle of the walls of blood vessels. The reflex activity of the autonomic nervous system is influenced by centres in the brain, for example the hypothalamus and in the brain stem.

Conduction of impulses in the autonomic fibres is slower than in the somatic component of the peripheral nervous system, since the axons are of a smaller diameter. Unlike the somatic motor system, there are two neurones between the central nervous system and the effector organ, so there is delay at the synapse between them. The junction between the two neurones is located in an autonomic ganglion. The preganglionic neurones originate in the brain stem or the spinal cord, and their fibres lie in cranial or spinal nerves.

The autonomic nervous system is divided into two divisions: the **sympathetic** and **parasympathetic**. The two divisions differ in their sites of origin in the brain and spinal cord (Figure 4.10). In addition, the neurotransmitter secreted by the postganglionic neurones of the sympathetic system is noradrenaline (norepinephrine) while all the other neurones are cholinergic. Many of the organs and glands are innervated by fibres of both the sympathetic and parasympathetic systems, which frequently have opposing effects. For example, parasympathetic fibres to the heart decrease the heart rate, whereas sympathetic fibres speed it up.

Sympathetic nervous system

Neurones of the sympathetic nervous system originate in the lateral horn of the grey matter of all the thoracic segments and the first two lumbar segments of the spinal cord. These preganglionic fibres lie in the spinal nerves T1 to L2 and synapse in one of the sympathetic ganglia lying on the bodies of the vertebrae. The postganglionic fibres link to the same spinal nerve, or pass

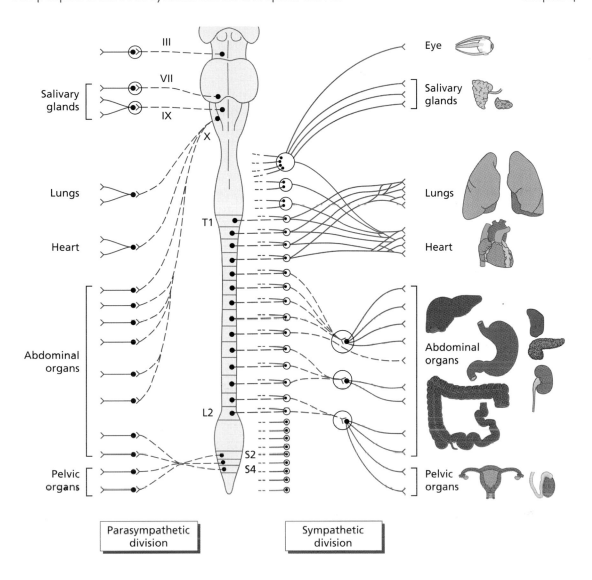

Figure 4.10 General plan of the autonomic nervous system in relation to the spinal cord and brain stem; sympathetic division on the right; parasympathetic division on the left.
- - - - - - - - represents preganglionic neurones.

up or down to other spinal levels via the chain of sympathetic ganglia located on either side of the vertebral column, from the base of the skull to the coccyx. This means that stimulation of the sympathetic nervous system can have a widespread effect in all regions of the body. Stimulation of the sympathetic nervous system prepares the body for action in the following ways:

- stimulation of cardiac muscle to increase the heart rate and the force of contraction of the heart muscle;

- constriction of the smooth muscle of blood vessels to regulate the blood pressure;
- relaxation of the smooth muscle of the walls of the bronchioles of the lungs to increase the ventilation volume;
- mobilisation of liver glycogen to raise the glucose level of the blood;
- dilatation of the pupil of the eye to allow more light to enter;
- stimulation of sweat glands in the skin to lose the extra heat generated from the muscles and to keep the body temperature constant.

The hypothalamus and the limbic system control activity in the sympathetic system in response to changes in the external and the internal environment (see Chapter 3). Sympathetic responses to emotional changes such as fear, anxiety and stress are also mediated via the hypothalamus.

Parasympathetic nervous system

The parasympathetic system acts in localised regions of the body, unlike the widespread response of the sympathetic. The preganglionic parasympathetic fibres are long and the ganglia are found near to the structure supplied. The postganglionic fibres are short and multibranching. There are two widely separated parts of the parasympathetic nervous system:

- the cranial division originates in motor fibres of the cranial nerves III, VII, IX and X;
- the spinal segments S2 to S4 contain preganglionic neurones in the lateral horn of the grey matter. Their axons form the pelvic splanchnic nerves which supply the descending colon and rectum, the bladder and the reproductive organs.

Practice note-pad 4C: spinal cord injury

Spinal cord injury may be associated with vertebral fracture due to falls, sporting injuries or road traffic accidents. The effects of damage to the spinal cord depend on the level and the extent of the injury or disease.

Partial damage of the spinal cord may create imbalance of muscle activity and muscle spasms, together with changes in sensation.

The effects of complete transection of the spinal cord depend on the level of injury:

- between C4 and T1: paralysis of all four limbs, quadriplegia (tetraplegia);
- mid-thoracic to L5: paralysis of the lower limbs, paraplegia;
- at C4: loss of diaphragm and intercostal muscle action, quadriplegia.

The parasympathetic division conserves and restores energy in the body in the following ways:

- decrease in both the heart rate and in the force of contraction of the heart muscle;
- constriction of the smooth muscle of the respiratory bronchioles;
- constriction of the pupil of the eye in response to bright light;
- stimulation of the smooth muscle and the glands of the digestive system.

Summary

- The peripheral nervous system connects the central nervous system to all parts of the body.
- Twelve pairs of cranial nerves exit the brain and 31 pairs of spinal nerves exit the spinal cord, each one branching to form peripheral nerves that enter the tissues of the body, for example muscles and glands.
- The somatic component of the spinal and peripheral nerves supplies the bones, muscles and skin. The axons of the visceral component supply the organs and glands of the body, for example the heart, lungs and digestive tract.
- A pair of spinal nerves emerges from each segment of the spinal cord. Each nerve has two roots that join to form a trunk passing between two adjacent vertebrae.
- The lower cervical and first thoracic spinal nerves branch and join, forming the brachial plexus supplying all the muscles and the skin of the upper limb. The lumbar and sacral nerves form the lumbar and sacral plexuses supplying all the muscles and the skin of the lower limb.
- The area of skin and the particular muscles supplied by one spinal nerve are known as a dermatome and a myotome, respectively.
- Activity is carried towards the central nervous system in the sensory or afferent axons lying in peripheral nerves. These are distinct from the motor or efferent nerve fibres that lie in the same peripheral nerve. Damage to a peripheral nerve produces loss of movement and sensation.
- The cranial nerves emerge in pairs from the brain in an irregular manner. Cranial nerves control the movements of the face in speech, mastication of food and the expression of emotion.
- Four of the cranial nerves are involved in the vestibulo-ocular reflex, which stabilises the gaze during head movement. Receptors in the inner ear detect the head movements and this information is transmitted to the brain stem via the vestibular VIII nerve. The vestibular nucleus links to the nuclei of the three cranial nerves that supply the muscles at the back of the eye.
- The autonomic nervous system is formed by the nerves that supply the organs and glands of the body, the blood vessels and the muscles at the base of the hairs in the skin. It is a motor system which is important in movement for its effects on the types of muscle found in the cardiovascular, respiratory and digestive systems.
- The sympathetic and parasympathetic divisions of this system have opposing actions on their target tissues and organs. Stimulation of the sympathetic system, controlled by the hypothalamus and limbic system in the brain, prepares the body for action. The parasympathetic system conserves and restores energy in the body by its action on the heart and the airways of the lungs. In the digestion of food, the parasympathetic system activates the smooth muscle and the glands of the alimentary tract.
- The peripheral nervous system is the structural framework for the conduction of activity originating in receptors to the brain and spinal cord. It also forms the final common pathway to muscles, glands and blood vessels. The way in which this activity is organised in the sensory and motor systems is considered in Section III, Chapters 11 and 12.

Section II

Anatomy of movement in everyday living

Joints, muscles and nerve supply

- Positioning movements: the shoulder and elbow
- Manipulative movements: the forearm, wrist and hand
- Nerve supply of the upper limb
- Support and propulsion: the lower limb
- Nerve supply of the lower limb
- Upright posture and breathing: the trunk

5

Positioning movements: the shoulder and elbow

Key terms

structure and function of the shoulder and elbow, movement and muscles of the shoulder and elbow

Conceptual overview

This chapter outlines the position, structure and function related to both the shoulder and elbow joints. The musculature relative to the shoulder and elbow joints will also be examined. Each joint is looked at in depth, detailing the different muscle groups and relating these to movement seen in everyday activities.

Tyldesley & Grieve's Muscles, Nerves and Movement in Human Occupation, Fourth Edition. Ian R. McMillan, Gail Carin-Levy.
© 2012 Ian R. McMillan, Gail Carin-Levy, Barbara Tyldesley and June I. Grieve. Published 2012 by Blackwell Publishing Ltd.

Introduction

The shoulder forms a foundation from which the whole of the upper limb can move. Acting like the cab of a crane, the shoulder allows the hand to be placed in all directions around the body, in the same way as the jib of a crane places its load. In upper limb function, the hand can be held high above the head, in front, behind, to the side and across the body, and touching the body. The role of the shoulder is to position the hand over this wide area.

The shoulder not only performs a wide range of movement but also anchors the arm to the trunk, supporting the weight of the upper limb as it moves. The main strut for this purpose is the clavicle, part of the shoulder (pectoral) girdle formed by the clavicle and scapula. When the hand performs precision movements, stability is provided by the joints of the girdle and all the muscles surrounding the shoulder. The shoulder joint is not part of the pectoral girdle but they are mutually dependent in all the movements of the upper limb. Figure 5.1 shows how both the humerus and the scapula both move when the arm is moved towards the vertical.

Movements at the elbow change the functional length of the upper limb, adjusting the distance of the hand from the body. Elbow flexion brings the hand towards the head and body for activities, such as washing, dressing, eating and drinking. Try splinting the elbow in extension to find out how much we depend on elbow flexion for daily activities. The opposite action of elbow extension takes the hand away from the body in reaching and grasping, and also enables the hand to push against resistance, for example sawing wood or pushing a swing door. A person with reduced lower limb function relies on the elbow extensors, together with shoulder muscles, to lift the body weight on the hands to rise from a chair.

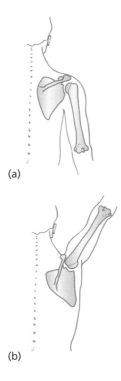

(a)

(b)

Figure 5.1   Posterior view of the scapula and humerus: (a) anatomical position; (b) arm vertical.

Movements of the shoulder, which involve the shoulder girdle and the shoulder joint, will be considered first, followed by the elbow. Upper limb movements depend on the co-operation of the shoulder and the elbow in positioning the hand.

PART I: THE SHOULDER

The shoulder (pectoral) girdle

Position and function

Reflective task

Look at the illustrations of the bones of the pectoral girdle in Appendix I. Use an articulated skeleton to examine: the clavicle linking the sternum and the scapula; the position of the scapula lying over the ribs; and the glenoid fossa of the scapula forming the socket for the head of the humerus.

The bones of the shoulder girdle are the clavicle and the scapula. The clavicle articulates at its medial end with the sternum of the thorax. The scapula is a large, flat triangular bone lying on the ribs, separated by a layer of muscle, in the posterior aspect of the thorax. The scapula is suspended by the muscles attached to its borders and surfaces so that it moves freely on the chest wall. The posterior surface of the scapula has a projecting spine which ends at the acromion process. The lateral end of the clavicle articulates with the acromion process. The head of the scapula lies laterally and has the glenoid fossa, a shallow concavity, for the articulation with the head of the humerus. From the upper part of the head, the coracoid process projects upwards and forwards to lie below the clavicle. The coracoid process provides a base for one of the proximal tendons of the biceps muscle lying on the anterior aspect of the arm.

All movements of the pectoral girdle involve both the clavicle and the scapula together. The movements of the scapula follow the shape of the ribs. The scapula is able to move freely on the thorax, because the muscles between the ribs and the scapula are covered by fascia which allows gliding movements. When the scapula moves on the chest wall, the glenoid fossa is turned to face in different directions, i.e. more directly forwards, backwards, upwards or downwards. This allows the humerus to move further in that particular direction and therefore increases the range of movement at the shoulder joint. If the shoulder girdle becomes fixed, all upper limb activites are restricted and compensation for the reduced range of movement can only be achieved by a shift of the whole body.

In summary, the functions of the shoulder girdle are:

- to anchor the upper limb to the trunk by means of the strut-like clavicle;
- to define the position of the shoulder joint and consequently the direction of the movements of the arm on the trunk;
- to increase the range of movement at the shoulder joint by changes in the angulation of the clavicle and in the position of the scapula on the chest wall.

Joints of the shoulder (pectoral) girdle

Two articulations are involved in the shoulder girdle. The **sternoclavicular joint** is a synovial joint between the medial end of the clavicle and the clavicular notch on the manubrium of the sternum. It is divided by an intra-articular disc of fibrocartilage joining the upper end of the clavicle to the first costal cartilge at its sternal end (Figure 5.2a). A strong costoclavicular ligament joins the medial end of the clavicle to the first rib, and the interclavicular ligament joins the medial ends of the right and left clavicles. The disc, together with the ligaments, prevents dislocation of the joint during falls on the outstretched arm or when a heavy load, for example a suitcase, is carried in the hand.

The **acromioclavicular joint** is a synovial joint that connects the lateral end of the clavicle with the acromion process of the scapula. The capsule is thickened by strong fibres both superiorly and inferiorly. The main factor stabilising the joint is the strong coracoclavicular ligament joining the lateral end of the clavicle to the coracoid process of the scapula (Figure 5.2b).

Reflective task

Palpate the sternoclavicular joint on a partner. Feel the rocking action of the clavicle on the sternum during shrugging the shoulders and folding the arms in front of the body. (A much reduced adjustment takes place at the acromioclavicular joint during these same movements.) Now ask your partner to move the arm in all directions at the shoulder joint. Note that movement at the sternoclavicular joint occurs each time the humerus moves.

Summary of the movements of the shoulder girdle

For the purpose of description, the movements of the shoulder girdle are divided as follows:

- **elevation**: the scapula moves upwards together with the lateral end of the clavicle. This movement is commonly described as 'shrugging the shoulders';
- **depression**: the scapula and lateral end of the clavicle move down to the resting position;
- **protraction**: the scapula moves laterally around the chest wall bringing the glenoid fossa to face more directly forwards. The vertebral border of each scapula (see Appendix I) moves further away from the spine;
- **retraction**: the scapula moves medially around the chest wall bringing the glenoid fossa to face more directly towards the side. The vertebral border on each scapula moves nearer to the spine;
- **lateral rotation**: the inferior angle of the scapula moves laterally and the glenoid fossa points upwards;
- **medial rotation**: the inferior angle of the scapula moves medially and the glenoid fossa returns to the resting position.

These movements of the shoulder girdle increase the range of movement at the shoulder joint. Elevation increases reaching upwards, while depression increases pointing downwards. Protraction takes the hand farther across the body to reach to the opposite side, and retraction takes the hand farther behind the body. Abduction or flexion of the arm, which takes the hand above the head, is increased in range by lateral rotation of the scapula.

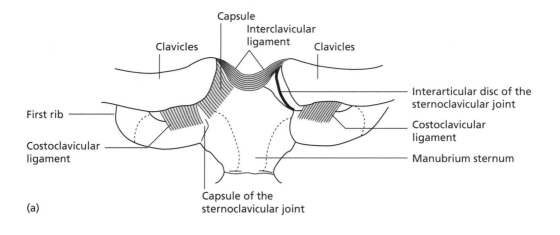

(a)

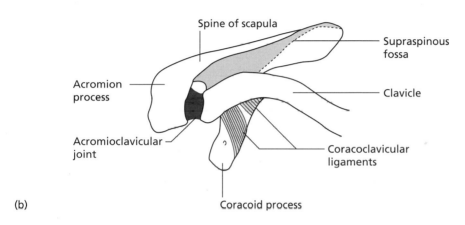

(b)

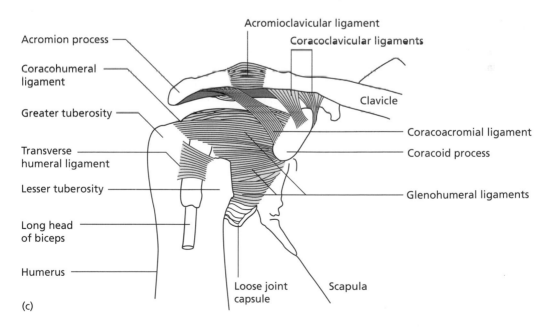

(c)

Figure 5.2 (a) Sternoclavicular joints, anterior view (left joint with capsule removed); (b) right acromioclavicular joint, superior view; (c) right glenohumeral joint, anterior view.

> **Reflective task**
>
> - Palpate the scapula on a partner whose horizontal arm swings round a wide circle forwards and backwards. Feel the movement of protraction as the arm swings across the front of the body, and retraction as it swings behind the body.
> - Lift the arm of a partner through the full range of abduction to reach above the head, then full adduction back to the side. Palpate the scapula during this action. Lateral rotation can be felt as the arm is raised, then medial rotation as the arm is lowered.

The shoulder (glenohumeral) joint

The bony articulation of the shoulder joint occurs between the head of the humerus and the shallow glenoid fossa on the lateral aspect of the scapula (Figure 5.2c). The glenoid fossa is deepened by a rim of fibrocartilage, the glenoid labrum. The head of the humerus is approximately one-third of a sphere, but only one-third of its surface area is in contact with the glenoid fossa during movement. The fibrous joint capsule is both thin and loose. The shape of the bony surfaces and the loose capsule both provide for a wide range of movement at the joint, but they present a poor prospect for stability.

Some support is given by two ligaments. The coracohumeral ligament extends from the coracoid process to the upper aspect of the greater tuberosity of the humerus. This ligament assists in holding the head of the humerus up to the glenoid fossa, but it is not entirely successful in this. An accessory ligament joins the coracoid and acromion processes to form an arch over the head of the humerus. This coracoacromial ligament prevents upward dislocation of the head of the humerus, for example in a fall on to the abducted arm.

Muscles join the humerus to the pectoral girdle around the anterior, posterior and superior aspects of the shoulder joint. These muscles suspend the upper limb from the pectoral girdle and also stabilise the shoulder joint. The tendon of the long head of the biceps muscle lies inside the shoulder joint from its origin on the superior part of the glenoid fossa. Lying in the groove formed between the greater and lesser tuberosities of the humerus, the tendon is surrounded by a synovial sheath, and emerges from the lower margin of the capsule to become the prominent anterior muscle of the arm.

Movements of the shoulder joint

The glenohumeral articulation is a synovial joint of the ball and socket type which has the greatest range of movement of all the joints of the body, together with a poor prospect for stability.

- **Flexion** movement carries the arm forwards and at an angle of 45 degrees to the sagittal plane.
- **Extension** is the return movement from flexion and continues to take the arm beyond the anatomical position.
- **Abduction** carries the arm sideways and upwards in the frontal plane. It depends on lateral rotation of the scapula beyond 30 degrees.
- **Adduction** returns the arm to the side.

- **Medial rotation** occurs about the long axis of the humerus, turning the anterior surface of the humerus medially. When the elbow is flexed, medial rotation at the shoulder takes the hand across the body as in folding the arms.
- **Lateral rotation** occurs about the long axis of the humerus, turning the anterior surface of the humerus laterally.

The movements of the shoulder joint, together with the pectoral girdle, are essential for the performance of all personal care and dressing activities.

Practice note-pad 5A: the shoulder joint

Subluxation of the shoulder occurs when the head of the humerus drops in the glenoid fossa. This may occur following a stroke when there is general weakness of all the muscles around the shoulder. Periarthritis is a painful condition of the shoulder caused by inflammation of the bursa below the acromion or of the synovial sheath in the bicipital groove, or the deposition of calcium in one or more of the rotator cuff muscles.

'Frozen shoulder' may result when the shoulder is not used due to pain or mild repeated trauma. Pain gradually increases over several months and then subsides, leaving stiffness which persists if untreated. All movements at the shoulder joint are limited at first and only return when the stiffness subsides.

Muscles of the shoulder region

The shoulder region has a large number of muscles which combine in various ways, grouping and regrouping in the performance of the movements of the upper limb. The muscles attached to the pectoral girdle anchor the scapula to the trunk, control the orientation of the glenoid fossa for movements at the shoulder joint, and stabilise the shoulder joint. Muscles with the latter function are known as the 'rotator cuff' muscles. Large triangular muscles, originating on the bones of the trunk and inserted into the humerus, act on the shoulder joint in its wide range of movement.

Muscles stabilising and moving the shoulder girdle

Muscles cross the anterior and posterior surfaces of the scapula, and are attached to its borders and processes. The muscles covering the anterior surface are sandwiched between the scapula and the ribs, and are loosely separated by connective tissue and fat, which allows the scapula to move freely on the chest wall. Four of the muscles moving the scapula originate from the vertebral column. It is important to understand clearly the position of the scapula in relation to the vertebral column, ribs and walls of the axilla, in order to appreciate the direction of pull of the muscles which turn the scapula in various directions.

There are six muscles attached to the triangular scapula that combine to produce these movements. The muscles are the **trapezius**, **levator scapulae**, **rhomboid major** and **minor**, **serratus anterior** and **pectoralis minor**. By pulling together in different combinations, these muscles can elevate, depress, protract, retract and rotate the scapula on the chest wall.

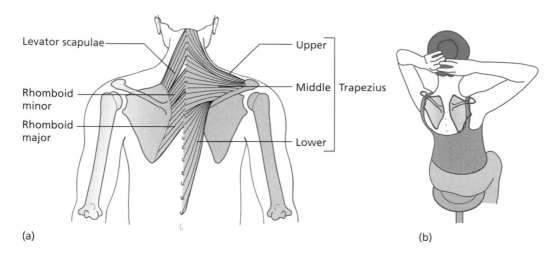

Figure 5.3   Trapezius, levator scapulae, rhomboid major and minor: (a) position; (b) reaching behind the head.

Trapezius

The two sides of the trapezius form a kite-shaped area of muscle, the most superficial muscle of the back. Each muscle is a triangle, with its base in the midline from the base of the skull down to the 12th thoracic spine (Figure 5.3a).

The upper fibres originate from the occipital bone of the skull and the ligamentum nuchae, which covers the cervical spines in the neck. The fibres pass downwards and forwards across the neck to the lateral end of the clavicle and continue on to the acromion of the scapula. Acting as a suspension for the pectoral girdle from the skull and neck vertebrae, contraction of these upper fibres lifts the shoulders in elevation. In addition, they give support to the shoulders when carrying heavy loads. The static work of the trapezius is felt when carrying heavy luggage or shopping.

The middle fibres pass horizontally from the upper thoracic spines to the length of the spine of the scapula. Contraction of these fibres pulls the scapula towards the spine and the scapula retracts. Activities involving this movement include reaching behind the head to comb the hair (Figure 5.3b) and to grasp a car seat-belt.

The lower fibres pass upwards from the lower thoracic vertebrae into a tendon that inserts into the base (medial end) of the spine of the scapula. Acting alone, these fibres will depress the shoulder when it has been raised. More important is the action of the lower fibres with the upper fibres to rotate the scapula, turning the glenoid fossa upwards during abduction of the arm.

Levator scapulae

The transverse processes of the first four cervical vertebrae provide the attachments for the levator scapulae, and the fibres descend to the vertebral border of the scapula above the spine (Figure 5.3a). The levator scapulae lies deep to the upper fibres of the trapezius and works with them to elevate the scapula.

Rhomboid major and minor

These two muscles form a continuous layer deep to the middle fibres of the trapezius, originating on the spines of the upper thoracic vertebrae, and insert into the medial border of the scapula (Figure 5.3a). The rhomboids can be considered as one muscle which pulls the scapula backwards in retraction.

Serratus anterior

This has a saw-toothed origin from the upper eight or nine ribs, clearly seen in male swimmers and boxers with powerful shoulder muscles. From this wide origin, the fibres wrap round the thorax and underneath the scapula to be inserted into the vertebral border of the scapula (Figure 5.4a).

The action of the whole muscle pulls the scapula forwards around the chest in protraction. This movement increases the forward reach of the upper limb and adds to the force of an action pushing forwards against resistance, such as a door (Figure 5.4b).

The lower fibres of the serratus anterior converge on the inferior angle of the scapula, and their action will rotate the scapula laterally to turn the glenoid fossa upwards to allow full abduction of the humerus. In lateral rotation, the serratus anterior works with the upper and lower fibres of the trapezius.

Reflective task

Look at an articulated skeleton to appreciate the exact position of the serratus anterior. Lying deep to the scapula, it separates the subscapularis from the chest wall.

Figure 5.5 shows the serratus anterior and the rhomboids seen in a transverse section across the thorax. Identify the vertebral border of the scapula and note how the serratus anterior and the rhomboids pull on the scapula in opposite directions to protract and retract the scapula, respectively.

Pectoralis minor

This is a small muscle lying in the anterior wall of the axilla. The fibres of the pectoralis minor ascend from the anterior surface of the third, fourth and fifth ribs, to be attached to the coracoid process of the scapula (Figure 5.6). By pulling on the coracoid process, the pectoralis minor can depress and protract the scapula in pushing movements. It can also assist in medial rotation of the scapula. The pectoralis minor lies deep to the pectoralis major, a large muscle acting on the shoulder joint, to be described later.

All the muscles attached to the clavicle and scapula combine in different ways to produce the movements of the pectoral girdle. The clavicle, spine and acromion of the scapula can be considered as two sides of a triangle, completed by a line across the root of the neck (Figure 5.7a). This triangle moves in elevation, depression, protraction and retraction, with the sternoclavicular joint acting as the pivot. The scapula itself is a triangle, which moves in the same directions as the upper triangle when pulled simultaneously at two of its angles. When three angles of the scapula are moved by muscle action, the scapula rotates, either medially or laterally (Figure 5.7b, c). The axis of rotation lies just inferior to the spine of the scapula, midway along its length.

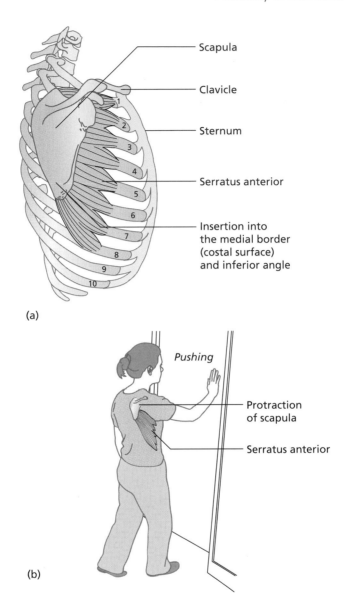

(a)

(b)

Figure 5.4   Serratus anterior: (a) position; (b) function, pushing a door.

Muscles stabilising the shoulder (glenohumeral) joint

The most effective provision of support for the joint is from the four muscles surrounding it and blending closely with the capsule. These muscle are the **supraspinatus**, **infraspinatus**, **teres minor** and **subscapularis**, which act like guy-ropes holding the humerus in contact with the scapula, and are known as the rotator cuff muscles. The lesser tuberosity of the humerus receives the sub-

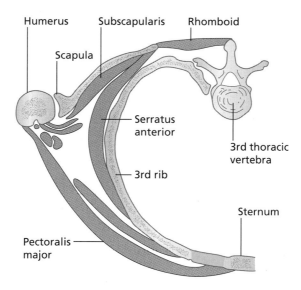

Figure 5.5 Transverse section of the thorax at the level of the third rib. Arrows show the direction of pull of the serratus anterior in protraction and the rhomboids in retraction of the scapula.

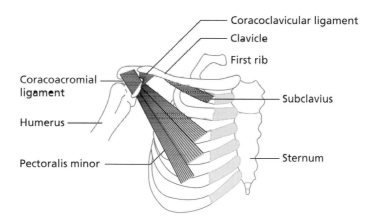

Figure 5.6 Pectoralis minor and subclavius, position.

scapularis tendon, covering the joint anteriorly (Figure 5.8a). The other three muscles are inserted into the greater tuberosity, with the supraspinatus superiorly, then the infraspinatus and teres minor below and posteriorly (Figure 5.8b). The absence of any additional support inferiorly means that dislocation is usually downwards and forwards, under its own weight as the arm hangs by the side, or during abduction movement.

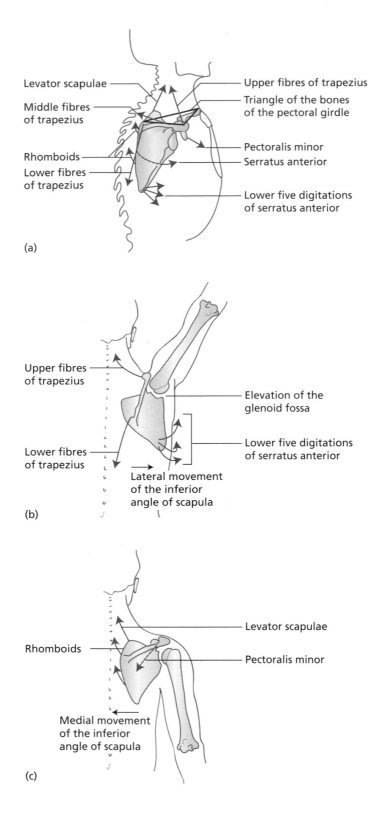

Figure 5.7 Direction of pull of the muscles of the shoulder girdle.

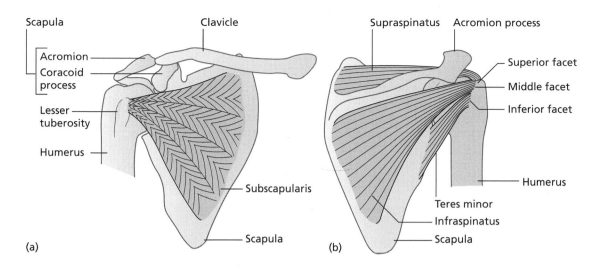

Figure 5.8   Right scapula and humerus to show the 'rotator cuff' muscles: (a) anterior view; (b) posterior view.

Reflective task

Observe the following functional activities, then record the directions of movement of the scapula and name the muscles involved.

(1)   Reach up to a high shelf.
(2)   Push open a door.
(3)   Reach behind to grasp a seat-belt in a car.
(4)   Turn over a page of a newspaper on a table.
(5)   Pull open a drawer.

The rotator cuff muscles have weak action as prime movers since their insertions are close to the joint, but they function as stabilisers in all movements of the shoulder joint. The supraspinatus initiates abduction of the shoulder before deltoid can exert its pull on the lateral shaft of the humerus. The other three muscles act as rotators of the humerus: subscapularis medially; infraspinatus and teres minor laterally.

Muscles acting on the shoulder joint

Three large muscles surrounding the glenohumeral joint move the joint through its wide range. Their attachments cover a wide area of the pectoral girdle and trunk, and converge to insert on to the humerus. The three muscles are the **deltoid**, **pectoralis major** and **latissimus dorsi**. The **teres major** and **coracobrachialis** are two other muscles acting on the shoulder joint that will be considered together.

Deltoid

The deltoid muscle gives the rounded shape to the shoulder and has the overall shape of an inverted triangle. The margins of the muscle can be clearly seen in athletes and swimmers. Lack of use after injury may lead to wasting, which gives the shoulder a 'squared' appearance.

Reflective task

- Lift a saucepan or book down from a high shelf and feel the continuous activity in the deltoid as the arm is raised and then lowered. If the deltoid was relaxed as the arm came down, the movement would be rapid and uncontrolled, and you would probably drop the book on the floor.
- Palpate the origin of deltoid in a partner with the arm relaxed by the side. Start anteriorly at the lateral end of the clavicle to feel the anterior fibres. Next cross the acromion process of the scapula where the middle fibres arise. Continue along the spine of the scapula to find the posterior fibres. All the fibres converge to insert on the lateral shaft of the humerus about half way down (Figure 5.9a).
- Inspect the skeleton to find the deltoid tuberosity formed by the pull of the deltoid on the humerus.

The deltoid is a powerful abductor of the arm, lifting the arm sideways and up above the head. It is also active when the arm is lowered back down to the side, working eccentrically to control the effect of gravity. All movements reaching forwards and above the head demand the deltoid muscle in action (Figure 5.9b).

The anterior fibres flex and medially rotate the humerus at the shoulder joint, while the posterior fibres extend and laterally rotate it. Both sets can work together to prevent forward and backward movement during abduction of the arm by the strong middle fibres. Part or all of the deltoid is used in most movements of the humerus on the scapula. The muscle also acts as a support sling for the shoulder, especially when the upper limb is carrying heavy loads such as a suitcase or shopping bag.

Pectoralis major

The pectoralis major is a large triangular muscle, the base of which lies vertically along the midline of the thorax and the apex is attached to the humerus. The lower border of the triangle can be felt in the anterior wall of the axilla. The main bulk of the muscle is difficult to observe in women as the breast covers some of its surface.

Reflective task

Press the hands together in front of the body to put the muscle into action. The muscle can now be palpated in the axilla by a partner.

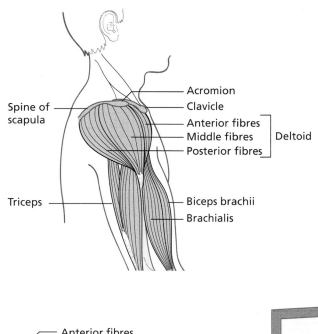

117

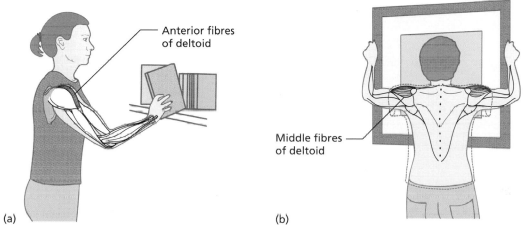

(a)   (b)

Figure 5.9   (a) Side view of the right shoulder showing the position of the deltoid muscle;
(b) functions of the deltoid: reaching forwards; reaching above the head.

The uppermost fibres of the pectoralis major arise from the clavicle medial to the anterior fibres
of the deltoid. The remainder of the base of the triangle is formed by fibres arising from the
anterior surface of the sternum and the costal cartilages of the first six ribs. All the fibres converge
to the insertion on the anterior humerus in the groove between the two tubercles (intertubercular
sulcus or bicipital groove), with the clavicular fibres lying superficial to the sternocostal fibres
(Figure 5.10a).

The clavicular fibres work with anterior fibres of the deltoid to flex the shoulder to a right angle.
The lower costal fibres work with the posterior deltoid to pull the arm downwards in extension.
Pulling down a window roller-blind is an extension movement against resistance. Acting as a

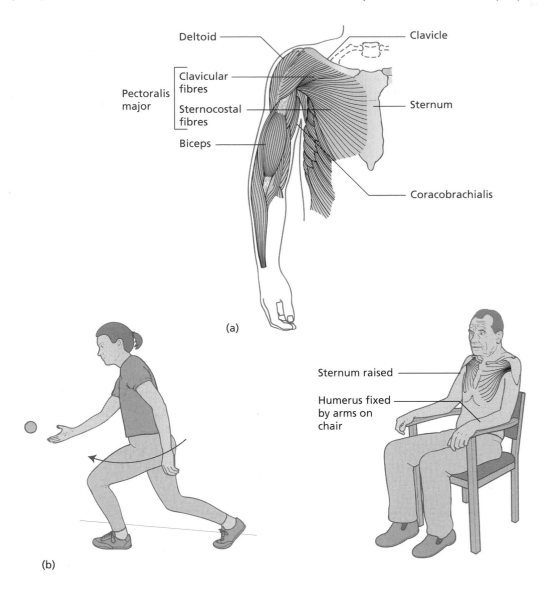

(a)

(b)

Figure 5.10   Pectoralis major: (a) position; (b) functions, throwing a ball and assisting breathing.

whole, the pectoralis major is an adductor and a medial rotator of the shoulder, drawing the arm across the body to place the hand on the opposite side, for example moving a saucepan or a book from the right side of the body to the left.

The pectoralis major is used to pull the arm forwards in throwing a ball (Figure 5.10b), javelin or discus. When the arm is taken backwards in tennis and squash, the pectoralis major draws the racket forwards to hit the ball in a forehand drive. Another function of the pectoralis major is to assist in deep breathing. When the humerus is fixed, the muscle pulls the sternum upwards and outwards to enlarge the thorax and draw more air into the lungs. Figure 5.10b shows the position of the arms used to assist breathing while sitting in a chair. (Two of the shoulder girdle muscles, serratus anterior and pectoralis minor, work with the pectoralis major in this position to increase the ventilation of the lungs.)

Latissimus dorsi

A shoulder muscle arising from a large origin in the lower back and thorax, the latissimus dorsi wraps round the trunk and converges towards the shoulder, forming the posterior wall of the axilla. (The pectoralis major and minor form the anterior wall.) The proximal attachment of the latissimus dorsi is by an aponeurosis from the spines of the lower six thoracic, all the lumbar, and the upper sacral vertebrae. Some fibres also arise directly from the posterior half of the iliac crest (Figure 5.11a). The uppermost fibres cross the inferior angle of the scapula, holding it down. From the wall of the axilla, the tendon passes underneath the glenohumeral joint to end on the anterior end of the humerus, in the floor of the bicipital groove.

> **Reflective task**
>
> Hold the arm up, palpate the posterior wall of the axilla, and work out how the tendon reaches the anterior aspect of the arm on the humerus.

The actions of the latissimus dorsi are extension, adduction and medial rotation of the shoulder joint. When the hand is above the head, the latissimus dorsi (working with the lower fibres of pectoralis major) pulls the arm downwards and backwards against resistance, as in pulling down a blind. Continuation of this movement together with medial rotation takes the hand behind the body, as in tieing an apron. Working statically, the latissimus dorsi adducts the arm against the body to hold a bag or file. In climbing, the hand is placed above the head, and the muscle works strongly to pull the trunk up towards the arm and lift the body upwards. Figure 5.11b shows these functions of the latissimus dorsi.

The latissimus dorsi is an important muscle for anyone with loss of function in the lower limb resulting from weak muscles or stiff joints. If the body cannot be raised from sitting by extension of the legs, the hands can be placed on the seat or arms of the chair, and the body lifted off the seat using the adduction action of the latissimus dorsi to hitch on the pelvis. Wheelchair patients rely heavily on this muscle to transfer from the chair to a bed or toilet seat. In crutch walking, the latissimus dorsi helps to support the weight of the body on the hands. The muscle can also be trained to lift one side of the pelvis, so that the leg clears the ground in the swing phase in walking, known as 'hip hitching', the method used to teach paraplegic patients in long leg calipers to walk.

Teres major and coracobrachialis

These are two strap-like muscles with a weaker individual action on the glenohumeral joint. The teres major is attached to the lower lateral border of the scapula and lies in the posterior wall of the axilla. The insertion is with the tendon of the latissimus dorsi on the anterior of the humerus. The two muscles act together on the glenohumeral joint.

The coracobrachialis originates from the coracoid process of the scapula and inserts into the rough area on the medial shaft of the humerus. The action of the coracobrachialis is flexion

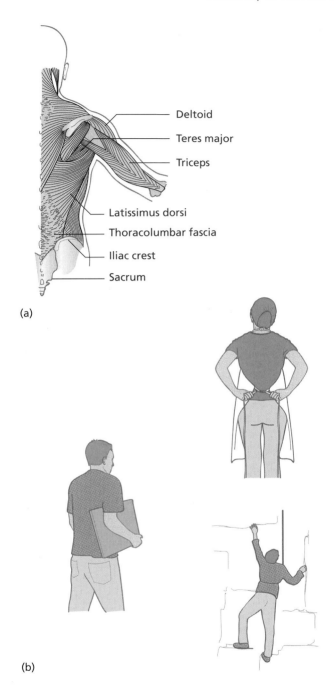

Deltoid

Teres major

Triceps

Latissimus dorsi

Thoracolumbar fascia

Iliac crest

Sacrum

(a)

(b)

Figure 5.11 Latissimus dorsi: (a) position; (b) functions, tieing an apron, holding a document case, pulling the trunk up towards the arm and therefore lifting the body upwards.

of the shoulder from the hyperextended position, i.e. humerus behind the trunk. There is evidence that the muscle functions to swing the arm forwards in walking and running. This muscle also adducts the arm on to the trunk when holding a newspaper or purse under the arm (Figure 5.11b).

PART II: THE ELBOW

Elbow position and function

The elbow is the hinge joint of the upper limb lying between the arm and the forearm. The shoulder carries the hand in all directions around the body, and the elbow places the hand in the correct position. Flexion movement at the elbow directs the hand towards the head and body in personal care and eating. The opposite extension movement moves the hand away from the body, increasing the length of the reach in all directions. Pushing activities, for example a wheelbarrow or wheelchair, involve static work for the elbow extensors.

Positioning movements of the upper limb involve the co-ordination of muscles of the elbow with the shoulder. When the hand is performing precision movements in front of the body, the flexors of the elbow combine with the flexors, adductors and medial rotators of the shoulder, and the protractors of the scapula. In reaching to grasp an object at the side of the body, the elbow extensors combine with the abductors and lateral rotators of the shoulder, and the retractors of the scapula. These commonly occurring patterns of movement over more than one joint are known as **synergies**. If the elbow movement is restricted, upper limb function is very limited, and the hand may only reach the mouth by moving the trunk towards it.

The elbow joint

The elbow is a synovial hinge joint moving through flexion and extension only.

> **Reflective task**
>
> Look at the humerus, radius and ulna illustrated in Appendix I.

The head of the radius and trochlear notch of the ulna articulate with the lower end of the humerus. The pulley-shaped trochlear surface at the lower end of the humerus and the trochlear notch of the ulna form the hinge of the elbow joint (see Chapter 2, Figure 2.3a). This close fit gives bony stability to the joint. The upper concave surface of the head of the radius slides over the capitulum of the humerus like a ball-bearing. The collateral ligaments arising from the epicondyles of the humerus form strong triangular bands that strengthen the capsule medially and laterally (Figure 5.12a, b). The shape of the articulating surfaces and the strong collateral ligaments both lead to a stable joint.

Within the capsule of the elbow joint there is a synovial joint between the proximal ends of the radius and ulna. This superior radioulnar joint, which plays no part in the function of the elbow, will be considered in Chapter 6.

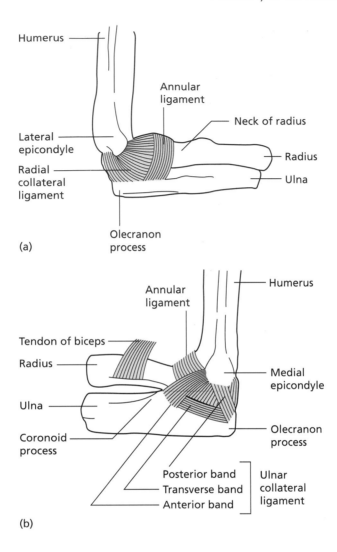

Figure 5.12   Right elbow joint: (a) lateral view: (b) medial view.

Movements of the elbow joint

- **Flexion** moves the forearm anteriorly to bend the elbow. The movement ends when the forearm contacts the arm.
- **Extension** returns the forearm to the anatomical position.

> **Reflective task**
>
> Watch the elbow in action during the following activities: using a saw or a hammer; lifting a tray from a table; eating with a fork; putting on a sweater.

Practice note-pad 5B: 'tennis elbow'

Pain in the area of the lateral epicondyle of the humerus may radiate widely due to repeated minor trauma to the muscles originating on the lateral epicondyle (wrist extensors). Pain occurs in rotational movements whereas flexion and extension of the elbow are normal.

Muscles moving the elbow

The muscles that move the elbow lie mainly in the arm above the elbow. They are found in the anterior and posterior compartments of the arm, which are separated on the lateral and medial sides by thick sheets of fibrous tissue, known as intermuscular septa. The **biceps brachii** and **brachialis** (flexors) lie in the anterior compartment; the **triceps brachii** and **anconeus** (extensors) lie in the posterior compartment. Two other muscles, found in the forearm, assist in elbow flexion. They are the **brachioradialis** and **pronator teres**.

Flexors of the elbow

Biceps brachii

The biceps muscle is the bulge in the arm that people use to demonstrate their muscle strength. The muscle is easy to see in the relaxed state in those who have done some weight training. The biceps has no attachment to the humerus. The origin of the biceps is by two tendons from the scapula. The long head is a tendon attached to the superior part of the glenoid cavity within the shoulder joint, and emerges from the capsule to lie in the intertubercular sulcus (bicipital groove) of the humerus. The short head is a tendon from the coracoid process of the scapula, closely connected to the tendon of the coracobrachialis. The tendons of the two heads join to form one muscle belly in the lower part of the arm, and the muscle inserts into the tuberosity on the medial side of the radial shaft just below the elbow. The tendon of insertion can be felt when the forearm rests on a table and the muscle is relaxed. A flat band of fibrous tissue, known as the bicipital aponeurosis, extends medially from the tendon and blends with the fascia covering the medial side of the forearm (Figure 5.13).

The flexor action of the biceps is obvious; contraction draws the radius towards the humerus. The muscle is most effective when the forearm is in the anatomical position (radius and ulna parallel). Working eccentrically, the biceps controls the lowering of the forearm and hand holding a tool or utensil (see Chapter 2).

The biceps also acts as a powerful muscle turning the forearm and hand to exert force on, for example, a door handle or screwdriver. This rotation movement of the forearm, known as supination, will be considered in Chapter 6. Pulling the cork from a bottle with a corkscrew uses both actions of the biceps, turning of the forearm followed by flexion. The biceps is the 'party muscle'!

Reflective task

Look at an articulated skeleton and turn the lower end of the radius and the hand into full pronation. Notice how the radial tuberosity has moved posteriorly. The pull of the biceps tendon will now rotate the proximal end of the radius back to the anatomical position, performing an unwinding action of the forearm.

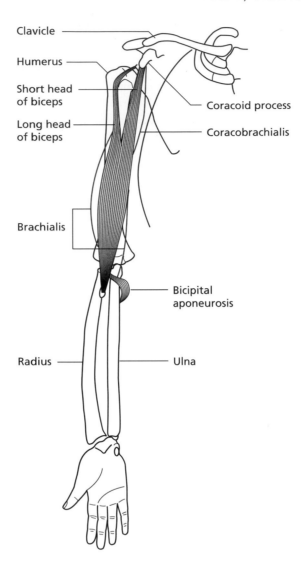

Figure 5.13   Biceps brachii, brachialis and coracobrachialis, anterior view of right arm.

Brachialis

The brachialis muscle lies deep to the biceps in the lower half of the arm. If the relaxed biceps is lifted and moved from side to side, the brachialis can be located below. The fibres of the brachialis arise from the anterior shaft of the humerus below the level of insertion of the deltoid. Passing over the anterior side of the elbow joint, the fibres insert by a broad tendon into the ulnar tuberosity below the coronoid process of the ulna (Figure 5.13).

The brachialis can flex the elbow efficiently in all positions of the forearm and hand. The ulna does not move in pronation and supination, so the direction of pull of the brachialis tendon always produces flexion. When the elbow flexors increase in size in response to weight training, the brachialis contributes most to the increase in muscle bulk.

Extensors of the elbow

Triceps brachii

The posterior compartment contains the three heads of the triceps. The long head is a broad tendon attached to the inferior part of the glenoid cavity, outside the capsule, but blended with it. (The long head of the biceps lies inside the joint.) The two other heads of the triceps arise from the shaft of the humerus. The lateral head takes origin from an oblique line below the greater tuberosity on the posterior shaft. The medial head is deep and attached to the lower posterior shaft of the humerus, corresponding to the origin of the brachialis anteriorly.

The long and lateral heads join to form one layer, which unites with the deep medial head, and all three end as a broad tendon inserted into the olecranon of the ulna (Figure 5.14a).

All extension movements involve the medial head; the other two heads are recruited when acting against resistance. It is the lateral head that becomes more obvious in the powerful triceps developed by the gymnast, weight-lifter and wheelchair athlete. The triceps provides all the power

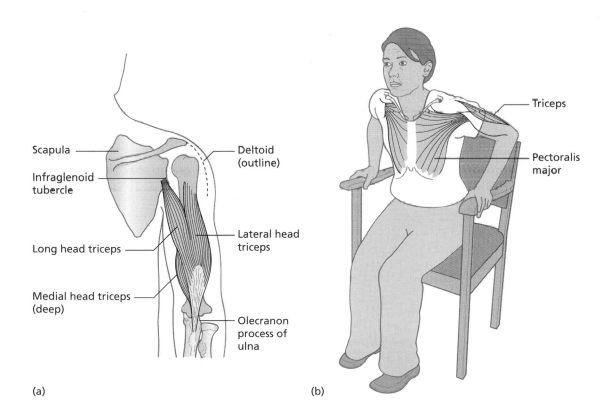

(a)   (b)

Figure 5.14   Triceps brachii: (a) position in posterior view of right arm, (b) acting with pectoralis major and latissimus dorsi to raise the body from sitting.

of the elbow in extension movements to reach above the head, and to push forwards and to the side. Figure 5.14b shows the use of the triceps with the pectoralis major to lift the body up from the sitting position if the muscles of the lower limb are weak.

Anconeus

This is the other posterior muscle that extends the elbow. This muscle is small and blends with the lower end of the triceps at the back of the elbow joint. The fibres of the anconeus originate on the lateral epicondyle of the humerus, and insert distal to the triceps on the olecranon of the ulna. Anconeus adds little to the total strength of elbow extension, but does contribute to the stability of the elbow joint.

Forearm muscles in elbow flexion

Brachioradialis

The brachioradialis is the most superficial muscle on the radial side of the forearm.

Reflective task

- Move the forearm to be at a right angle to the arm and turn the hand to face medially. Flex the elbow and offer resistance with the other hand.
- Palpate the brachioradialis in a position parallel to the long axis of the radius.

The brachioradialis originates from the ridge above the lateral epicondyle of the humerus. The fibres pass down the lateral side of the forearm, and the tendon inserts into the radius just above the styloid process at the wrist (Figure 5.15a, b). In the anatomical position, the muscle can only pull the head of the radius closer to the capitulum of the humerus. When the radius is rotated to bring the styloid process in line with the middle of the elbow joint (the midprone position), the brachioradialis is able to flex the elbow in a powerful way. The midprone position is frequently adopted to allow the strong leverage to aid flexion, e.g. using a hammer or saw, or lifting a baby (Figure 5.15c) or heavy boxes. Working statically, the brachioradialis holds the elbow in flexion to support loads, for example books or the handle of a bag over the forearm.

Pronator teres

The pronator teres is another forearm muscle that helps in flexion of the elbow. It arises from the medial epicondyle of the humerus with the wrist and finger flexors. (The brachioradialis origin is above the lateral epicondyle of the humerus with the wrist extensors.) The fibres of the pronator teres cross obliquely below the elbow joint to be inserted into the lateral shaft of the radius about half way down. When the forearm is in the anatomical position (radius and ulna parallel), the pronator teres has a weak action on elbow flexion. When all the elbow flexors are in action, the pronator teres counteracts the tendency for the biceps to supinate the arm.

Figure 5.15b shows both the brachioradialis and pronator teres. They will be considered again in Chapter 6 with the forearm muscles.

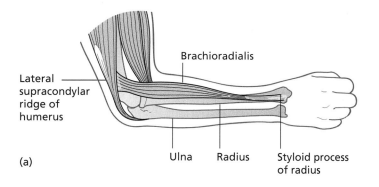

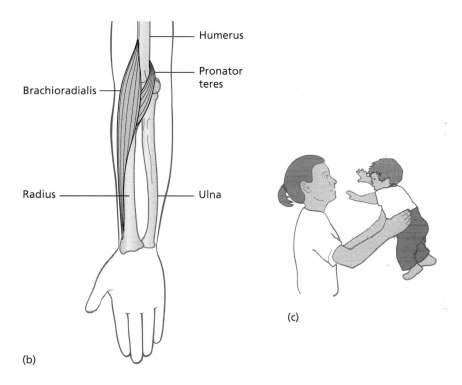

Figure 5.15 Brachioradialis in the right forearm: (a) lateral view in midprone position; (b) anterior view with pronator teres; (c) lifting and holding a baby.

Summary of the shoulder and elbow in functional movements

(1) **Reaching forwards**:
   - protraction of the scapula: serratus anterior, pectoralis minor;
   - flexion of the shoulder joint: deltoid (anterior fibres), pectoralis major (clavicular fibres), coracobrachialis;
   - extension of the elbow: triceps.

(2) **Pulling back towards the body (from forward reach)**:
- retraction of the scapula: rhomboids, trapezius (middle fibres);
- extension of the shoulder joint: deltoid (posterior fibres), latissimus dorsi;
- flexion of the elbow: biceps, brachialis.

(3) **Reaching across the body**:
- protraction of the scapula: serratus anterior, pectoralis minor;
- flexion, adduction and medial rotation of the shoulder joint: deltoid (anterior fibres), pectoralis major, subscapularis;
- extension of the elbow: triceps.

(4) **Reaching behind the body**:
- retraction of the scapula: rhomboids, trapezius (middle fibres);
- extension and lateral rotation of the shoulder joint: deltoid (posterior fibres), infraspinatus, teres minor;
- extension of the elbow: triceps.

(5) **Lifting the trunk on the arms (from a seat)**:
- depression of the scapula: trapezius (lower fibres), pectoralis minor;
- extension and adduction of the shoulder joint: latissimus dorsi, teres major;
- extension of the elbow: triceps.

The performance of positioning movements of the shoulder and the elbow can be seen in reaching for a box of cornflakes in a cupboard above head height (Figure 5.16) and then pouring the flakes into a bowl.

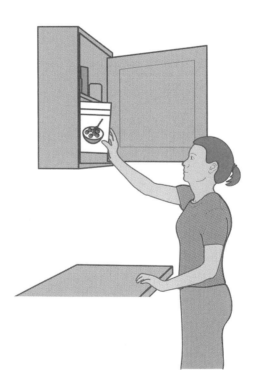

Figure 5.16   Positioning movements of the shoulder and elbow.

Summary

- The shoulder girdle, formed by the clavicle and scapula, anchors the upper limb to the trunk.
- The scapula, moving freely on the posterior wall of the thorax, orientates its position in the direction of shoulder movement. The muscles moving the scapula originate on the bones of the thorax and cross the scapula to be attached to its borders and processes.
- The shoulder joint, between the scapula and the humerus, is the synovial ball and socket type with a wide range of movement.
- The stability of the shoulder joint relies on the four rotator cuff muscles that surround the joint.
- Three large triangular muscles, the deltoid, pectoralis major and latissimus dorsi, combine in different ways to move the shoulder joint in all directions. These movements allow the hand to be placed in front, behind and to the side of the body, as well as above the head.
- The elbow forms the hinge joint between the arm and the forearm.
- The elbow flexor and extensor muscles lie on the anterior and posterior aspects of the upper arm, respectively. Flexion movement brings the hand towards the head and body. Extension movement increases the length of reach of the upper limb.
- Combined action of the shoulder and the elbow carries the hand to all positions around the body. The exact orientation of the hand depends on the movements of the forearm and wrist, which will be considered in Chapter 6.

6

Manipulative movements: the forearm, wrist and hand

Key terms

structure and function of the forearm, wrist and hand; muscles and movement of the forearm, wrist and hand; types of grip

Conceptual overview

This chapter outlines the structure and functions related to the forearm, wrist and hand. The musculature of the forearm, wrist and hand will be examined in detail. Specific types of grips of the hand are explored in detail relative to their role in gripping during everyday occupations.

Tyldesley & Grieve's Muscles, Nerves and Movement in Human Occupation, Fourth Edition. Ian R. McMillan, Gail Carin-Levy.
© 2012 Ian R. McMillan, Gail Carin-Levy, Barbara Tyldesley and June I. Grieve. Published 2012 by Blackwell Publishing Ltd.

Introduction

The forearm and wrist provide the base for the fine skilled movements of the fingers and thumb. Objects and tools must be held in a particular orientation for their functional use. A cup full of coffee will soon be spilled if it cannot be held upright. This depends not only on the grip of the fingers and thumb on the handle of the cup but also on the position of the forearm and the stability of the wrist. The hand must also be orientated accurately on to surfaces when the hand explores the environment.

Many manipulative tasks involve the bilateral activity of the two hands working together. The two hands may be performing similar movements, as in rolling pastry or pressing the keys of a computer keyboard. At other times, one hand may provide stability while the other hand makes precise movements, for example in stirring the contents of a saucepan, unscrewing the top of a jar or sewing.

Fine movements of the fingers and thumb are performed by the intrinsic muscles of the hand. These muscles also depend on forearm muscles for their strength and for the fixation of their proximal attachments. Together, the forearm, wrist and hand form an interdependent system for the performance of manipulative movements.

Functions of the forearm and wrist

The forearm and wrist co-operate in the orientation of the hand in space.

The **forearm**:

- enables the hand to grip handles and hold objects in any orientation in the performance of functional activities;
- allows the hand to function as a tactile sense organ by contact with all surfaces.

The **wrist**:

- lifts the hand to a functional position by counteracting the effect of gravity tending to pull the hand into flexion or ulnar deviation;
- stabilises the relative positions of the hand and forearm during manipulative movements.

The combination of the movements of the forearm and the wrist means that the hand is joined to the arm by a virtual joint that moves in all axes.

The forearm

In the anatomical position, the radius and the ulna are parallel. When movement occurs in the forearm the radius rotates and crosses over the ulna. This movement of the radius carries the hand with it.

When the elbow is flexed, the radius and ulna are parallel, and the palm of the hand faces upwards. The movements of the forearm are:

- **pronation**: turns the hand to face downwards and the radius and ulna are crossed;
- **supination**: turns the hand to face upwards and the radius and ulna are parallel again.

The **midprone** position is when the hand faces inwards or medially. This is the functional position of the hand.

When pronation and supination are limited, for example after fractures of the forearm, there is considerable loss of hand function.

> **Reflective task**
>
> - Find handles and rails in different positions, i.e. vertical, horizontal, at an angle. Grip each one and notice how the position of the forearm changes in each position to allow the hand to grip.
> - Grip the vertical handle of a teapot or jug and then tip to pour out the contents. Note how the grip remains the same while the tipping is done by pronation and supination of the forearm.
> - Turn a tap or a round door-knob. The fingers and thumb exert pressure on the tap, while the forearm movement provides the power to turn it.

Radioulnar joints

The movements of pronation and supination occur at synovial pivot joints found at the proximal and distal ends of the radius and ulna. In between, the shafts of the two bones are held together by an interosseous membrane, a fibrous joint of the syndesmosis type (Figure 6.1a).

The **superior (proximal) radioulnar joint** lies between the head of the radius and the radial notch on the ulna. The joint lies inside the capsule of the elbow joint, but its movements are entirely independent. The radius is held in contact with the ulna by the annular ligament (lined by a thin layer of cartilage), which surrounds the head of the radius and is firmly attached to the margins of the radial notch on the ulna (Figure 6.1b). The capsule of the elbow joint blends with the annular ligament so that the radius can rotate independently within this ring whatever the angulation of the elbow joint may be.

The **inferior (distal) radioulnar joint**: the lower end of the radius pivots round the head of the ulna, and is held in contact with it by a disc of fibrocartilage. This disc joins the styloid process of the ulna to the ulnar notch of the radius (Figure 6.1c). The joint has a thin loose capsule, but the bones are held together by the articular disc and the interosseous membrane above.

All the muscles involved in pronation and supination are inserted into the radius, which then moves around the fixed ulna. The supinators, inserted into the radius, can also assist other muscles to move the elbow, e.g. the biceps brachii is also an elbow flexor, and the supinator helps in extension of the elbow.

Pronation puts the palm of the hand flat on a surface, or tips forwards a vessel held in the hand (Figure 6.2a). Strong pronation and supination movements are needed to use a screwdriver or a corkscrew (Figure 6.2b).

Supination is more powerful than pronation, and so most screws have a right-handed thread.

The brachioradialis, already described with the elbow flexors in Chapter 5, can move the forearm to the midprone position from full pronation or full supination.

Muscles producing pronation and supination

Two forearm muscles are active in **pronation**: the pronator teres and pronator quadratus.

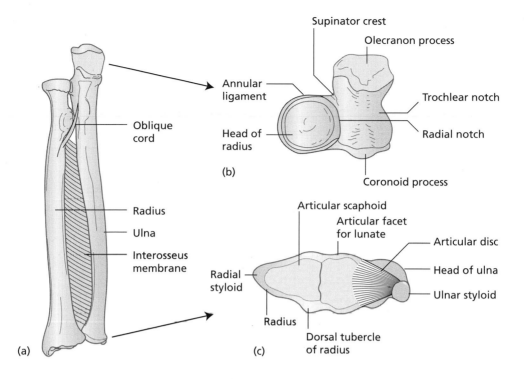

Figure 6.1 Right radioulnar joints: (a) middle, anterior view; (b) proximal; (c) distal.

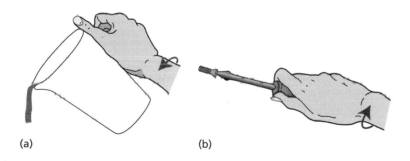

Figure 6.2 Activites involving pronation and supination: (a) pouring from a jug – pronation; (b) turning a screw – supination.

The **pronator teres** (Figure 6.3a), which crosses the anterior forearm from the medial side of the elbow to half way down the lateral shaft of the radius has already been described in Chapter 5, with the elbow flexors.

The **pronator quadratus** (Figure 6.3a) is a deep muscle of the forearm just above the wrist. Its fibres pass transversely between the lower anterior shafts of the radius and ulna. The muscle is deep to the flexor tendons which pass into the hand. When force is applied to the outstretched

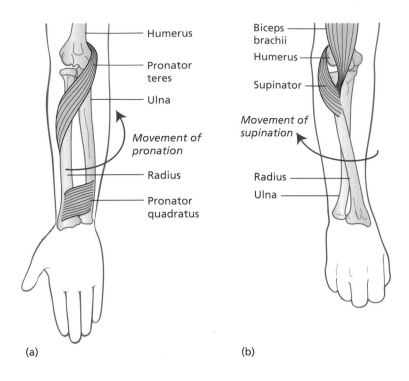

Figure 6.3   Muscles and movements of (a) pronation and (b) supination. Right forearm and hand.

hand in pushing or falling, the pronator quadratus prevents separation of the radius and ulna. Many pronation movements are made with the pronator quadratus alone, the pronator teres being recruited for extra power against resistance.

The two muscles active in **supination** are the biceps brachii and supinator.

The **biceps brachii** (Chapter 5, Figure 5.13) makes all supination movements against resistance. Its tendon pulls on the radial tuberosity just below the elbow to rotate the radius to the position parallel with the ulna. The attachments and action of biceps have already been described in Chapter 5 with the elbow flexors.

The **supinator** (Figure 6.3b) is a deep posterior muscle of the forearm which is involved in slow, unopposed movements of supination, such as when the arm hangs by the side. This muscle is covered by the long extensors of the wrist and fingers. The origin of the supinator is from the lateral epicondyle of the humerus and adjacent areas of the ulna. A short flat muscle, its fibres wrap round the proximal end of the radius close to the bone and insert into the upper end of the shaft.

The wrist

The wrist region is concerned with movements of the carpus of the hand on the distal ends of the radius and ulna of the forearm. The range of movement is increased by the movement of the carpal bones on each other, particularly between the proximal and distal rows.

Joints and movements of the wrist

Reflective task

Look at the illustrations of the radius, ulna and the bones of the hand in Appendix I. Use an articulated sleleton of the hand to identify the eight carpal bones arranged in two rows.

The wrist joint is composed of the joints between the carpal bones (intercarpal joints) and the radiocarpal articulation between the forearm and the proximal row of carpals. The intercarpal joint between the two rows of carpals is known as the midcarpal joint. The main movement at the wrist occurs at the radiocarpal and midcarpal joints.

The **radiocarpal joint** is formed by the concave distal end of the radius and an articular disc over the ulna articulating with a reciprocally convex surface formed by the three carpal bones in the proximal row, i.e. scaphoid, lunate and triangular (triquetral). This joint is an ellipsoid type allowing movement in two directions (see Chapter 2, Figure 2.3c). The articular surface of the radius and ulna is shown in Figure 6.1c.

The **midcarpal joint** lies between the proximal and distal row of carpals, i.e. distal surfaces of the scaphoid, lunate and triquetral, with proximal surfaces of the trapezium, trapezoid, capitate and hamate. The joint cavity is continuous between the two rows of carpals and extends between the individual bones. (The fourth bone in the proximal row, the pisiform, does not take part in either of the joints.)

The capsule of the radiocarpal joint, strengthened by ligaments, extends to cover the midcarpal joint. Both joints are strengthened on each side by the ulnar and radial collateral ligaments (Figure 6.4).

The **movements** at the joints of the wrist are flexion, extension, abduction (radial deviation) and adduction (ulnar deviation).

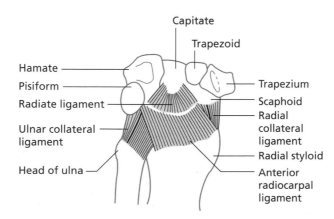

Figure 6.4   Right wrist (radiocarpal) joint, anterior aspect.

There is no active rotation of the wrist about a longitudinal axis. Remember that rotation of the hand on the forearm occurs at the radioulnar joints of the forearm, i.e. pronation and supination movements.

Radiographs of the wrist in action show that all the carpals move as well as the radiocarpal articulation. In some movements, the scaphoid, for instance, may move as much as 1 cm. The radiocarpal joint contributes most to extension and adduction, while the midcarpal joint moves further in flexion and abduction. All the joints act together as a single mechanism for wrist movement.

Reflective task

- Place the supinated hand (palm upwards) on a flat surface in a relaxed position. Notice the slight flexion and deviation to the ulnar side.
- Look at an articulated skeleton to see the shape of the lower end of the radius extending further on the dorsal side and laterally at the styloid process, which accounts for the position of the hand.
- Lift the hand and move the wrist into flexion, extension, abduction (radial deviation) and adduction (ulnar deviation). Note the range of each of these movements. You will see that the hands move further in flexion than extension, and more easily in ulnar deviation than radial deviation.
- Compare your own range of these wrist movements with those of other people. Notice the difference in range between individuals, but the relative amounts for each movement are usually the same.

Since there is a variation in range of movement in normal subjects, the assessment of an injured wrist should be done by comparing it with the normal wrist of the same person and not with the 'average' wrist.

Practice note-pad 6A: fractures of the forearm and wrist

A common mechanism of forearm and wrist fracture is a fall on to the outstretched hand. This causes:

- Colles' fracture when the lower broken ends of bone are displaced backwards; or
- Smith's fracture when only the radius is fractured and the distal fragment displaces forwards.

A fall on the hand with the wrist in full extension may fracture the scaphoid. The scaphoid bone fractures across its waist, and the proximal fragment may die due to poor blood supply. This avascular necrosis may produce persistent pain and weakness of the wrist.

Muscles moving the wrist

The muscles arranged around the wrist combine in different ways to produce the movements of flexion, extension, abduction and adduction. If the wrist is viewed in cross-section, the flexor and extensor tendons involved in wrist movement can be seen around the oval shape of the carpus. The tendons pull on the carpus in different combinations, like the strings of a marionette, to produce all the movements of the wrist.

The two anterior muscles, active in **flexion** of the wrist, are the **flexor carpi ulnaris** and **flexor carpi radialis**. The palmaris longus is another wrist flexor that lies between the other two, but it is absent in 15% of people. All three muscles have a common origin on the medial epicondyle of the humerus, and form the superficial layer of muscles in the anterior forearm.

The flexor carpi ulnaris is attached to the pisiform bone and on to the base of the fifth meta-carpal. The flexor carpi radialis lies deep to the muscles at the base of the thumb as it crosses the wrist and ends at the bases of metacarpals 2 and 3 (Figure 6.5a).

The palmaris longus has a long thin tendon that inserts into the palmar aponeurosis, a layer of dense fibrous tissue below the skin of the palm, considered in more detail later in the chapter.

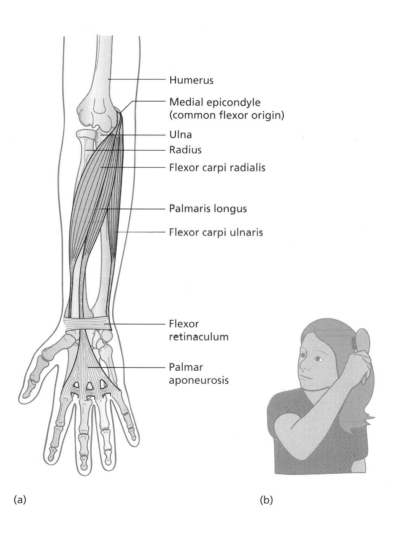

Humerus

Medial epicondyle
(common flexor origin)

Ulna

Radius

Flexor carpi radialis

Palmaris longus

Flexor carpi ulnaris

Flexor
retinaculum

Palmar
aponeurosis

(a)   (b)

Figure 6.5 Flexors of the wrist: (a) position in the superficial layer of the anterior right forearm; (b) combing the hair.

> **Reflective task**
>
> Make a fist and flex the wrist to see the flexor tendons appear on the anterior aspect. The palmaris longus is in the midline and flexor carpi ulnaris medial to it, attached to the pisiform. The flexor carpi radialis laterally may be more difficult to find.

A functional use of the wrist flexors can be seen in Figure 6.5b, where they are used to counteract the resistance offered by the hair on the comb.

Three posterior muscles, active in **extension** of the wrist, are the **extensor carpi ulnaris** and the **extensor carpi radialis longus and brevis** (Figure 6.6a). The long radial extensor takes origin on the ridge above the lateral epicondyle of the humerus with brachioradialis, already described in Chapter 5. The other two muscles are attached to the lateral epicondyle which is the common

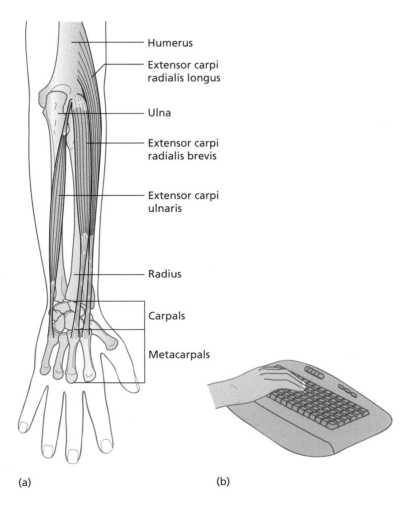

Humerus
Extensor carpi radialis longus
Ulna
Extensor carpi radialis brevis
Extensor carpi ulnaris
Radius
Carpals
Metacarpals

(a)   (b)

Figure 6.6 Extensors of the wrist: (a) position in the posterior right forearm; (b) hand held with extended wrist to use a keyboard.

extensor origin. All three muscles pass down the posterior side of the forearm and insert at the wrist following the same pattern as the flexors: extensor carpi radialis longus into metacarpal 2; extensor carpi radialis brevis into metacarpal 3; and extensor carpi ulnaris into metacarpal 5.

> **Reflective task**
>
> Make a fist and extend the wrist to see the extensor tendons on the posterior side. Extensor carpi radialis brevis is more central and may be difficult to feel, as it is crossed by tendons of muscles passing to the thumb.

In the use of the pronated hand, e.g. pressing keys of a typewriter or piano (Figure 6.6b), the wrist extensors are active to lift the weight of the hand against gravity. Weakness of these muscles leads to 'wrist drop'. In strong gripping by the whole hand, the wrist extensors act as synergists to counteract flexion of the wrist by the long finger flexors.

Abduction and **adduction** of the wrist is achieved by contraction of the flexor and extensor muscles on the radial and ulnar sides, respectively. See Figure 6.7 for the position of the tendons around the wrist. Contraction of the flexor carpi ulnaris and extensor carpi ulnaris muscles adducts the wrist, often known as ulnar deviation. Similarly, contraction of the flexor carpi radialis and extensor carpi radialis longus and brevis together will result in abduction of the wrist or radial deviation.

Figure 6.7 shows the positions of the tendons of the wrist flexors and extensors arranged around the wrist. Note that the flexors insert into the anterior or palmar side, and the extensors insert into the posterior or dorsal side. A strong and stable wrist in the midprone position of the forearm is used in operating many tools, for example a saw. When the muscles around the wrist are weak, the hand falls into ulnar deviation when holding the tool.

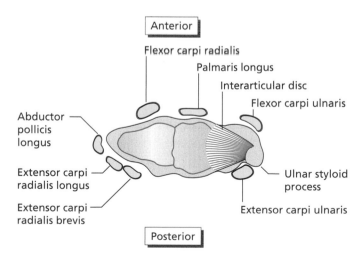

Figure 6.7 Position of the wrist flexors and extensors around the distal end of the radius and ulna, inferior view.

> **Reflective task**
>
> Hold a mug of coffee or large tool, e.g. a hammer, in the hand. Note that the forearm is in the midprone position and the weight of the mug or tool is tending to pull the wrist into ulnar deviation. The abductors (radial deviators) of the wrist must work statically to hold the position.

Functions of the hand

The hand performs fine movements of the fingers and thumb to operate small tools and keyboards. The intrinsic muscles of the hand combine to make the small movements of the fingers and the thumb required in skillful activites, for example writing, texting using a mobile phone, painting and playing musical instruments.

The hand is the mechanism to grasp handles and large tools while the upper limb moves them in space. In all gripping movements, the thumb is placed opposite to the fingers in different ways depending on the size and shape of the object. The wrist is important in gripping by providing a stable base for the hand, and by directing the pull of the tendons of the forearm muscles acting on the fingers and thumb. Grasping activites also involve release movements to let go or set down, using the opposing group of muscles to those that make the grip.

The hand is also a sense organ. The skin of the hand, particularly the palm and the fingertips, is richly supplied with receptors, and a large area of the somatosensory cortex in the brain (see Chapter 3) processes information from them. All gripping activities involve the continuous monitoring of activity in the tactile and pressure receptors in the hand. For example, in writing, accurate formation of the letters depends on the correct pressure of the fingers on a pen, and the hand on the paper. Response from receptors in the skin of the hand is important to protect it from injury. Trauma or pathological changes in the bones and joints of the wrist may damage sensory fibres in the nerves passing over them and affect hand sensation.

> **Reflective task**
>
> Try writing with a pen whilst wearing a thin pair of rubber gloves.

Further processing of all the sensory information in the brain allows us to 'recognise' objects held in the hand without seeing them. This is known as stereognosis (see Chapter 3).

Finally, the hand is used in communication and in the expression of emotion. Watch how people use their hands as they greet each other, or chat in a group. Hands are used to complement and reinforce the spoken word in a conscious way, or may be used unconsciously in 'body language'.

In summary, the functions of the hand are:

- the performance of fine manipulative movements;
- to grasp and release objects and tools;
- as a sense organ for the exploration of the environment and recognition of objects;
- in the communication and expression of emotion.

Movements of the hand: fingers and thumb

The movements of the hand are performed by muscles that originate partly in the hand (intrinsic muscles) and partly in the forearm (extrinsic muscles), passing over the wrist into the hand. The hand performs complex and precision movements in the manipulation of utensils, tools and equipment in daily living. The increased use of electrically powered equipment in the home and in the workplace has reduced the need for the hand to exert great power, but has introduced a greater variety of precision movements required to operate switches and controls.

A large number of muscles, originating in both the forearm and the hand, is inserted into the fingers and the thumb. Most of the tendons of these muscles pass over several joints, and the combinations of different directions of pull of the tendons allow the fingers to move in a variety of ways.

- The five digits are numbered 1–5 from lateral (thumb) to medial.
- The fingers are identified by name: index finger, middle finger, ring finger, little finger.
- The central axis of the hand extends through the third metacarpal and the third (middle) finger.
- When the fingers separate, the other fingers move away from the central axis (Figure 6.8).
- The names of muscles moving the fingers include 'digitorum', while those moving the thumb include 'pollicis'. Thenar muscles are associated with the thumb, and hypothenar muscles are associated with the little finger.

Joints of the fingers and thumb

The main joints are identified in Figure 6.9.

The **metacarpophalangeal** (MCP) joints, commonly known as the knuckles, are formed by the articulations of the heads of the metacarpals with oval concavities at the base of the proximal phalanges. The thumb, as well as the four fingers, has an MCP joint. The MCP joints of the fingers are synovial ellipsoid, biaxial joints. Each MCP joint of the fingers has a strong palmar ligament,

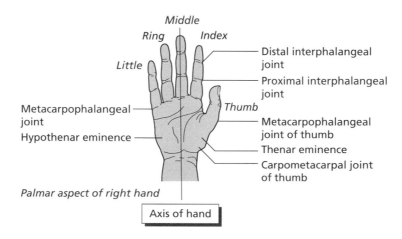

Figure 6.8 Palmar view of the right hand; location of the joints.

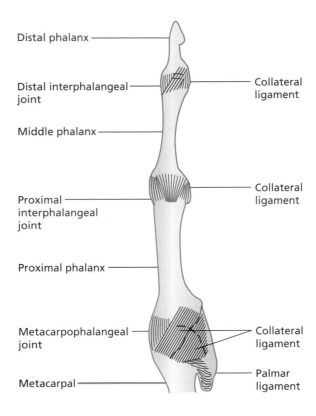

Distal phalanx

Distal interphalangeal joint

Middle phalanx

Proximal interphalangeal joint

Proximal phalanx

Metacarpophalangeal joint

Metacarpal

Collateral ligament

Collateral ligament

Collateral ligament

Palmar ligament

Figure 6.9   Joints of the finger; lateral view.

which is attached firmly to the phalanx but loosely to the metacarpal bone. The palmar ligaments of these four joints are connected by a deep transverve ligament, which holds the heads of the metacarpals together to form the body of the palm of the hand. The collateral ligaments are bands present on each side of the joints (Figure 6.9). The movements of the MCP joints allow the fingers to flex and extend, abduct and adduct. In abduction, the fingers move away from the middle finger, which forms the central axis of the hand.

The **interphalangeal** (IP) joints are the articulations between two phalanges. Each finger has two interphalangeal joints, known as proximal (PIP) joints and distal (DIP) joints. The thumb has one IP joint. They are all synovial hinge joints with collateral ligaments (Figure 6.9). These joints allow flexion and extension movements only.

The **carpometacarpal joint of the thumb** is a synovial saddle joint. This joint is formed between the base of the first metacarpal and the trapezium, the most lateral bone in the distal row of carpals. The distal surface of the trapezium is scooped out in two directions like a saddle on which the metacarpal moves (see Chapter 2, Figure 2.3f). The loose capsule surrounding the joint is strengthened by lateral, anterior and posterior ligaments. The shape of this articular surfaces, combined with a loose capsule, allows the thumb considerable mobility.

Movements of the thumb

The movements of the thumb occur principally at the carpometacarpal joint. The MCP and IP joints of the thumb are hinge joints which increase the range of flexion and extension of the thumb.

In the resting position of the thumb, the first metacarpal (thumb) is medially rotated.

> **Reflective task**
>
> Look at the pad of the thumb when the hand is in a relaxed position on a flat surface with the palm upwards. Note that the thumb is facing across the palm at right angles to it.

From this position with the pad of the thumb facing medially, the movements of the thumb are described at right angles to those of the fingers.

- **Flexion** of the thumb carries it across the palm in a plane at right angles to the thumb nail (Figure 6.10b).
- **Extension** is the return movement from flexion and continues into the 'hitch a lift' position (Figure 6.10d). In full extension of the thumb, the oblique pull of the long extensor of the thumb can, in some people, pull the first metacarpal into lateral rotation so appearing to provide a 'flat' hand.
- **Abduction** takes the thumb away from the palm of the hand and at right angles to it (Figure 6.10a).
- **Adduction** is the return movement from abduction, which pulls the thumb back towards the palm of the hand.

Opposition is a unique movement that brings the thumb into contact with each of the fingers. This movement is possible because the first metacarpal is able to rotate on the trapezium both medially and laterally. Opposition is the combined movements of flexion, medial rotation and adduction to bring the thumb into contact with any of the fingers. Figure 6.10c shows the thumb in opposition to the flexed fingers. The thumb can, however, be opposed to the fingers in a variety of ways to form different types of grip. This will be considered later in the chapter.

> **Reflective task**
>
> - Look at your own hand. Starting at the base of the hand, notice the flexure line of the wrist, and then feel the shafts of the metacarpals on the back of the hand. Identify the MCP joints at the knuckles and check the movements that occur at these joints – flexion, extension, abduction and adduction. Identify the PIP and DIP joints and check the movements – flexion and extension only.
> - Palpate the first metacarpal bone of the thumb, which moves independently of the other metacarpals.
> - Move the thumb through all the directions described above and feel how all the movement occurs at the carpometacarpal joint.

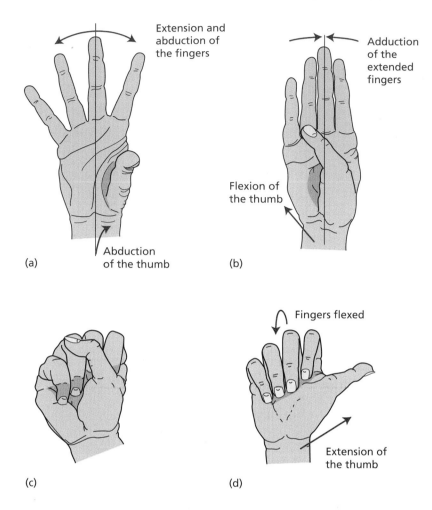

Figure 6.10   Positions of the right hand seen in palmar view: (a) fingers extended and abducted – the open hand; (b) fingers extended and adducted, thumb flexed; (c) fingers flexed, thumb in opposition – the closed hand; (d) fingers flexed, thumb extended.

Muscles moving the hand: fingers and thumb

During many functional activities, the hand closes round an object to grasp and manipulate it in various ways. The fingers are flexed and adducted; the thumb is in opposition (Figure 6.10c). The hand also opens to prepare for gripping or to release an object and set it down (Figure 6.10a).

Reflective task

Open the hand. Notice how the fingers and thumb abduct as they extend in opening the hand. Close the hand. Notice how the fingers and thumb adduct as they flex to close the hand.

The muscles moving the hand will be described under three headings based on the functional use of the hand:

- muscles closing the hand;
- muscles opening the hand;
- muscles producing fine precision movements of the fingers and thumb.

Closing the hand

The muscles closing the hand lie in the anterior part of the forearm deep to the wrist flexors, and in the palm of the hand.

Forearm muscles

The forearm muscles that close the hand are: the flexor digitorum superficialis, the flexor digitorum profundus and the flexor pollicis longus.

The **flexor digitorum superficialis** originates at the medial side of the elbow with the wrist flexors, i.e. from the medial epicondyle of the humerus. The origin of the muscle continues diagonally across the bones below the elbow, attached to the coronoid process of the ulna and the anterior shaft of the radius (Figure 6.11a).

The **flexor digitorum profundus** lies deep to the superficialis and takes origin from the anterior and medial shaft of the ulna (Figure 6.11b).

The **flexor pollicis longus** also lies deep to the superficialis and is attached to the anterior shaft of the radius (Figure 6.11b). The flexor digitorum profundus and flexor pollicis longus appear as one muscle in the deep layer on the anterior part of the forearm covering the radius, the ulna and the interosseus membrane in between them.

All three muscles pass down the anterior forearm to the wrist, where the two muscles that insert into the fingers each divide into four tendons. Each of these tendons passes through the palm and over the palmar surface of each finger, where the flexor digitorum superficialis divides to insert into the sides of the middle phalanx. This allows the deeper flexor digitorum profundus tendon to pass on to insert into the distal phalanx. (See Figure 6.19, which shows how these two muscles insert into each finger.) The tendon of flexor pollicis longus turns laterally to reach the thumb and insert into the base of the distal phalanx.

The three muscles together flex all the joints of the fingers and the thumb. The tendons of the index, ring and little fingers diverge from the axis of the hand from wrist to fingertip. This means that as the fingers flex, they also adduct towards each other.

Muscles of the hand

Five intrinsic muscles of the hand also assist the forearm muscles in closing the hand, acting on the thumb and little finger.

The **flexor pollicis brevis** and **opponens pollicis** move the thumb and lie in the thenar eminence of the hand. The **flexor digiti minimi** and **opponens digiti minimi** are comparable muscles in the hypothenar eminence below the little finger.

The **adductor pollicis** lies deep in the palm of the hand, covered by the long flexor tendons and the flexor policis brevis.

Figure 6.12 shows these five muscles.

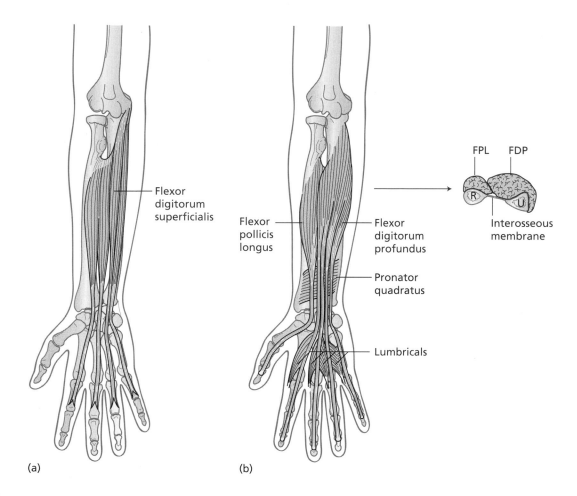

Flexor digitorum superficialis

Flexor pollicis longus

Flexor digitorum profundus

Pronator quadratus

Lumbricals

FPL   FDP

R   U

Interosseous membrane

(a)   (b)

Figure 6.11   Flexors of the fingers and thumb in the right forearm and hand: (a) flexor digitorum superficialis (middle layer); (b) flexor digitorum profundus and flexor pollicis longus (deep layer).

A band of fibrous tissue known as the flexor retinaculum crosses the palmar side of the carpal bones over the long flexor tendons. The thenar and hypothenar muscles originate from this retinaculum.

The flexor digiti minimi is inserted into the base of the proximal phalanx of the little finger, and the flexor pollicis brevis is attached to the proximal phalanx of the thumb.

The opponens muscles are attached to the length of the shaft of the metacarpal bone of their corresponding little finger or thumb. During the opposition movement of the thumb, the shaft of the first metacarpal is rotated about its axis by the pull of the opponens pollicis. At the same time, the flexor draws the thumb across and towards the palm. The opponens digiti minimi increases the bulk of the medial border of the hand in a cupping movement used to grasp a round knob, such as the round head of the gear lever of a car.

The adductor pollicis is attached along a wide origin in the centre of the palm on the shaft of the third metacarpal and has a second head from the capitate bone. This muscle forms the web of the thumb and inserts into the proximal phalanx of the thumb on the ulnar side. The adductor

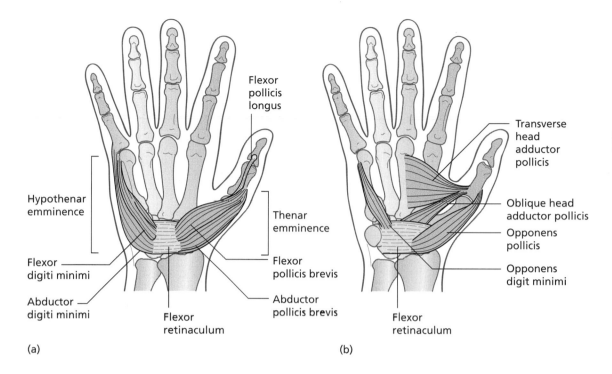

Figure 6.12 Thenar and hypothenar muscles in the palm of the right hand: (a) superficial layer; (b) deep layer.

pollicis acts strongly to draw the thumb towards the hand in pinching movements between the thumb and index finger.

Connective tissues of the hand

The connective tissue in the palm of the hand plays an important role in the protection and binding of the muscles and tendons, so that smooth movement in the correct direction is achieved. Three particular sites will be described: the flexor retinaculum, the palmar aponeurosis and the flexor tendon sheaths.

The long finger flexors of the forearm enter the hand over the anterior side of the wrist. They are held in position by a band of fibrous tissue called the **flexor retinaculum**. This also provides a base for the attachment of the thenar and hypothenar muscles.

Reflective task

Look at the skeleton of the hand and note how the carpal bones form a trough on the palmar side for the long flexor tendons. Look at the arrangement of the carpal bones and find four raised bony points on either side of this trough. These are: the pisiform and the hook of the hamate medially, and the tubercle of the scaphoid and crest of the trapezium laterally. These are the points for the attachment of the flexor retinaculum.

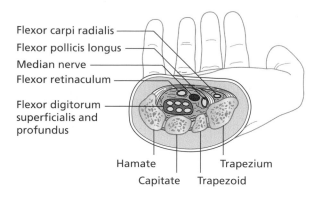

Flexor carpi radialis
Flexor pollicis longus
Median nerve
Flexor retinaculum
Flexor digitorum superficialis and profundus

Hamate   Trapezium
Capitate   Trapezoid

Figure 6.13 Section through the carpus to show the carpal tunnel.

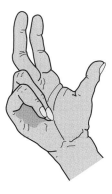

Figure 6.14 Right hand with Dupuytren's contracture.

The flexor retinaculum stretches across the carpal bones, converting the trough into a tunnel known as the carpal tunnel (Figure 6.13). Note that the exact position of the flexor retinaculum is across the base of the hand, i.e. under the heel of the hand, and not in the position of a bracelet around the wrist.

The **palmar aponeurosis** is a triangular sheet of fibrous tissue covering all the long muscle tendons of the palm. The apex is joined to the flexor retinaculum at the wrist and receives the insertion of the palmaris longus, if this muscle is present (see Figure 6.5a). The sides of the triangle blend with the fascia covering the muscles of the thumb and little finger, and the sheet ends at the base of the fingers. The palmar aponeurosis is anchored to the metacarpals and to the deep transverse palmar ligament.

Practice note-pad 6B: Dupuytren's contracture

This condition occurs when there is shrinkage of the fibrous tissue in the palmar aponeurosis, usually on the ulnar side. The little and ring fingers are pulled down so that they flex into the palm of the hand (Figure 6.14).

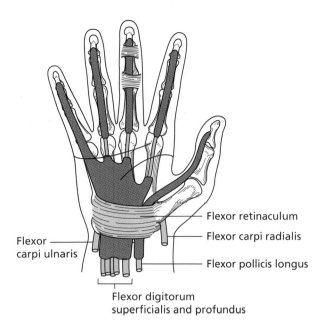

Figure 6.15 Tendon sheaths of the long flexor tendons in a palmar view of the right hand.

Practice note-pad 6C: occupational overuse syndrome

Tenosynovitis is an inflammation of the synovial sheaths around the tendons of muscles, when there is swelling due to an accumulation of fluid. This may be due to overuse, for example any repetitive movement. For example, the tendons passing through the carpal tunnel at the wrist are confined to a narrow space so that any increase in fluid compresses the median nerve, causing pain, loss of sensation and muscle weakness. This is known as **carpal tunnel syndrome**. It occurs sometimes in pregnancy, in middle-aged women and in rheumatoid arthritis.

As the long flexor tendons pass through the carpal tunnel and up over the palmar surface of each finger, they are wrapped in a double layer of synovial membrane known as a **tendon sheath** (Figure 6.15). Each tendon sheath is held in position on the palmar surface of the bones of the finger by fibrous bands forming tunnels. These fibrous bands are also joined to the palmar aponeurosis and are thin over the IP joints to allow flexibilty of the fingers.

Opening the hand

The muscles opening the hand lie in the posterior part of the forearm, and in the thenar and hypothenar groups.

Forearm muscles

The forearm muscles that open the fingers are the extensor digitorum, the extensor indicis and the extensor digiti minimi (Figure 6.16).

The **extensor digitorum** and the **extensor digiti minimi** originate with the wrist extensors from the lateral epicondyle of the humerus. The **extensor indicis**, a deep muscle, takes origin on the posterior border of the ulna. The tendons formed from these three muscles pass posteriorly over the wrist held down by a band of fibrous tissue, the extensor retinaculum. On the dorsal side of the hand, the extensor digitorum divides into four. The extensor indicis lies adjacent to the index finger tendon of the extensor digitorum and blends with it. The extensor digiti minimi lies medial to the other tendons and blends with the little finger tendon of the extensor digitorum (Figure 6.16). The tendons of the muscles insert into the dorsal surface of the fingers via a complex arrangement of fibrous tissue known as the dorsal extensor expansion. This will be described in more detail later in the chapter.

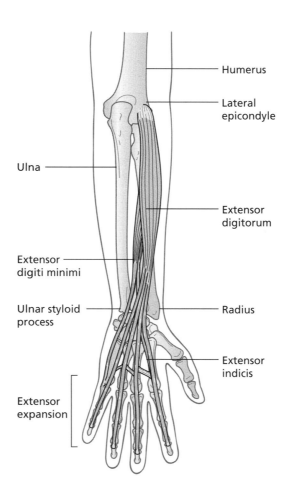

Figure 6.16   Extensors of the fingers in the posterior right forearm.

Reflective task

- Palpate the extensor tendons as they pass over the posterior side of the wrist and on to the back of the hand.
- Observe how the long extensor tendons can be seen on the back of the hand when it is opened. Notice how the tendons are close together at the level of the wrist. The tendons of the index, ring and little fingers diverge away from the central axis of the hand to reach the fingers. The pull of the extensor tendons, therefore, abducts as well as extends these three fingers.

Three forearm muscles act in separating the thumb when opening the hand: the abductor pollicis longus, the extensor pollicis longus and the extensor pollicis brevis.

The three muscles originate from the posterior shaft of the radius and ulna as follows: the **abductor pollicis longus** from the upper shaft of the radius and ulna; the **extensor pollicis longus** from the shaft of the ulna below; and the **extensor pollicis brevis** from the shaft of the radius below.

All three muscles pass deep to the extensor digitorum and become superficial on the radial side of the wrist to reach the thumb (Figure 6.17). At the base of the thumb they form the borders of the 'anatomical snuffbox'. These long muscles of the thumb are called the deep outcropping muscles of the forearm, since they begin deep in the posterior forearm and emerge near to the surface on the radial side of the wrist. Each muscle inserts into a different bone in the thumb: the abductor pollicis longus inserts into the first metacarpal, the extensor pollicis brevis into the proximal phalanx; and the extensor pollicis longus into the distal phalanx.

Reflective task

Observe the 'anatomical snuffbox' by extending the thumb with the wrist extended. A depression appears bounded by tendons below the thumb. Palpate the abductor pollicis longus and extensor pollicis brevis lying together in the same boundary of the 'snuffbox'. The other dorsal boundary is formed by the tendon of the extensor pollicis longus, which uses the dorsal tubercle of the radius to change direction at the wrist.

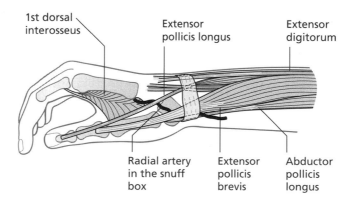

Figure 6.17   The 'anatomical snuffbox'; radial side of the right wrist and hand.

Muscles of the hand

Two intrinsic muscles of the hand assist the forearm muscles in opening the hand, acting on the thumb and the little finger. The abductor pollicis brevis lies in the thenar eminence, and the abductor digiti minimi lies in the hypothenar eminence. Both of these muscles originate at the flexor retinaculum at the palmar side of the base of the hand (see Figure 6.12).

The **abductor pollicis brevis** is inserted into the base of the proximal phalanx of the thumb on the lateral side (see Figure 6.12a). Note that the thumb faces inwards at right angles to the palm, so that when the abductor pollicis brevis contracts, it draws the thumb away from the palm (see Figure 6.10a). From this fully abducted position, the opponens pollicis can pull on the shaft of the first metacarpal, so turning the pad of the thumb to face the pads of the fingers, forming a precision grip.

The **abductor digiti minimi** originates from the flexor retinaculum and pisiform bone, and inserts into the base of the proximal phalanx of the little finger on the medial side (see Figure 6.12a).

The action of opening the hand is important in releasing a grip and in placing an object on a surface. A young baby can grasp a toy in the hand, but drops it randomly. At a later stage, when co-ordination between opposing groups of muscles has developed, the child can then put the toy down precisely as the hand opens.

Precision movements of the fingers and thumb

The fingers and thumb perform a variety of skilled movements. Alternate action of flexors and extensors at all the joints of the fingers is required to press the keys of a keyboard. When the fingers and thumb grip a pen or paintbrush, fine movements of the distal joints manipulate the pen or brush over the paper. Dressing skills, especially doing up buttons, demand precision movements of the hand. Many work skills, for example assembling electronic equipment, also require accurate movements of the fingers and the thumb.

The nervous system co-ordinates precision movements in the two hands together. The hand is represented by large areas in both the somatosensory and the primary motor cortex of the brain. The ability to perform highly skilled co-ordinated movements in both hands is seen in playing many musical instruments (Figure 6.18).

Three sets of intrinsic muscles deep in the palm of the hand are important in precision movements: the lumbricals, the dorsal interossei and the palmar interossei (Figures 6.19, 6.20).

The **lumbricals** are four small muscles that originate from the tendons of flexor digitorum profundus, the deepest long finger flexor in the palm (Figure 6.19). Each muscles passes in front of the MCP joint of the corresponding finger, passes backwards on the radial side of this joint, and inserts into the dorsal surface of the finger on the radial side. The detail of the insertion will be considered later with the description of the dorsal extensor expansion of the fingers.

The actions of the lumbricals are flexion of the MCP joints and extension of the IP joints. They link the long flexor tendons in the palm to the long extensor insertion on the dorsal side of the fingers. In this way, they act as a bridge between the two, which balances the flexion and extension movements of the fingers. There is evidence that the lumbricals are active in all fine movements of the fingers.

The **interosseous muscles** lie in the spaces between the metacarpal bones. There are two layers of interosseous muscles (Figure 6.20). The dorsal layer is the most superficial on the back of the hand. The palmar layer lies between the dorsal layer and the lumbricals.

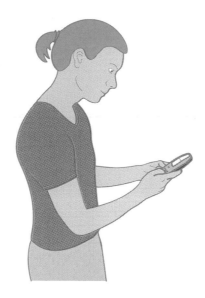

Figure 6.18   Bilateral manipulative movements.

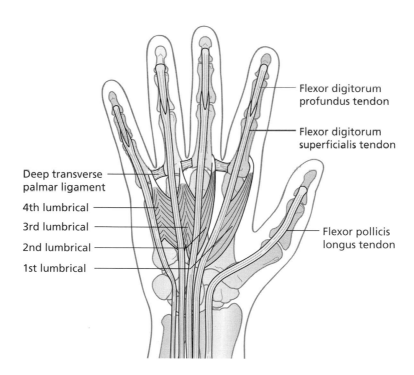

Figure 6.19   Lumbrical muscles; position in a palmar view of the right hand.

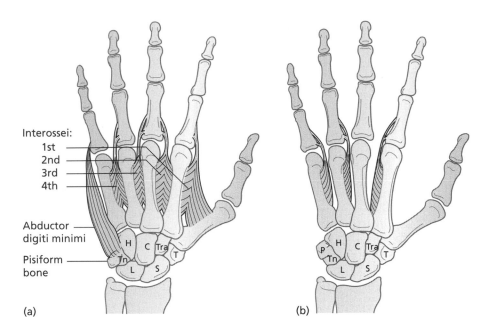

Interossei:
1st
2nd
3rd
4th

Abductor
digiti minimi

Pisiform
bone

(a)   (b)

Figure 6.20   Interosseous muscles in a palmar view of the right hand: (a) dorsal interossei and abductor digiti minimi; (b) palmar interossei.

The four **dorsal interossei** originate from the sides of adjacent shafts of metacarpals 1–5, deep to the extensor tendons. The position of these muscles is best understood from a diagram (Figure 6.20a). Note that the two lateral (thumb side) dorsal interossei pass on the radial side of the MCP joints of the index and middle fingers; the medial two muscles pass on the ulnar side of the MCP joints of the middle and ring fingers. The tendons of all four muscles reach the dorsal surface of the fingers to blend with the outer bands of the extensor hood of the index, middle and ring fingers, just beyond the level of the MCP joints (Figure 6.21a).

Action of all four dorsal interossei will spread the fingers away from the central axis of the hand. The middle finger has two dorsal intersseous muscles, and therefore can abduct from the central axis to either side. The attachment of each tendon into the dorsal surface of the finger means that each muscle will also assist in extension of the DIP joints.

The dorsal interossei can be palpated between the shafts of the metacarpal. When these muscles are wasted, owing to nerve damage, the skin sinks between the metacarpals and the back of the hand looks like a skeleton.

The three **palmar interossei** lie on the palmar side of the dorsal interossei. The position of these muscles can be seen in Figure 6.20b. Each is attached to one side of a metacarpal shaft, and is inserted into the outer band of the dorsal expansion of the same finger. From their attachments it can be seen how they will draw the fingers together in adduction when they contract.

One way to remember the actions of the two sets of interossei is by the initials: Dorsal ABduct (DAB); Palmar ADduct (PAD).

Both the dorsal and the palmar interossei co-operate with the lumbricals in flexion of the MCP joint and extension of the IP joints.

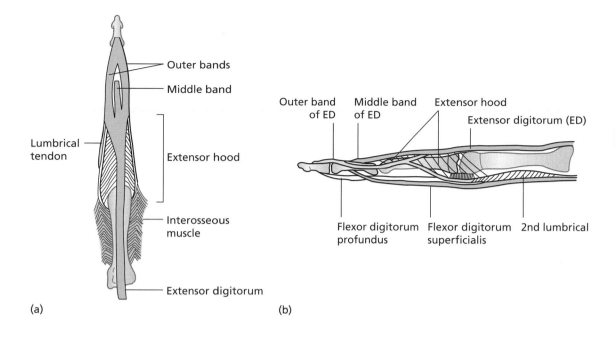

Figure 6.21   Dorsal digital expansion and extensor hood of the right middle finger: (a) dorsal view; and (b) side view (second dorsal interosseous removed).

Practice note-pad 6D: rheumatoid hand

The fingers of the hand may be seen to be angled towards the ulnar side at the MCP joints. This ulnar drift deformity is due to subluxation of the proximal phalanx within the MCP joint capsule, particularly the index and middle fingers. The MCP joints are swollen and painful. It is important to maintain the strength of the first dorsal interosseous muscle to keep the fingers in alignment.

Dorsal (extensor) digital expansion of the fingers

The insertion of muscles on to the dorsal surface of the fingers is a complex system of fibrous bands known as the dorsal digital expansion or extensor hood. The extensor digitorum, the lumbricals and the interossei are inserted into it.

The tendon of extensor digitorum divides into three as it crosses the MCP joint. The middle band is inserted into the base of the middle phalanx, and the outer bands are inserted into the base of the distal phalanx (Figure 6.21a). The outer bands receive the insertions of the lumbricals and the interossei. Fine transverse fibres spread out from the middle band to form a movable extensor hood over the proximal phalanx and the head of the metacarpal (Figure 6.21a, b). The base of the hood extends to be attached to the deep transverse palmar ligament. This extensor hood prevents any bowstring of the extensor tendon.

Each lumbrical lies on the palmar side of the metacarpal at first, and then crosses the MCP joint to insert into the outer band of the dorsal expansion on the radial side. In this way the lumbricals can flex the MCP joint and extend the IP joints of each finger.

The interossei lie in parallel with the metacarpals and are held down by the extensor hood at the MCP joint. The interossei pull on the outer band of the dorsal expansion to produce abduction and adduction of the fingers. The attachment of the interossei to the dorsal digital expansion means that they also assist the lumbricals in flexion of the MCP joints and extension of the IP joints.

The functional significance of the dorsal digital expansion is to allow the complex movements of the fingers to occur. Activities such as writing involve simultaneous flexion of some joints and extension of others. A balance between flexor and extensor muscle activity is required to produce this. All the precision movements of the hand result from a variety of combinations of movements at the joints of the fingers and the thumb.

Reflective task

- Look at the palmar side of a hand skeleton and at your own hand. Work out how the lumbricals begin in the palm with the long flexor tendons, and end on the dorsal side of each finger, passing round the thumb side of the MCP joint.
- Draw a line on the hand for the main axis through the middle finger and work out how the dorsal and palmar interossei are positioned around it.
- Palpate the first dorsal interosseous muscle by abducting the index finger while the thumb is in abduction.

Practice note-pad 6E: finger deformity

Rheumatoid arthritis

- **Swan neck deformity**: hyperextension of the PIP joint and flexion of the DIP joint caused by rupture of the tendon of flexor digitorum profundus and the pull of the lumbricals on the outer bands of the extensor expansion.
- **Trigger finger**: a flexor tendon may become trapped at the entrance to its sheath. The cause may be thickening of the tendon sheath, or the swelling and/or nodules around the tendons. The finger lies in flexion, and it has to be extended passively by the other hand, when it straightens with a snap. The ring and middle fingers are most commonly affected.

Trauma to the finger

- **Mallet finger**: due to injury to the outer bands of the extensor expansion proximal to the DIP joint by a ball travelling at speed which hits the tip of the finger. Active extension of the DIP is absent, but passive movement is normal.
- **Button-hole deformity**: caused by lesion to the middle band of the extensor expansion by a direct cut or burn. The PIP remains flexed by the outer bands of the extensor expansion being drawn forwards until they lie anterior to the fulcrum of the joint and there is no extensor to act upon the joint to extend it.

> **Reflective task**
>
> - Look at the dorsal side of the right middle finger and Figure 6.21a. Locate the position of the dorsal digital expansion and the insertion of extensor digitorum by three bands. A lumbrical is inserted into the outer band on the radial side. A dorsal interosseus muscle is inserted into the outer band on each side.
> - Look at the side view of the right middle finger and Figure 6.21b. Work out where the tendons of the extensor digitorum, flexor digitorum superficialis and flexor digitorum profundus each insert into the finger.

Types of grip

The hand is used in a variety of ways to grasp and hold handles, tools, levers and so on. The different types of grip made by the hand in daily activities involve particular movements at the various joints of the hand, and the combination of activity in muscle groups in the forearm and hand. The ability to grip various objects is an important part of the assessment of the damaged hand.

> **Reflective task**
>
> Observe the different ways that people use their hands to grip objects over a whole day, while dressing, cooking, eating, travelling, working and during leisure.

The type of grip selected depends upon the shape of the object to be grasped, what one wants to do with it and the texture of its surface. Naming all the different types of grip is a difficult task when the hand is used in such a wide variety of ways, and individuals approach each method of grasp according to their own style of working.

There are two main types of grip: power grips and precision grips.

Power grips

In the power grips all of the fingers are flexed round an object (Figure 6.22). The thumb is curled round in the opposite direction to press against, or meet the fingers around the object. All of the muscles that close the hand are active. Both the thenar and hypothenar muscles keep the hand in contact with the object grasped.

The hypothenar muscles are important to stabilise the medial side of the palm against a handle, and the muscles of the fingers and the thumb grip the object firmly. The wrist extensors are active to give a stable base for the gripping action; they increase the tension in the long finger flexors and prevent them from acting on the wrist as well. As the hand grips harder, the wrist extensors increase their activity.

The power grips bring the maximum area of sensory surface of the fingers, thumb and palm into contact with the object being grasped, so that feedback from the receptors of the hand ensures that exact pressure and control are being exerted on the handle or tool.

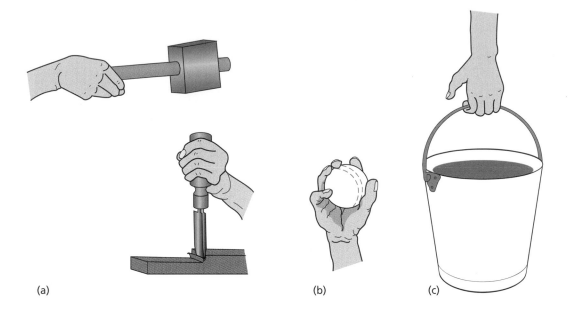

Figure 6.22   Power grips: (a) cylinder; (b) ball; (c) hook.

The power grip is the most primitive grasping movement. One of the primary reflexes of the newborn baby is finger flexion in response to touching the palm. By 6 months, the whole hand can form a palmar grasp with the thumb in opposition. Exertion of power by the finger flexors requires the additional group action of the wrist extensors and elbow stability, which does not develop until later. By the fifth year the child can grip strongly with each hand individually.

The unique feature of the power grip is to hold an object firmly so that it can be moved by the more proximal joints of the upper limb, such as the shoulder, elbow or radioulnar joints. For example the hand grasps a door handle, but it is the elbow and shoulder muscles that press it down, and the muscles acting on the radioulnar joints that turn the knob. The hand moulds itself to the shape of the object grasped in the power grip before the power is exerted to move it.

The **cylinder grip** is used for handles that lie at right angles to the forearm, such as a racket, a jug handle or the handbrake of a car. The skin of the palmar surface of the fingers and the palm curves round the handle, and the thumb lies in opposition over the fingertips.

Where a tool or object, such as a hammer, screwdriver or trowel, is being used in line with the forearm the fingers flex around the handle in a graded way with maximum degrees of flexion in the little finger and least in the index finger. The thumb lies either over the fingertips or along the handle of the tool being grasped. The wrist is ulnar deviated and the maximum area of skin of the palm, thenar and hypothenar eminences is in contact with the handle of the tool. This is a grip giving considerable control, together with powerful manipulation of the tool (Figure 6.22a).

The **ball grip** encompasses circular knobs, balls and the top of mugs or jam jars (Figure 6.22b). The fingers and thumb adduct on to the object and sometimes the palm of the hand is not involved.

The **hook grip** is used for carrying a suitcase, bucket or shopping bag by the side of the body with a straight elbow and wrist. Only the flexed fingers are used in this grip, the thumb is not involved (Figure 6.22c). Following a median nerve lesion (see Chapter 7) the thumb cannot be opposed and the hook grip is the only power grip possible.

Precision grips

The hand in the precision grip holds an object between the tips of the thumb and one, two or three fingers, e.g. holding a pencil or small tool. The intrinsic muscles of the hand are now involved, in co-operation with the long flexors and extensors of the digits. The hand is positioned by the wrist and forearm, and the gripping is performed by the muscles acting on the joints of the fingers and thumb.

The precision grip is a more advanced manipulative movement than the power grip, appearing around 9 months of age in child development. Coordination of the flexor/extensor mechanism of the fingers is essential for grasping a small object and moving it precisely.

The digits have serially arranged joints to perform these manipulative movements. The thumb has three joints: the first carpometacarpal (CMC) joint, the MCP joint and the interphalangeal (IP) joint. Each finger also has three joints: the MCP joint, the PIP joint and the DIP joint. It is the variety of movements at all these joints that combines to execute the different precision grips. The lumbrical and interosseus muscles form the balancing forces between the long finger flexors and extensors, and the intrinsic muscles of the thumb bring the pad of the thumb into opposition.

- The **plate grip**: the MCP joints of the fingers are flexed with the IP joints extended; the thumb is opposed across the palmar surface of the fingers. The grip is used when holding a plate or another object that needs to be kept horizontal (Figure 6.23a). An alternative name is the lumbrical grip.
- The **pinch grip**: the MCP and PIP joints of the index finger are flexed and the finger meets the opposed thumb. The DIP is pushed into extension in the finger and thumb. The pinch grip may include the middle finger. The grip is used to hold and manipulate small tools, for example a sewing needle (Figure 6.23b) or a small screwdriver. This is also known as the pad-to-pad grip.
- The **key grip**: the extended thumb is held on the radial side of the index finger (Figure 6.23c). This is also known as the lateral grip.
- The **pincer grip**: all the joints of the index finger are flexed and the fingertip is brought into contact with the tip of the abducted thumb (Figure 6.23d). The grip is used to pick up small items, for example beads or pins. This is also called the tip-to-tip grip.

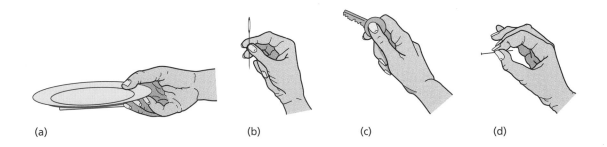

(a)   (b)   (c)   (d)

Figure 6.23   Precision grips: (a) plate; (b) pinch; (c) key; (d) pincer.

Summary of muscles of the forearm and intrinsic muscles of the hand

The muscles of the forearm and hand have been described in three functional groups. For revision purposes, the muscles will now be grouped in their anatomical position with notes on common points of origin to assist the learning of the attachments of the individual muscles.

Muscles of the forearm

Anterior

- Superficial layer: pronator teres, flexor carpi radialis, palmaris longus, flexor carpi ulnaris (common flexor origin is the medial epicondyle of the humerus).
- Middle layer: flexor digitorum superficialis.
- Deep layer: flexor digitorum profundus, flexor pollicis longus, pronator quadratus.

Posterior

- Superficial layer: brachioradialis, extensor carpi radialis longus and brevis, extensor digitorum, extensor digiti minimi, extensor carpi ulnaris, anconeus (common extensor origin is the lateral side of the elbow).
- Deep layer: supinator, abductor pollicis longus, extensor pollicis longus and brevis, extensor indicis (origins from the posterior surface of the radius and ulna).

The 12 posterior muscles can be divided into the following:

- three act on elbow and radioulnar joints: brachioradialis, supinator and anconeus;
- three act to extend the wrist: extensor carpi ulnaris, extensor carpi radialis longus and brevis;
- three act to extend the fingers: extensor digitorum, extensor indicis and extensor digiti minimi;
- three act on the thumb: extensor pollicis longus and brevis, abductor pollicis longus.

Intrinsic muscles of the hand

Palmar

- Thenar muscles: flexor pollicis brevis, abductor pollicis brevis and opponens pollicis (some include adductor pollicis).
- Hypothenar muscles: flexor digiti minimi, abductor digiti minimi and opponens digiti minimi.

The six thenar and hypothenar muscles all originate on the flexor retinaculum at the base of the hand. The three thenar muscles are the mirror image of the three hypothenar muscles. The opponens muscles of the two eminences are deep as they are inserted into the metacarpal shafts.

Deep muscles of the palm

Lumbricals, palmar interossei, dorsal interossei, adductor pollicis.

Summary

- The forearm, wrist and hand form an interdependent system for the performance of manipulative movements. The forearm orientates the hand to a functional position.
- In the anatomical position the radius and ulna are parallel; the forearm is supinated.
- The movement of pronation carries the lower end of the radius over the ulna so that the bones are crossed, with the radius lying anterior to the ulna. The hand moves with the radius so that the palm now faces backwards or downwards.
- The return movement is supination, which turns the hand forwards or upwards. These movements occur at the superior and inferior radioulnar joints in the forearm.
- The main functional position of the hand is midprone, when the hand faces medially.
- The movements of pronation and supination allow the hand to hold objects and tools at any angle in their use, and to place the hand accurately on surfaces in the environment.
- The wrist joint forms the articulation between the hand and the forearm.
- Active movements at the wrist are flexion, extension, abduction and adduction. The range of these movements is extended by the midcarpal joint between the proximal and distal row of carpals in the hand.
- The main function of the wrist is to stabilise the position of the forearm and hand during manipulative movements, particularly counteracting the effect of gravity pulling the hand into flexion or ulnar deviation.
- The functions of the hand are the performance of manipulative movements, grasping and releasing objects; sensing objects in reaching space for their recognition and use; communication and the expression of emotion.
- Movements of the fingers occur at the metacarpophalangeal and interphalangeal joints. The thumb moves principally at the carpometacarpal joint (saddle type), where the movement of opposition brings the thumb into contact with each of the fingers.
- The muscles that close the hand in gripping movements lie in the anterior compartment of the forearm and the palm of the hand. The opposing groups of muscle, lying in the posterior compartment of the forearm and the palm of the hand, open the hand in releasing movements.
- Precision movements of the fingers and thumb are performed by the deep (intrinsic) muscles of the palm of the hand.
- Gripping activities performed by the hand are divided into power grips, when all the fingers are flexed around objects; and precision grips, when an object is held between the tips of the thumb and one, two or three fingers. The two main types of grip are further divided into types that relate to the shape of the surface grasped and the relative positions of the fingers and thumb.

7

Nerve supply of the upper limb

Key terms

structure and location of the brachial plexus, branches in the upper limb, muscles supplied by the branches of the brachial plexus

Conceptual overview

This chapter outlines the significance and location of the brachial plexus and the branches that pass into the upper limb. The terminal branches are named and muscle groups innervated by those branches are identified. Movements associated with those mucscle groups are discussed in activities of daily living. The functional effects of nerve damage are also highlighted.

Tyldesley & Grieve's Muscles, Nerves and Movement in Human Occupation, Fourth Edition. Ian R. McMillan, Gail Carin-Levy.
© 2012 Ian R. McMillan, Gail Carin-Levy, Barbara Tyldesley and June I. Grieve. Published 2012 by Blackwell Publishing Ltd.

Introduction

Upper limb function depends on five roots of origin of spinal nerves in the neck. These spinal roots branch and join in a complex manner forming the brachial plexus, which passes over the first rib and under the clavicle to reach the axilla. There, five nerves emerge and pass down the limb to supply all of the structures in the arm, forearm and hand. Traction injuries to the upper limb can tear the roots from the spinal cord. If all of the roots are involved, upper limb function is lost. The brachial plexus is also vulnerable to pressure in the axilla.

The brachial plexus

The position and plan of the brachial plexus are shown in Figures 7.1 and 7.2. The plexus is derived from five spinal segments, C5–C8 and T1. Three trunks are formed by the upper two and the lower two roots joining. These three trunks pass downwards and laterally between two muscles of the neck: the scalenus anterior and medius (see Chapter 10, Figure 10.7). The trunks meet the axillary artery and continue with it behind the clavicle. Each trunk then divides into anterior and posterior divisions to deliver the nerves to the anterior and posterior aspects of the limb, respectively. The six divisions continue through the axilla where they combine to form three cords lying behind the pectoralis minor muscle (see Chapter 5, Figure 5.6) and surrounding the axillary artery. The posterior divisions form the posterior cord, and the anterior divisions form the medial and lateral cords.

The posterior cord terminates in the posterior extensor nerve of the upper limb. The medial and lateral cords terminate in the flexor nerves of the upper limb. At the lower part of the axilla, the three cords split into the five terminal branches which enter the arm (Figure 7.2).

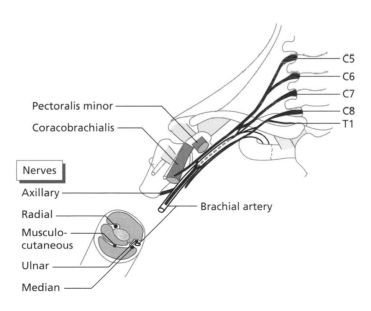

Figure 7.1   Position of the brachial plexus.

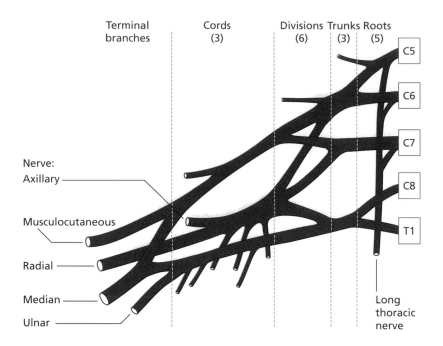

Figure 7.2   Plan of the brachial plexus showing the origin of the terminal branches.

Reflective task

Look at the articulated skeleton to identify the exact position of the brachial plexus, starting at the cervical vertebrae, passing over the first rib under the clavicle, to the axillary region below the shoulder joint.

Practice note-pad 7A: brachial plexus lesions

The brachial plexus may be damaged in a variety of ways:

(1)   at birth;
(2)   by traction injuries to the neck;
(3)   by traction on the outstretched hand;
(4)   through compression in the axilla, for example in 'Saturday night palsy', when a person goes to sleep in an armchair with one arm hanging over the edge of the chair.

The resulting loss of function is variable. The upper roots C5 and C6 may be damaged with resultant loss of function in the abductors and flexors of the shoulder, and flexors and extensors of the elbow. The arm cannot be lifted from the side, and hangs in a position of adduction, medial rotation, pronation and finger flexion: this is known as Erb's paralysis or the 'waiter's tip' position.

Damage to the lower roots (C7, C8 and T1) produces weakness of the intrinsic muscles of the hand, especially on the medial side, which is the ulnar or 'power' side. This is known as Klumpke's paralysis.

Terminal branches of the brachial plexus

There are five terminal branches of the brachial plexus. The movements that are activated by each of the five nerves can be summarised as follows:

- **axillary nerve**: shoulder movement;
- **radial nerve**: extension of the elbow, wrist, fingers and thumb;
- **musculocutaneous nerve**: flexion of the elbow;
- **median nerve**: flexion of the wrist and fingers, opposition of the thumb;
- **ulnar nerve**: fine manipulative movements of the fingers.

The five nerves enter the arm. The axillary nerve terminates at the shoulder. The other four nerves continue through the arm and on to the forearm, where the radial and the median nerves divide into two. The muscular branches of the musculocutaneous nerve terminate at the elbow, and those of the radial nerve end at the wrist. The median, ulnar and radial nerves (cutaneous branch only) enter the hand.

Look at Figure 7.2 to see how the radial nerve originates from all the roots of the plexus, and the ulnar nerve from the lower roots (C8 and T1).

Axillary nerve: shoulder movement

The **axillary nerve** nerve is important in all movements that lift the arm away from the side of the body, since it supplies the deltoid muscle and teres minor (Figure 7.3). From the posterior cord, the axillary nerve branches backwards under the capsule of the shoulder joint, and winds round the surgical neck of the humerus to supply the whole of the deltoid muscle. A branch to the teres minor continues as a cutaneous nerve supplying the skin over the deltoid muscle.

The other muscles moving the shoulder (except for the trapezius) are supplied by direct branches of the plexus in the neck.

Practice note-pad 7B: axillary nerve lesion

Fracture of the neck of the humerus or subluxation of the shoulder joint may damage the axillary nerve. The resulting loss of function is the inability to abduct the arm away from the body.

Radial nerve: posterior extensor nerve

The radial nerve is the largest branch of the brachial plexus, formed as the continuation of the posterior cord (Figure 7.3). In the arm, the radial nerve supplies the whole of the triceps muscle. The nerve is essential for extension movement of the elbow, since the triceps is the only muscle capable of this movement with any power (see Chapter 5).

In front of the lateral epicondyle of the humerus at the elbow, the nerve divides into two.

- The **superficial terminal branch** continues along the lateral side of the forearm under the brachioradialis. Just above the wrist, the nerve pierces the deep fascia to supply a variable area of skin over the dorsal surface of the hand on the thumb side (Figure 7.4).

166

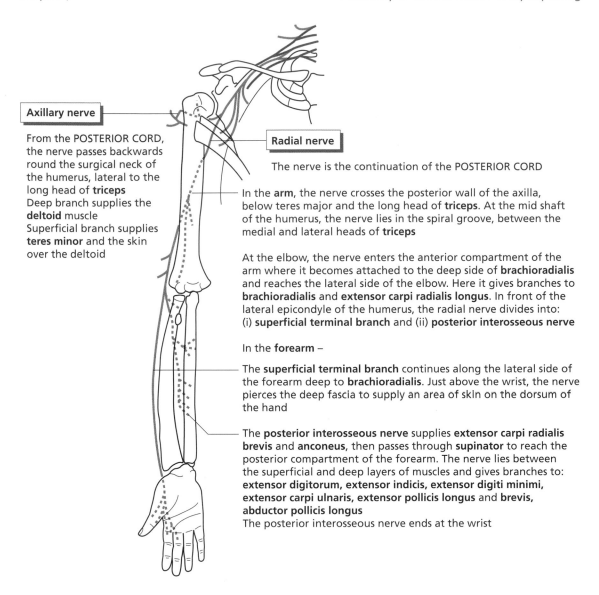

Axillary nerve

From the POSTERIOR CORD, the nerve passes backwards round the surgical neck of the humerus, lateral to the long head of **triceps**
Deep branch supplies the **deltoid** muscle
Superficial branch supplies **teres minor** and the skin over the deltoid

Radial nerve

The nerve is the continuation of the POSTERIOR CORD

In the **arm**, the nerve crosses the posterior wall of the axilla, below teres major and the long head of **triceps**. At the mid shaft of the humerus, the nerve lies in the spiral groove, between the medial and lateral heads of **triceps**

At the elbow, the nerve enters the anterior compartment of the arm where it becomes attached to the deep side of **brachioradialis** and reaches the lateral side of the elbow. Here it gives branches to **brachioradialis** and **extensor carpi radialis longus**. In front of the lateral epicondyle of the humerus, the radial nerve divides into:
(i) **superficial terminal branch** and (ii) **posterior interosseous nerve**

In the **forearm** –

The **superficial terminal branch** continues along the lateral side of the forearm deep to **brachioradialis**. Just above the wrist, the nerve pierces the deep fascia to supply an area of skin on the dorsum of the hand

The **posterior interosseous nerve** supplies **extensor carpi radialis brevis** and **anconeus**, then passes through **supinator** to reach the posterior compartment of the forearm. The nerve lies between the superficial and deep layers of muscles and gives branches to: **extensor digitorum, extensor indicis, extensor digiti minimi, extensor carpi ulnaris, extensor pollicis longus** and **brevis, abductor pollicis longus**
The posterior interosseous nerve ends at the wrist

Figure 7.3   Axillary nerve and radial nerve: course and distribution, right anterior view.

- The **posterior interosseous nerve** supplies the extensor muscles in the forearm, ending at the wrist, where it supplies all of the joints of the wrist.

   The radial nerve as a whole supplies all of the extensor muscles of the arm and forearm. The nerve has no motor role in hand function. Extension movements of the elbow are important for reaching above the head. Extension of the wrist is important in maintaining the functional position of the hand (Figure 7.5a) for all movements of the fingers and thumb.

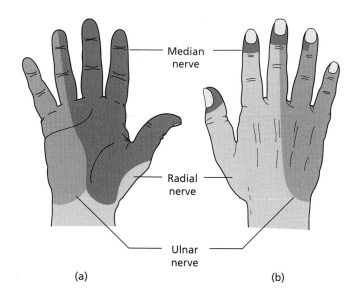

Figure 7.4   Areas of skin supplied by the radial, median and ulnar nerves: (a) palmar; (b) dorsal.

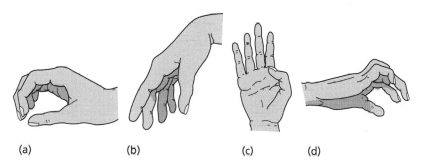

Figure 7.5   Positions of the right hand: (a) functional position of the normal hand; and after damage to (b) the radial nerve – 'wrist drop'; (c) the median nerve – 'ape hand'; (d) the ulnar nerve – 'claw hand'.

Practice note-pad 7C: radial nerve lesion

Injuries to the radial nerve most commonly occur as a complication of the fracture of the **midshaft of the humerus,** where the radial nerve lies in the radial groove (Figure 7.3). This injury results in 'wrist drop' (Figure 7.5b), the hand cannot be lifted against gravity and the power grip is weak. The resulting weakness leads to an inability to reach up to a high shelf or to push against resistance, e.g. a door.

Injury at the **elbow,** which may occur as a complication of supracondylar fracture of the humerus, causes weak extension of the fingers and the thumb, particularly at the MCP joints.

Injury at the **wrist,** due to laceration or burns, only results in a small area of sensory loss on the dorsum of the hand over the first dorsal interosseus muscle.

> **Reflective task**
>
> Watch the hand and forearm of people doing activities such as making a cup of tea and eat-ing with a knife and fork. Note the position of the wrist during the movements. If the wrist could not be held in extension, the hand would drop under its own weight and the weight of any object held in it.

168

Musculocutaneous and median nerves: anterior flexor nerves

There are two terminal branches of the lateral cord of the brachial plexus that are important for flexion movements of the upper limb. The musculocutaneous nerve supplies the elbow flexors; and the median nerve supplies the wrist, fingers and thumb flexors, working in co-operation with the ulnar nerve.

The **musculocutaneous nerve** pierces the coracobrachialis, and then passes down the arm between the biceps and brachialis. The nerve supplies these three muscles, which can be remembered by the initials BBC. At the elbow, the nerve becomes cutaneous at the lateral side of the tendon of biceps, to become the nerve to the skin on the lateral side of the forearm (Figure 7.6).

The **median nerve** is formed from the lateral and medial cords of the brachial plexus. The course and distribution of the median nerve can be seen in Figure 7.7. There are no branches of the median nerve in the arm, it is a nerve of the the forearm and hand only. A communicating branch with the musculocutaneous nerve in the arm is present in some individuals. At the elbow, the median nerve lies anteriorly and medial to the tendon of biceps.

In the forearm, branches are given off to four flexor muscles of the wrist and fingers. A deep branch, the **anterior interosseus nerve**, lies on the interosseous membrane between the radius and ulna, and supplies the two deep flexor muscles of the fingers and thumb, and the pronator quadratus lying above the wrist. Note that the median nerve supplies all of the flexors in the forearm except for the flexor carpi ulnaris and the medial half of the flexor digitorum profundus (to the ring and little finger).

In the **hand**, the median nerve passes underneath the flexor retinaculum and through the carpal tunnel, lying on top of the tendons of long finger flexors. In the hand the median nerve supplies the three thenar muscles and first two lumbricals, and the skin over the palmar surface of the thumb, index and middle fingers, continuing over the fingertips to the dorsal side (Figure 7.4a, b).

The median nerve is essential for hand function. In gripping movements, the median nerve supplies the muscles that flex the fingers round an object or handle, and also the thenar muscles which bring the thumb into opposition to the fingers. Gripping also relies on tactile sensation in the skin of the palm of the hand, which is supplied by the median nerve on the side of the thumb, index and middle fingers.

The ulnar nerve: fine movements of the fingers

The **ulnar nerve** is a continuation of the medial cord of the brachial plexus. Figure 7.8 shows the course and distribution of the ulnar nerve. There are no branches of the ulnar nerve in the arm.

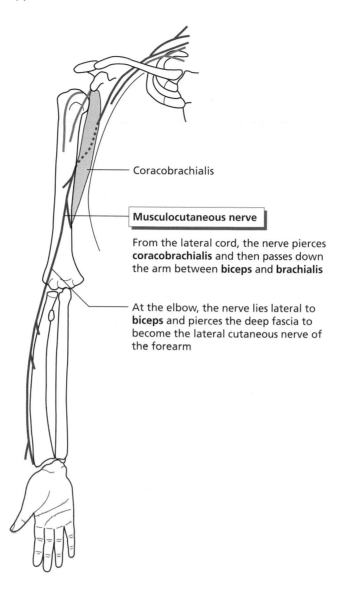

Coracobrachialis

Musculocutaneous nerve

From the lateral cord, the nerve pierces
coracobrachialis and then passes down
the arm between **biceps** and **brachialis**

At the elbow, the nerve lies lateral to
biceps and pierces the deep fascia to
become the lateral cutaneous nerve of
the forearm

Figure 7.6   Musculocutaneous nerve: course and distribution, right anterior view.

Reflective task

- Pull your thumb back and to the side of the palm of your dominant hand by winding a bandage round the wrist and round the thumb. Now try to use your hand in everyday activities to experience the problems when the thumb cannot be opposed to the fingers.
- Wear a thin plastic glove with the ring and little fingers cut away on your dominant hand during hand activities. You will then experience the effects of loss of skin sensation in median nerve injury.

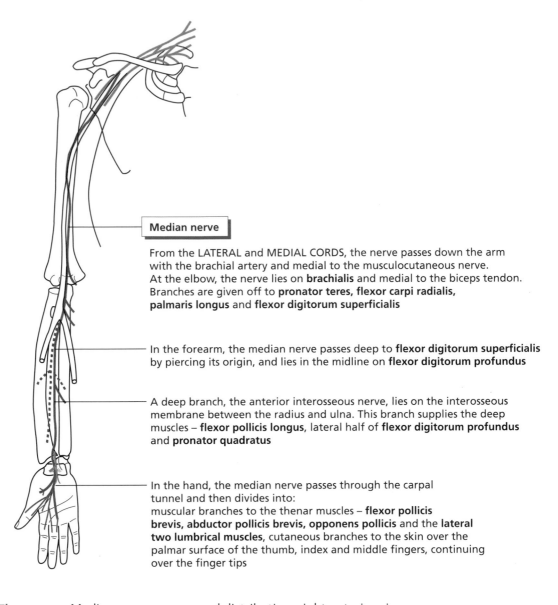

Median nerve

From the LATERAL and MEDIAL CORDS, the nerve passes down the arm
with the brachial artery and medial to the musculocutaneous nerve.
At the elbow, the nerve lies on **brachialis** and medial to the biceps tendon.
Branches are given off to **pronator teres, flexor carpi radialis,
palmaris longus** and **flexor digitorum superficialis**

In the forearm, the median nerve passes deep to **flexor digitorum superficialis**
by piercing its origin, and lies in the midline on **flexor digitorum profundus**

A deep branch, the anterior interosseous nerve, lies on the interosseous
membrane between the radius and ulna. This branch supplies the deep
muscles – **flexor pollicis longus**, lateral half of **flexor digitorum profundus**
and **pronator quadratus**

In the hand, the median nerve passes through the carpal
tunnel and then divides into:
muscular branches to the thenar muscles – **flexor pollicis
brevis, abductor pollicis brevis, opponens pollicis** and the **lateral
two lumbrical muscles**, cutaneous branches to the skin over the
palmar surface of the thumb, index and middle fingers, continuing
over the finger tips

Figure 7.7   Median nerve: course and distribution, right anterior view.

The course of the nerve in the forearm and hand is apparent when the inside of the elbow is
bumped. Banging the funny bone gives a tingling sensation down the inside of the forearm and
on to the little finger.

In the forearm, the ulnar nerve supplies the flexor carpi ulnaris and the medial half of the flexor
digitorum profundus. These are the anterior muscles of the forearm that are not supplied by the
median nerve.

At the wrist, the nerve lies medially and passes over the flexor retinaculum. Two cutaneous
nerves are given off at, or above, the wrist to supply the skin over the palmar and dorsal sides of
the medial hand, and the ring and little fingers (Figure 7.4).

Practice note-pad 7D: median nerve lesion

The appearance of the hand in median nerve lesions is often called ape or monkey hand (Figure 7.5c). The thenar eminence is wasted and the thumb is drawn backwards in line with the fingers, due to unopposed action of extensor pollicis longus. The loss of function of the lateral two lumbricals leads to flattening of the lateral side of the palm. The MCP joints are drawn into extension and the IP joints into slight flexion.

The most usual site of damage is at the **wrist**. Then the thumb is unable to oppose, and this, together with the loss of sensation from the fingertips makes many gripping movements difficult.

If the nerve is damaged at the **elbow**, there is added loss of finger flexion, particularly the index and middle fingers, which also affects gripping. It is the precision grips that are most affected by median nerve damage.

In **carpal tunnel syndrome**, the median nerve is compressed in the carpal tunnel at the wrist by increase in pressure from the swelling of flexor tendon sheaths or carpal joints. It can be very painful, and the loss of sensation and muscle weakness lead to clumsiness and dropping objects.

In the hand, the terminal branches supply all of the intrinsic muscles not supplied by the median nerve. All of the interossei (palmar and dorsal) are innervated by the ulnar nerve, the medial two lumbricals, the muscles of the little finger and the adductor pollicis lying deep in the palm. It is the movements and sensation of the medial side of the hand that depend on the ulnar nerve.

The ulnar nerve is important for keyboard operators, musicians and all those who need fine co-ordinated movements of the fingers. The power grips are dependent on the ulnar nerve to stabilise the medial side of the hand around the handle of a tool. In grasping large objects, the fingers depend on the ulnar nerve for abduction of the fingers by the interossei to spread the hand over the object before closing on it.

The ulnar and the median nerves co-operate in hand function for movements of the fingers and the thumb, and for sensory feedback from the skin of the palm.

Practice note-pad 7E: ulnar nerve lesion

The ulnar nerve is most frequently damaged when the hand is put through glass, as when falling through a window. The ulnar nerve is in a vulnerable position when the hand is out-strechted to 'break a fall'. The appearance of the hand in ulnar nerve lesions is known as 'claw hand' (Figure 7.5d). The ring and little fingers curl in a flexion deformity, with hyper-extension at the MCP joints, owing to paralysis of the medial two lumbricals. Loss of the dorsal interossei means the fingers cannot be separated. The web between the thumb and index finger, formed by the adductor pollicis and the first dorsal interosseous muscle, is wasted.

The ulnar and median nerves may be damaged together in severe laceration of the wrist. The result is impairment of total hand function, with loss of all grips.

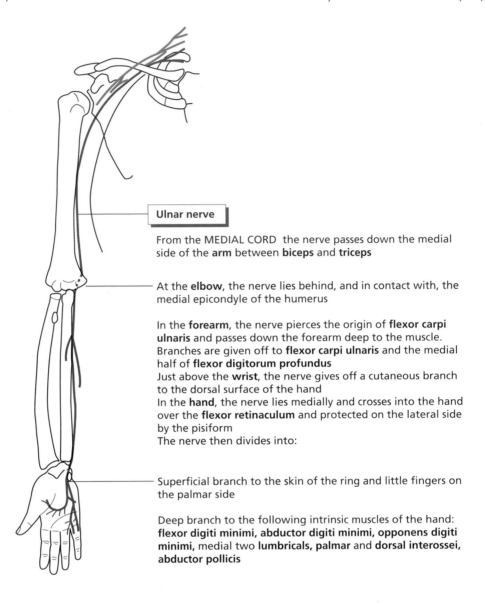

Ulnar nerve

From the MEDIAL CORD the nerve passes down the medial side of the **arm** between **biceps** and **triceps**

At the **elbow**, the nerve lies behind, and in contact with, the medial epicondyle of the humerus

In the **forearm**, the nerve pierces the origin of **flexor carpi ulnaris** and passes down the forearm deep to the muscle. Branches are given off to **flexor carpi ulnaris** and the medial half of **flexor digitorum profundus**
Just above the **wrist**, the nerve gives off a cutaneous branch to the dorsal surface of the hand
In the **hand**, the nerve lies medially and crosses into the hand over the **flexor retinaculum** and protected on the lateral side by the pisiform
The nerve then divides into:

Superficial branch to the skin of the ring and little fingers on the palmar side

Deep branch to the following intrinsic muscles of the hand: **flexor digiti minimi, abductor digiti minimi, opponens digiti minimi**, medial two **lumbricals, palmar** and **dorsal interossei, abductor pollicis**

Figure 7.8   Ulnar nerve: course and distribution, right anterior view.

Outline of the direct branches from the brachial plexus

The five terminal branches of the brachial plexus supply all of the muscles moving the elbow, forearm, wrist and hand. The muscles of the shoulder (excluding the deltoid and teres minor, which are supplied by the axillary nerve) receive direct branches from the plexus.

The **suprascapular nerve** is a branch of the trunk formed by the upper roots (C5 and C6) that supplies the two posterior rotator cuff muscles, the supraspinatus and infraspinatus.

Direct branches from the posterior cord supply the muscles of the posterior wall of the axilla: the subscapularis, the teres major and the latissimus dorsi. A branch from the lateral cord supplies the pectoralis major, which forms the anterior wall of the axilla.

Two branches of the medial cord form separate cutaneous nerves to the skin on the medial side of the arm and forearm. A third branch supplies the pectoralis minor and the lower fibres of the pectoralis major.

The trapezius is the only muscle attached to the scapula that is not supplied by a branch of the brachial plexus. The spinal root of the spinal accessory nerve (cranial nerve XI) branches to the anterior of the trapezius.

Spinal segmental innervation of the upper limb

In the embryo, as the upper limb grows out from the sides of the trunk, the nerve from the central segment C7 grows down towards the end of the limb (Figure 7.9a). The spinal nerves from the upper segments of the plexus, C5 and C6, supply the skin of the lateral border of the limb, the shoulder muscles and the elbow flexors. The lower segments, C8 and T1, supply the medial border of the limb. This means that the dermatomes and myotomes (see Chapter 4) lie in order down the lateral side of the limb, across the hand and up the medial side (Figure 7.9b).

In the prediction of the effects of spinal cord injury it is important to relate the spinal segmental level to the muscles and the areas of skin supplied. Motor and sensory loss occurs below the level

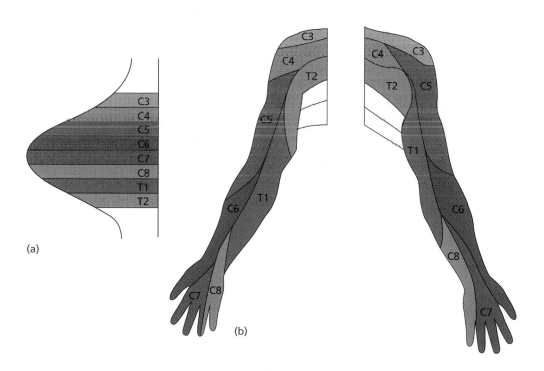

Figure 7.9 Distribution of spinal segments C5 to T1 to the skin of the upper limb: (a) limb bud in the embryo; (b) anterior and posterior views of dermatomes in the adult.

of the lesion in the spinal cord (Practice note-pads 4C and 11A). In general, the nerves supplying the muscles of the shoulder originate from the upper segments (C5 and C6), and those concerned with movements of the fingers are derived from the lower segments (C8 and T1). (See Appendix II, Tables A2.2 and A2.3.)

Summary

- The nerve supply of the whole of the upper limb is derived from five segments (C5–C8 and T1) of the spinal cord in the region of the neck.
- The roots of the spinal nerves emerging from these segments join and branch in a complex manner as they pass over the first rib and under the clavicle, forming the brachial plexus.
- In the axilla, the brachial plexus ends with the formation of five terminal branches: the axillary, radial, musculocutaneous, median and ulnar nerves.
- Direct branches from the plexus supply all of the shoulder muscles, except for the deltoid, teres minor and trapezius.
- The course and distribution of the five upper limb nerves are summarised in Figures 7.3, 7.6, 7.7 and 7.8.
- The main functions of these nerves related to the muscles that they supply are as follows:
  - The axillary nerve is important in all activities where the hand is at head height or above.
  - The radial nerve provides elbow extension, maintains the functional position of the hand by wrist extension, and releases the hand from gripping by extension of the fingers and thumb.
  - The musculocutaneous nerve activates the muscles to bring the hand towards the head and body.
  - The median nerve is active in gripping movements of the fingers and thumb.
  - The ulnar nerve is involved in fine manipulative movements of the fingers, and in the stability of the ulnar side of the hand in power grips.
- The cutaneous supply in the hand protects the hand from injury by hot surfaces.

8

Support and propulsion: the lower limb

Key terms

structure and function of the pelvis, thigh, leg and foot; gait and lower limb muscles

Conceptual overview

This chapter deals with the functions of the lower limb and their role in support and movement. The bones, joints and movements will be examined in detail. The performance of locomotion will be examined in relation to different activities when transferring from one position to another.

Tyldesley & Grieve's Muscles, Nerves and Movement in Human Occupation, Fourth Edition. Ian R. McMillan, Gail Carin-Levy.
© 2012 Ian R. McMillan, Gail Carin-Levy, Barbara Tyldesley and June I. Grieve. Published 2012 by Blackwell Publishing Ltd.

Introduction

The lower limbs are the supporting pillars when we stand. A pillar must have strength and must not collapse under the weight above. The bones, joints and muscles together convert the lower limb into a stable support which is linked to the trunk by the pelvic girdle. The pillar is divided into segments, the thigh, leg and foot. The segments are linked by joints, the hip, knee, ankle and joints of the foot, which can adjust to the changes that occur in the line of weight through the limbs as the head and trunk move above. The muscles around the joints counteract the effects of gravity and any external forces that disturb the balance of the body.

Locomotor movements require the lower limbs to support the weight of the head, arms and trunk above while the body is propelled forwards. The limbs perform repetitive movements of one limb in support while the other limb swings forward. This alternation of swing and support means that each limb as a whole must combine strength with mobility. The pattern of movement must also adapt to walking sideways, up and down slopes and different textures of the ground.

In functional activities, for example getting out of bed and getting up from a chair, the lower limbs are active in transferring the body from one position to another. Weakness of muscles or loss of joint mobility makes these transfer activities difficult and the upper limb then has to compensate (see Chapter 5, Figure 5.14b).

Information from pressure receptors in the skin of the sole of the foot and from the proprioceptors in all the muscles of the lower limb plays an important role in maintaining the balance of the upright body. Feedback from these receptors maintains an economical pattern of locomotion.

In summary, the overall functions of the lower limb are to provide:

- transfer of the body from lying to sitting, to standing;
- support for the head, arms and trunk in all upright positions and movements;
- propulsion in walking, running and climbing stairs;
- sensory information for posture and balance.

Joints and movements of the pelvis, thigh and leg

The pelvis forms the link between the vertebral column and the thigh for the transmission of the body weight downwards from the trunk to the hip and knee joints, and on to the feet. The joints of the thigh and the leg combine to give stability for support of the upright body and adequate range of movement for the limb as a whole.

Movements at the hip allow the thigh to move in the frontal, sagittal and transverse planes. The knee, like the elbow, moves mainly in one plane (sagittal), and allows shortening of the lower limb so that the foot can clear the ground in walking. The ankle is important in placing the foot on different surfaces of the ground for support and then initiating the propulsion of the body forwards.

> **Reflective task**
>
> Stand and move your lower limbs in three planes (sagittal, frontal and transverse). Note the movements at the hip, knee and ankle joints, and contrast the range of each with the corresponding upper limb joints.

The pelvic girdle: position and function

The pelvis or pelvic girdle is an irregular ring of bone composed of the two innominate bones and the sacrum formed by five fused vertebrae. Each innominate bone is made up of the ilium, ischium and pubis, which fuse at the socket for the hip joint. The ilium extends upwards and ends at the iliac crest, which can be felt when placing 'hands on hips'. The ischium lies inferiorly and ends with a roughened ischial tuberosity, which can be felt when sitting upright on a hard seat. The pubis on either side meets in the midline to complete the ring of bone anteriorly. The sacrum articulates superiorly with the fifth lumbar vertebra at the lumbosacral joint.

> **Reflective task**
>
> Look at the illustrations of the pelvis in Appendix I. Use an articulated skeleton to identify: the sacrum of the vertebral column; the two innominate bones that meet in the midline; and the socket (acetabulum) for the head of the femur. Trace how the body weight is transferred from the vertebral column to the femur via the pelvis.

The stability of the pelvis is provided by strong ligaments binding the innominate bone to the sacrum anteriorly and posteriorly. The bony pelvis provides a base for the attachment of muscles of the trunk and the hip. The anterior abdominal muscles end in an aponeurosis which is thickened inferiorly to form the inguinal ligament, extending from the anterior end of the iliac crest to the pubis in the midline. This forms an anatomical space for the passage of nerves and blood vessels from the trunk to the thigh anteriorly.

The bony pelvis, together with the muscles lying across its floor (see Chapter 10), support and protect the reproductive organs, the bladder and the rectum. During childbirth, the pelvis adapts to increase the diameter of the canal for the passage of the head of the baby.

Joints of the pelvis

The **sacroiliac joint** between the sacrum and the ilium of the innominate bone is a joint that is part synovial and part fibrous. The ear-shaped irregular joint surfaces, on the posterior medial part of the ilium and the upper lateral side of the sacrum, fit closely. The joint is bound by anterior and posterior ligaments. The thin joint cavity often becomes fused by fibrous bands with age. The two innominate bones join anteriorly at the **pubic symphysis**, a secondary cartilaginous joint.

Only limited gliding movements are possible at these joints. Mobility has been sacrificed for the stability required to resist the high level of forces on the pelvis in walking, running and jumping.

Movements of the pelvis as a whole change the tilt of the innominate bones. The ilium moves forwards and the ischium moves backwards in anterior forward tilting of the pelvis. The reverse occurs in backward tilting. The posterior muscles of the hip and the anterior abdominal wall produce these movements (see Chapter 10). Pelvic tilting also occurs in response to the tension in the hamstring muscles, which originate on the ischial tuberosities and pass down the posterior aspect of the thigh to the knee.

The hip joint

The hip joint, like the glenohumeral joint at the shoulder, is a synovial joint of the ball and socket type, but there the similarities end. The shoulder joint is designed for mobility, but the hip joint has to fulfil two functions, those of mobility and stability. The socket of the hip joint is formed by the acetabulum, meaning 'little vinegar cup'. The acetabulum lies at the side of the pelvis and is a deep, outwards-facing cup surrounded by a rim of fibrocartilage, known as a labrum. The head of the femur forms the ball, which is two-thirds of a sphere. When the ball is in the socket, the labrum curves inwards beyond the equator of the head of the femur to grip it and help to hold it in place.

The hip joint has a strong capsule that includes most of the femoral neck. The capsule is further strengthened by very strong ligaments anteriorly, and by small half rotator cuff muscles posteriorly. ThFe iliofemoral ligament is the strongest in the body; it is Y-shaped, passing across the front of the joint (Figure 8.1). This ligament limits the range of extension of the hip and therefore can be used to support the trunk on the lower limb. Stability is also assisted by circular fibres within the capsule, called the orbicular fibres, which give the capsule a 'waist', so increasing the suction effect of the cup on the head of the femur (Figure 8.1).

The **movements** of the hip joint are as follows:

- **Flexion** carries the thigh forwards in the sagittal plane, as in the leg swing in walking and lifting the foot on to the step above in climbing stairs.
- **Extension** is the return movement from flexion and continues beyond the anatomical position to place the foot behind the body. Extension raises the body from sitting to standing, and up on to the step above in climbing stairs.
- **Abduction** carries the thigh sideways in the frontal plane to step to the side.
- **Adduction** is the return movement from abduction and also carries the foot across the body.
- **Medial** and **lateral rotation** turn the femur inwards and outwards. These movements turn the foot inwards and outwards as there is no rotation at the knee.

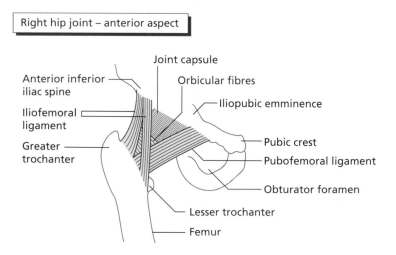

Figure 8.1 Hip joint, right anterior view.

The knee joint

The knee is a large, complex synovial joint, which may be called an atypical hinge joint. The main axis of movement flexes and extends the leg on the thigh, but there is some rotation at the knee when the knee is flexed and the foot is off the ground.

The rounded condyles of the femur articulate with the shallow, saucer-shaped condyles of the tibia. Note that the fibula is not included in the joint. A fibrocartilaginous semicircular disc, known as a meniscus, lies on each of the tibial condyles (Figure 8.2a). The menisci have four important functions within the knee: (i) to increase congruence between the femur and the tibia; (ii) to act as shock absorbers as the body weight falls on to the tibial plateau; (iii) to assist in weight bearing across the joint; and (iv) to aid lubrication by the circulation of synovial fluid within the knee joint.

The knee joint has strong collateral ligaments, and an obique ligament that passes posteriorly across the joint. The medial collateral ligament is a broad band, the posterior margin of which is attached to the medial meniscus. The lateral collateral ligament is a round cord which is mobile and not attached to the capsule or the lateral meniscus. Anteriorly, the knee joint is strengthened by the tendon of the anterior muscle of the thigh (quadriceps) as it passes over the patella to be inserted into the anterior tubercle of the tibia (Figure 8.2b).

Reflective task

Feel the front of the knee joint and locate the patella. Three fingers' breadth below the lower border of the patella you will feel a large lump. This is the anterior tubercle of the tibia where the quadriceps is inserted.

Within the knee joint, there are two further very important ligaments. These are attached to the centre of the tibial plateau and pass upwards to attach within the intercondylar notch of the femur (Appendix I). They appear to cross one another and so they are called the cruciate ligaments (Figure 8.2a). The position of the cruciate ligaments in the centre of the joint means that they prevent the femur rolling off the tibia. The cruciate ligaments also form a fulcrum for the 'locking action' of the knee, which occurs when the femur rotates slightly medially at the end of full extension.

The **movements** of the knee joint are as follows:

● **Flexion** is the movement in the sagittal plane that bends the leg towards the thigh. The knee flexes when the leg is lifted up to the next step in climbing stairs, and when sitting in a crouched position or cross-legged.

180

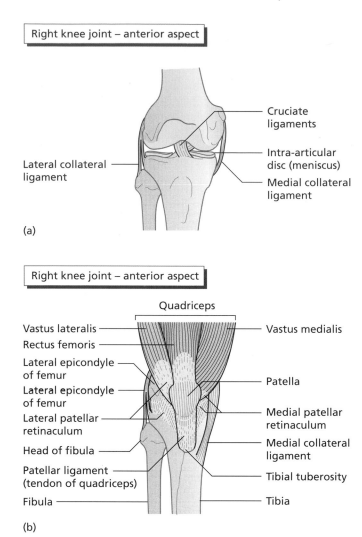

Figure 8.2   Knee joint, right anterior view: (a) patella, capsule and quadriceps removed; (b) intact.

- **Extension** straightens the leg from the flexed position to the anatomical position. When the foot is fixed by the ground, there is some rotation at the end of the range into full extension, and at the start of flexion, owing to the shape of the condyles of the femur.

Practice note-pad 8B: meniscal and ligament injuries of the knee

Twisting injuries of the knee may occur in sport, particularly football. The following damage may occur:

- The medial meniscus tears and splits through its length. The torn portion sometimes becomes displaced and lodged between the femur and the tibia.
- The medial ligament is most commonly torn, and in severe cases the anterior cruciate ligament is involved as the tibia rotates laterally. Less commonly, the lateral ligament is torn, and the posterior cruciate ligament tears when the tibia is forced backwards in relation to the femur.

The ankle joint

Reflective task

Look at the illustrations of the tibia, fibula and the bones of the foot seen in medial and lateral view in Appendix I.

The ankle joint is a synovial hinge joint. The articular surfaces of the ankle joint are the upper surface of the talus bone of the foot and the inferior surface of the tibia. The weight-bearing surfaces are the curved trochlear of the talus and the reciprocal shallow notch of the tibia. Stabilising surfaces are the medial malleolus of the tibia and the lateral malleolus of the fibula, which provide a firm grip on the sides of the talus, creating a bony mortice and tenon joint.

The medial collateral ligament (also known as the deltoid ligament) is very strong and fan-shaped (Figure 8.3a). Its attachment to the navicular bone of the foot makes it an important support mechanism for the medial arch of the foot. The lateral ligament has three bands binding the lower end of the fibula to the talus and the calcaneum (Figure 8.3b).

The **movements** of the ankle joint are described with reference to the neutral position, which is the position of the foot in the normal standing position, when the foot makes a right angle with the leg.

Dorsiflexion is when the foot is drawn upwards towards the leg (Figure 8.4). Dorsiflexion of the ankle lifts the toes clear of the ground when the leg is swinging forwards in walking or kicking a ball.

Plantar flexion when the movement is in the opposite direction from the neutral position (Figure 8.4). Plantar flexion lifts the heel off the ground to give propulsion forwards in walking, and upwards in standing on the toes. The ankle is least stable in the plantar flexed position.

Reflective task

- Sit with the foot off the ground. Start with the foot at right angles to the leg. MOVE the ankle through dorsiflexion (toes up) and then plantar flexion (toes down).
- Stand upright and lift the body up on to the toes. Note how this is a plantar flexion movement at the ankle.

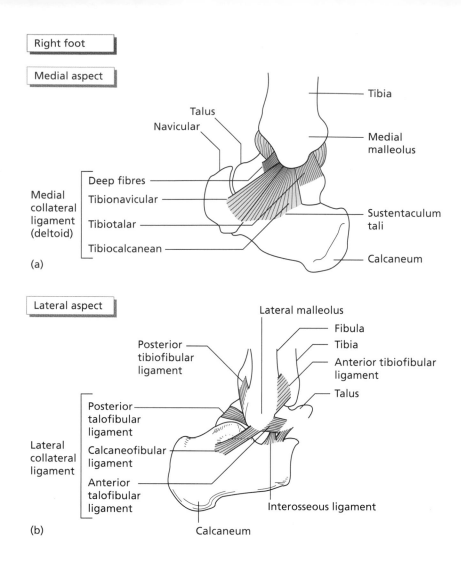

Tibia

Talus

Navicular

Medial malleolus

Deep fibres

Tibionavicular

Medial collateral ligament (deltoid)

Tibiotalar

Tibiocalcanean

Sustentaculum tali

Calcaneum

(a)

Lateral aspect

Lateral malleolus

Fibula

Posterior tibiofibular ligament

Tibia

Anterior tibiofibular ligament

Talus

Posterior talofibular ligament

Lateral collateral ligament

Calcaneofibular ligament

Anterior talofibular ligament

Interosseous ligament

(b)

Calcaneum

Figure 8.3 Ankle joint, right: (a) medial view; (b) lateral view.

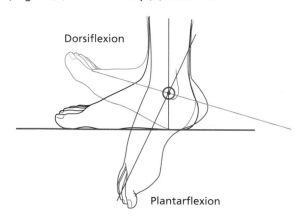

Dorsiflexion

Plantarflexion

Figure 8.4 Movements of the ankle: dorsiflexion and plantar flexion.

183

> **Practice note-pad 8C: ankle injuries**
>
> In injury to the ankle, the foot is usually twisted and turns inwards, which tears the lateral ligament (Figure 8.3b). More severe injury causes a fracture of the fibula (Pott's fracture) when the lateral malleolus is pushed off the talus. In some cases both malleoli are fractured.

Muscles of the thigh and leg in support, swing and propulsion

The muscles of the leg and thigh will be described under three headings related to their function in support, swing and propulsion.

The **support** muscles convert the lower limb into a pillar, either single or double, in standing, walking and negotiating stairs.

The muscles involved in **swing** carry the lower limb forwards, backwards, sideways or upwards while the opposite limb is in support.

Propulsion muscles exert forces on the ground to propel the body horizontally or upwards in walking, jumping or climbing stairs.

Support

There is a remarkable economy of muscle activity involved in standing upright on two legs. The joints of the lower limb are in a close-packed position when standing, and stability depends largely on the tension of the ligaments around the joints. Two particular structures are important.

The anterior ligament of the hip joint, the **iliofemoral ligament** (Figure 8.1) is important in resisting the tendency for the trunk to fall backwards on the lower limbs when the line of the body weight falls behind the hip joint. Little activity is required in the hip flexors and extensors. The paraplegic with paralysed hip muscles learns to place the hips well in front of the line of gravity and relies entirely on the tension in the iliofemoral ligament for stability at the hips in standing (Figure 8.5a).

The **iliotibial tract** (also known as the fascia lata) is a band of dense fascia that extends across the hip and knee on the lateral side of the thigh. In standing, the tension in a small muscle, known as the tensor fascia lata, which originates on the anterior superior spine of the ilium and inserts into the iliotibial tract, keeps the hip and knee extended, with the help of the gluteus maximus, the large superficial muscle of the buttock (Figure 8.5b).

People rarely stand to attention like guardsmen on parade, but adopt changing positions of 'slack standing' with the knees slightly flexed and the weight shifting from one leg to the other.

> **Reflective task**
>
> Watch people standing at a bus stop, queueing for tickets at a station, or talking in groups. Note the variety of lower limb position. Shop assistants, teachers, nurses and surgeons spend long periods standing. The constant shifting of position reduces fatigue in any one muscle group, and also aids the return of blood to the heart by the pumping action of leg muscles.

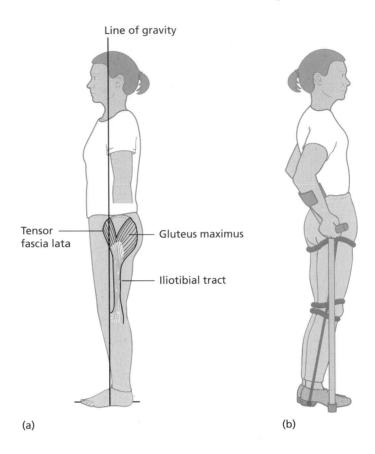

Line of gravity

Tensor — fascia lata

Gluteus maximus

Iliotibial tract

(a)   (b)

Figure 8.5 Upright standing: (a) iliotibial tract, line of gravity; (b) paraplegic standing.

Muscles of the hip in single support

In standing on one leg, the muscles around the hip of the supporting leg are active to move the body weight over the supporting leg; and to prevent the pelvis from dropping on the unsupported side.

The adductor group of muscles on the inside of the thigh contracts to shift the pelvis over the supporting leg. At the same time, the tendency for the pelvis to drop is counteracted by activity in the abductors of the hip in the supporting leg. Figure 8.6a shows the position of the abductors and adductors in the supporting leg. Contraction of the abductors will pull on the pelvis and keep it level. Further tilt of the pelvis gives added clearance for the raised foot.

The **abductors** of the hip are the **gluteus medius** and **gluteus minimus**.

Two fan-shaped muscles lie deep to the gluteus maximus, the largest muscle of the buttock. Gluteus medius and minimus originate from the outer surface of the ilium, and both muscles insert into the greater trochanter of the femur (Figure 8.7).

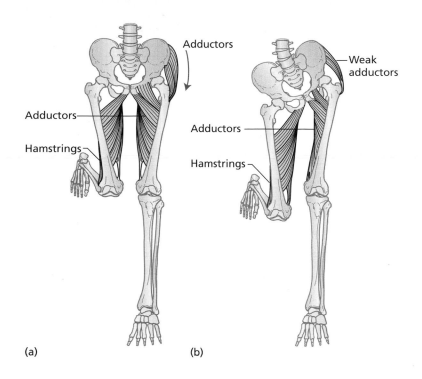

(a)   (b)

Figure 8.6   Single support: (a) action of the hip abductors and adductors to keep the pelvis level; (b) Trendelenburg's sign.

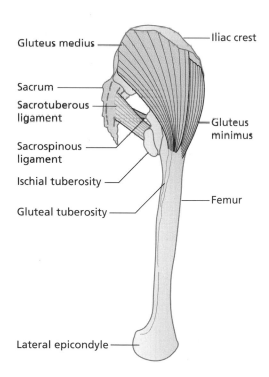

Figure 8.7   Gluteus medius and minimus, lateral view of the right hip.

> **Reflective task**
>
> Stand some distance from a long mirror, and take a few steps slowly. Note: if the right leg is off the ground, the right side of the pelvis is unsupported and could drop to the right, and so the left abductors must contract. For the next step, the opposite abductor muscles contract. (There is also a muscle of the trunk involved, the quadratus lumborum, and this will be described in Chapter 10.)

> **Practice note-pad 8D: Trendelenburg's sign**
>
> Problems of the hip, e.g. congenital dislocation, fracture of the neck of the femur or paralysis of hip abductors, produce an abnormal pattern of walking. The hip drops to the opposite side when weight is taken on to the affected hip: this is known as Trendelenburg's sign (Figure 8.6b).

The **adductors** of the hip are a group of five muscles lying on the inner side of the thigh (Figure 8.8). In the various positions of the hip joint, the individual muscles of the adductor group can

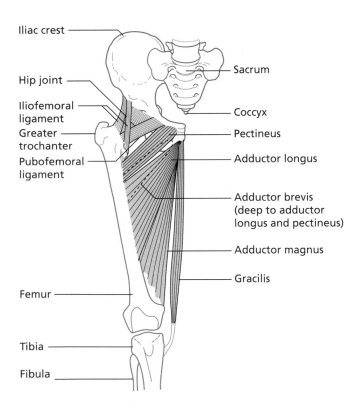

Figure 8.8   Adductor group of the hip, right anterior view.

also act as flexors, extensors and rotators. Strong adduction of the thigh is not very significant to everyday activities except when riding a bicycle or a horse, when contraction of the adductors keeps you on the saddle. When standing on an unstable platform, the adductors act with the abductors to keep the body weight over the feet.

The names of the adductors of the hip are **adductor magnus**, **adductor longus**, **adductor brevis**, **pectineus** and **gracilis**. The adductors originate from the anterior surface of the body of the pubis, extending medially on to the superior and inferior ramus. The adductor magnus is the most posterior muscle of the group, and its origin extends back to the ischial tuberosity. From the small area of origin, the muscles fan out to insert into the full length of the posterior shaft of the femur. The posterior fibres of the adductor magnus pass vertically down to the adductor tubercle, just above the medial side of the knee. The gracilis is a strap muscle lying medially in the group and ends below the knee.

The lower limb as a single support demands more stability at the **knee** and the **ankle**. The quadriceps muscle on the front of the thigh extends the knee (see section on Propulsion later in chapter) and the muscles around the ankle keep the balance of the leg over the foot.

Reflective task

Watch a partner in bare feet stand on one leg. Notice any changes in the level of the pelvis, and the side-to-side movement of the foot taking place just below the ankle joint.

Swing

Leg swing can occur when one leg is free to move while the opposite leg is supporting the body weight. The movements of the free leg swing the limb to place the foot forwards, upwards or to the side.

Reflective task

Stand on one leg and swing the free leg in all directions. Think about the daily activities that use these movements. How does the leg swing in: (i) walking; (ii) climbing stairs; (iii) stepping into the bath; (iv) getting into a car; and (v) getting on to a bicycle?

The muscles involved in swinging the leg forwards are:

- the **hip flexors** combined with abductors and rotators;
- the **knee flexors**;
- the **ankle dorsiflexors**.

Flexors of the hip

The main hip flexors are the iliacus and psoas, usually grouped together and called iliopsoas, assisted by the sartorius, the rectus femoris and the tensor fascia lata.

The **iliopsoas** originates in the abdomen. The fibres of the psoas are attached to the transverse processes, bodies and discs of the lumbar vertebrae. The iliacus takes origin from the inner surface

188

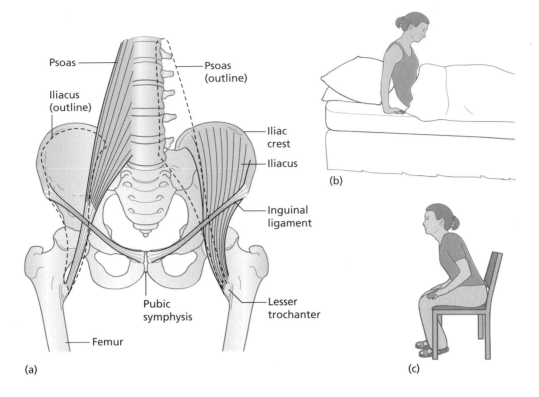

(a)

(b)

(c)

Figure 8.9 Iliacus and psoas: (a) position, anterior view of pelvis and hip; (b) sitting up from lying; (c) preparing to stand from sitting.

of the ilium on the iliac fossa. The two muscles leave the abdomen together, passing under the inguinal ligament, over the front of the hip joint, and insert into the lesser trochanter of the femur (Figure 8.9a).

> **Reflective task**
>
> Sit with the trunk slightly forwards. Place the hand at the waist between the lower ribs and iliac crest, with the fingers across the lower back. Raise the foot off the ground and feel the activity in the psoas just lateral to the vertebral column. The bulk of the muscle you are feeling lies posteriorly, but remember that its tendon passes over the anterior side of the hip joint to reach the femur.

The iliopsoas is active in sitting up from lying. The insertion on the femur is fixed in the extended leg and the contraction of the iliopsoas pulls on the ilium of the pelvis and the lumbar spine to lift the trunk upright (Figure 8.9b). In preparing to stand up from sitting, the iliopsoas pulls the trunk forwards to bring the centre of gravity forwards over the foot base before extending to

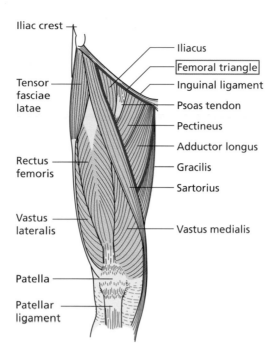

Iliac crest

Iliacus

Femoral triangle

Inguinal ligament

Tensor fasciae latae

Psoas tendon

Pectineus

Adductor longus

Rectus femoris

Gracilis

Sartorius

Vastus lateralis

Vastus medialis

Patella

Patellar ligament

Figure 8.10   Sartorius and quadriceps femoris, right anterior.

upright (Figure 8.9c). The iliopsoas contracts in climbing stairs to lift the leading leg upwards on to the next step.

The **sartorius** is a long, thin, strap-like muscle that crosses the anterior thigh (Figure 8.10). When the hip and the knee are flexed, the lateral rotation action at the hip produced by the sartorius is important. The overall actions of the sartorius put the limb into the cross-legged position, as adopted by the early tailors (hence the name). The same movement is used to draw up the lower limbs in swimming and in yoga.

The **rectus femoris** is part of the quadriceps group of muscles described under knee extensors. The **tensor fascia lata** originates on the ilium and is inserted into the iliotibial tract (Figure 8.5).

Abductors and rotators of the hip

The abductors of the hip, the gluteus medius and gluteus minimus, are involved in swinging the leg to the side. Walking includes considerable side-stepping to avoid obstacles. In sitting, the hip abductors are used to swing the thigh from one chair to another, or from a car seat to prepare to stand.

There are six small lateral rotator muscles arranged close to the hip joint, in a similar way to the rotator cuff muscles of the shoulder. The six muscles lie across the posterior side of the hip joint deep to the gluteus maximus. The names of the muscles are: piriformis, obturator internus, gemellus superior, gamellus inferior, quadratus femoris and obturator externus. Detailed attachments of these muscles can be found in standard anatomy textbooks. Since there is no significant rotation at the knee and ankle, the hip rotators are important in positioning of the feet, for example turning the toes outwards.

Flexors of the knee

The knee flexors in leg swing lift the foot clear of the ground. The muscles active in flexion of the knee are the hamstring group at the back of the thigh. The three hamstring muscles are the biceps femoris, the semimembranosus and the semitendinosus. The medial part of the adductor magnus also acts as a hamstring.

190

> **Reflective task**
>
> Feel the tendons of the hamstrings in the fold of the knee in the sitting position. Two tendons lie medially (semimembranosus and semitendinosus), and one tendon can be felt laterally (biceps femoris).

All three **hamstrings** originate on the ischial tuberosity of the pelvis (Figure 8.11). The biceps femoris also has a short head of origin from the linea aspera of the femur, and passing laterally to the knee, both heads are inserted into the head of the fibula. The semimembranosus begins

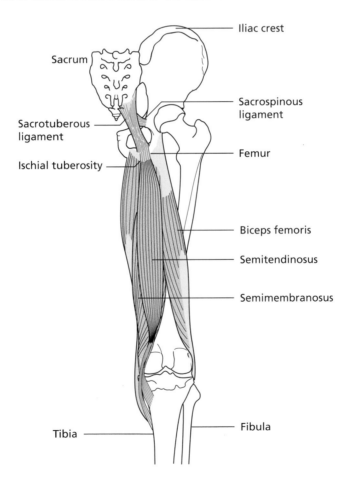

Figure 8.11   Hamstring muscles, right posterior.

as a flat tendon that forms one-third of its length, and the muscle fibres insert by a thick tendon behind the medial condyle of the tibia. The semitendinosus begins as muscle fibres and becomes tendinous two-thirds of the way down the thigh, to insert into the tibia on the medial side below the knee.

When the trunk leans forwards, the ischial tuberosities (origin of the hamstrings) are carried upwards and backwards in relation to the hip. The hamstring muscles can then be felt stretching in the thigh. Contraction of the hamstrings from this position extends the hip, and the trunk is raised to the upright position.

Dorsiflexors of the ankle

The ankle dorsiflexors counteract the weight of the foot, which tends to drop during the swing, and lifts the toes clear of the ground. The individual muscles in the group of dorsiflexors are the tibialis anterior, the extensor hallucis longus and the extensor digitorum longus (Figure 8.12).

The **tibialis anterior** is attached to the anterolateral shaft of the tibia and inserts on the medial side of the foot into the medial cuneiform and the base of the first metatarsal. The **extensor hallucis longus** originates on the shaft of the fibula and inserts into the distal phalanx of the big toe. The **extensor digitorum longus** has fibres attached to the shafts of the tibia and fibula and the interosseous membrane in between. The common tendon passes over the front of the ankle and divides into four, each inserting via an extensor expansion to the toes, in a similar way to the

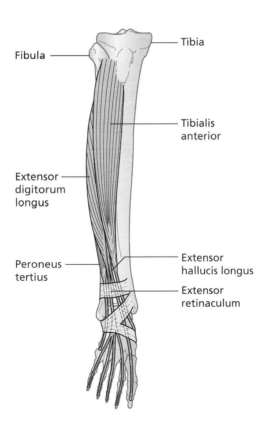

Figure 8.12   Anterior tibial group of muscles, right anterior.

> **Reflective task**
>
> - Palpate the bulge of muscles below the knee and lateral to the shin. Lift the toes upwards by dorsiflexing the ankle and feel the group in action. Tibialis anterior is the most superficial muscle that can be felt.
> - Observe the three tendons passing over the front of the ankle: the tibialis anterior medially adjacent to the medial malleolus, then the extensor hallucis longus going to the big toe, and the extensor digitorum longus laterally. Compare with Figure 8.12.

extensors of the fingers. A fifth tendon is sometimes present, which is the tendon of peroneus tertius, inserting into the base of the fifth metatarsal.

Two transverse bands of fascia over the anterior side of the leg above the ankle hold the tendons of the dorsiflexors in position during movements of the ankle (Figure 8.12).

Propulsion

So far, movements of the lower limb in support and swing have been described. This section will look at the muscles of the thigh and leg that exert force against the ground to move the body forwards and upwards.

Muscle groups used in propulsion movements are:

- the **hip extensors**;
- the **knee extensors**;
- the **ankle plantar flexors**.

Extensors of the hip

The main hip extensor is the **gluteus maximus** (Figure 8.13). The most superficial muscle of the gluteal group, the gluteus maximus is the largest muscle in the body. It can be seen when lying prone or standing upright, forming the curve of the buttocks. The gluteus maximus extends the hip to lift the body in standing up from sitting and in climbing stairs.

The extensive origin of the gluteus maximus spreads from the posterior corner of the iliac crest across the posterior side of the sacrum and coccyx, with some fibres attached to the fascia of the lower back (thoracolumbar fascia) and to the sacrotuberous ligament of the pelvis. All of the fibres pass downwards and laterally over the posterior side of the hip joint. The main insertion of the muscle is into the iliotibial tract, with the remaining fibres passing deeply to attach to the gluteal tuberosity on the posterior shaft of the femur.

The hamstring muscles (see earlier section on Swing) also have an extensor action at the hip, particularly when the trunk is flexed forwards. The hamstrings are often damaged in athletes in the explosive propulsion movement from the position of leaning forwards at the starting blocks.

Extensors of the knee

The knee extensors are the quadriceps femoris group, composed of four muscles on the anterior of the thigh. The individual muscles are: the rectus femoris, the most superficial in the midline;

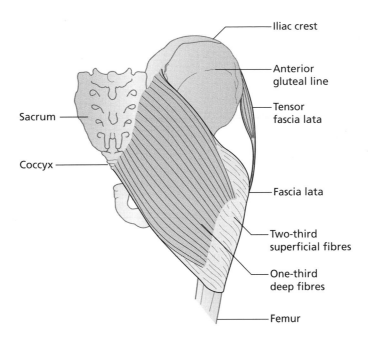

Figure 8.13   Gluteus maximus, right posterior.

the vastus medialis on the medial side; the vastus lateralis on the lateral side; and vastus inter-medius, which lies deep to the rectus femoris. These muscles can be clearly seen in athletes and footballers, when the vasti in particular become enlarged in response to weight training.

> **Reflective task**
>
> Sit on a chair and put your hands on the top of your thighs. Now stand up slowly and feel the quadriceps in action. Pause in standing and feel the tension decrease. Then sit down slowly to feel the quadriceps in action again. The muscle is working concentrically to extend the knee and lift the body upwards, then working eccentrically against gravity as the knee flexes and the body lowers to the seat of the chair again.

The **quadriceps** group can be seen in anterior view in Figure 8.10, with the exception of the vastus intermedius which lies deep to the rectus femoris.

The rectus femoris is the only part of the quadriceps that passes over the hip joint. This muscle is attached by two heads, one from the anterior inferior iliac spine and the other from just above the acetabulum. The three vastus muscles surround the shaft of the femur. The vastus medialis begins posteriorly on the spiral line and down the medial side of the linea aspera. The fibres wrap round medially to approach the knee. The vastus lateralis is attached posteriorly to the lateral side of the linea aspera and wraps round the lateral side of the femoral shaft. The vastus inter-medius originates on the anterior and lateral shaft of the femur. In the transverse section of the thigh in Figure 8.14, the quadriceps can be seen around three sides of the shaft of the femur.

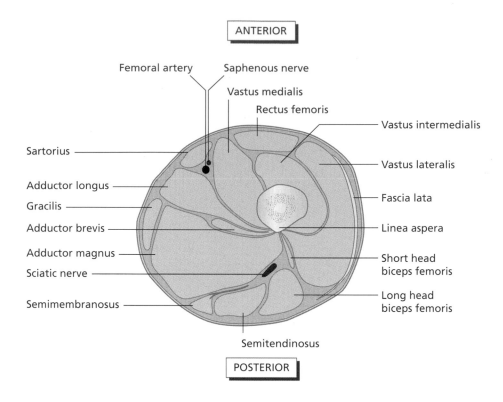

ANTERIOR

Femoral artery — Saphenous nerve

Vastus medialis

Rectus femoris

Vastus intermedialis

Sartorius

Vastus lateralis

Adductor longus

Fascia lata

Gracilis

Adductor brevis

Linea aspera

Adductor magnus

Short head biceps femoris

Sciatic nerve

Long head biceps femoris

Semimembranosus

Semitendinosus

POSTERIOR

Figure 8.14 Relationship of the muscles of the thigh, transverve section of the right thigh at the upper third level.

All four muscles of the quadriceps meet at the patella on the front of the knee, and insert by a common tendon, the ligamentum patellae, to the anterior tubercle of the tibia. The ligamentum patellae provides extra stability for the knee joint on the anterior side where the capsule is absent. The lower horizontal fibres of the vastus medialis prevent lateral displacement of the patella at the end of knee extension.

The quadriceps group is a powerful extensor of the knee, and the rectus femoris alone has a weak flexor action on the hip. Acting with the gluteus maximus, the quadriceps raise the body from sitting and squatting. When the knees are flexed at an angle less than a right angle, the quadriceps has to develop a force of 4–5 times body weight to hold the position. The knees are under great stress when the body is raised from a low squat position, since the line of body weight is some distance from the knee joint (Figure 8.15) (see also Chapter 2).

When the knee is injured, or after a period of bed rest, the quadriceps wastes very rapidly. The strength of this muscle is restored by lying supine and lifting one leg at a time with the knee held in extension.

Plantar flexors of the ankle

The ankle plantar flexors raise the heel from the ground and lift the body upwards or forwards in a 'push-off' movement. The calf muscles, attached by the Achilles tendon to the heel, are active in this movement.

194

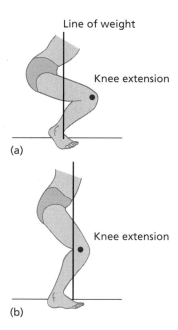

Line of weight

Knee extension

(a)

Knee extension

(b)

Figure 8.15   Change in the line of gravity in moving from (a) low squat to (b) high squat.

Reflective task

Stand on your toes and feel the calf muscles contracting. The muscles are also working eccentrically when you lower your heels to the ground.

When the calf muscles are weak, the spring and lift of the lower limb is lost.

The gastrocnemius and soleus, which form the calf of the leg, are the superficial muscles active in plantar flexion of the ankle (Figure 8.16a).

The **gastrocnemius** is attached by two heads to the posterior surface of the femur, one above each femoral condyle. The **soleus** attaches below the knee, across the soleal line on the posterior shaft of the tibia, and to the head and shaft of the fibula. Both muscles join to form the very strong Achilles tendon attached to the posterior surface of the calcaneum. The length of the calcaneum behind the axis of the ankle joint gives good leverage to the calf muscles. There is a small muscle, the plantaris, lying between the gastrocnemius and the soleus. The short belly of this muscle originates above the lateral condyle of the femur, near to the lateral head of the gastrocnemius, and becomes a thin tendon just below the knee joint. The tendon passes down the length of the calf to insert on to the calcaneum in the Achilles tendon.

The **flexor digitorum longus**, **flexor hallucis longus** and **tibialis posterior** are the deep plantar flexors lying underneath the gastrocnemius and soleus. The names of the two long flexors are related to their action on the toes, and they originate on the posterior shaft of the tibia and fibula (hallucis to the fibula, and digitorum to the tibia). The tibialis posterior lies deep to these two and originates on the shaft of both the tibia and the fibula. The tendons of all three muscles pass

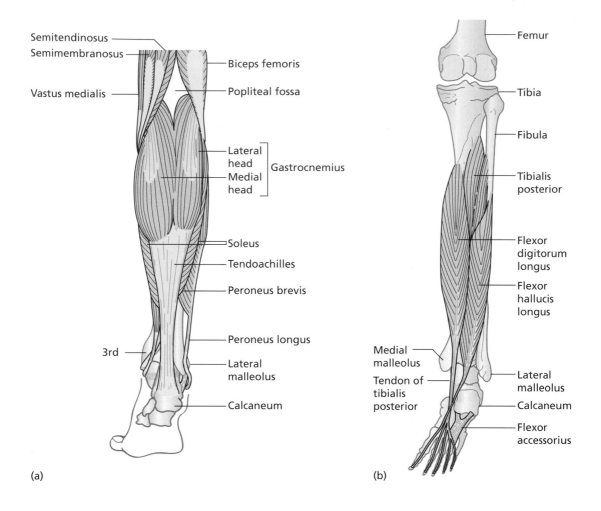

Femur

Tibia

Fibula

Tibialis posterior

Flexor digitorum longus

Flexor hallucis longus

Lateral malleolus

Calcaneum

Flexor accessorius

Medial malleolus

Tendon of tibialis posterior

Semitendinosus
Semimembranosus

Biceps femoris

Popliteal fossa

Vastus medialis

Lateral head
Medial head } Gastrocnemius

Soleus

Tendoachilles

Peroneus brevis

Peroneus longus

3rd

Lateral malleolus

Calcaneum

(a)   (b)

Figure 8.16 Ankle plantar flexors, right posterior: (a) superficial, gastocnemius and soleus; (b) deep muscles.

round the medial side of the ankle to enter the sole of the foot and insert on the plantar surface of the bones of the foot (Figure 8.16b).

> ### Practice note-pad 8E: avulsion of the Achilles tendon
>
> The Achilles tendon may sustain spontaneous avulsion (severing), with a feeling of being struck just above the heel and an inability to tiptoe. This occurs in tennis players and athletes who rely on thrust at the ankle, and sometimes in middle age when the tendon has degenerated.

Functions of the foot

The foot is a relatively small area that makes contact between the body weight and the ground. The surface of the ground may be rough, smooth, hard, soft, level or sloping, and the sole of the foot has to be able to accommodate all of these. The weight of the body above compresses the parts of the foot in different directions and the foot resists this deformation.

Another feature of the foot is flexibility and strength to provide spring and lift during movement. At each step in walking, 60% of the time is spent supporting the body weight and providing momentum for moving the body forwards. In walking up stairs and jumping, strong propulsive forces must be generated by the ankle and transmitted through the foot to lift the body upwards. The skin of the sole of the foot monitors the pressure on it exerted by the position of the upright body above and the variations in the surface of the ground below. This information is transmitted to the brain via the somatosensory system, and adjustments to posture are made to keep the body in balance. In this way, the foot is one of the factors that regulate the posture of the body (see Chapter 11).

In summary, the functions of the foot are:

- to accommodate to variations in the supporting surface during standing and locomotion;
- to provide spring and lift in body movement;
- to provide sensory information for the regulation of body posture in standing and moving.

Joints and movements of the foot

> **Reflective task**
>
> Look at the bones on the foot seen in lateral and medial view in Appendix I.

The **ankle joint** between the lower end of the tibia and fibula, articulating with the convex trochlear surface of the talus, moves the foot in dorsiflexion and plantar flexion.

There are two important joints between the tarsal bones that move the foot in other directions.

The **subtalar joint** is formed by a concave facet on the undersurface of the talus, articulating with a convex surface on the upper surface of the calcaneum. Strong ligaments unite the bones, particularly an interosseous ligament that acts as a fulcrum for movements of the foot on the leg.

The **midtarsal joint** is formed by the articulations between the talus, calcaneum and navicular medially, together with that between the calcaneum and the cuboid laterally. This forms an irregular joint extending from one side of the foot to the other. The subtalar and midtarsal joints co-operate in the movements of the foot.

The **movements of the foot** that occur between the tarsal bones are known as **inversion** and **eversion** (Figure 8.17).

In inversion, the foot turns so that the sole faces inwards when the foot is off the ground, the medial border is raised and the lateral border is depressed. This movement shifts the body weight to the lateral side of the foot when weight bearing.

In eversion, the opposite movement occurs. The sole of the foot faces outwards, with the lateral border raised and the medial border depressed, when the foot is off the ground. This movement shifts the weight towards the medial side of the foot in weight bearing.

197

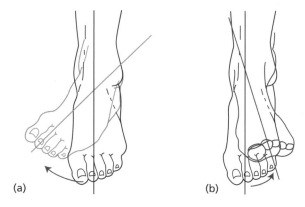

(a)   (b)

Figure 8.17   Movements of the foot: (a) inversion; (b) eversion.

Most of the movement in inversion and eversion occurs at the subtalar joint. This joint also allows the side-to-side adjustment of the line of gravity in standing. The midtarsal joint is more important in anterior to posterior adjustments in the upright posture. Inversion and eversion are important when putting the foot down on sloping ground or on an irregular surface.

> **Reflective task**
>
> Remember how difficult it is to walk on loose shingle, on a rocky hillside or down the aisle of a moving train.

The movements of the **toes** occur at the metatarsophalangeal and the interphalangeal joints. Movements of flexion, extension, abduction and adduction occur at the metatarsophalangeal joints at the ball of the foot. The abduction and adduction movements are seen clearly in the feet of a baby, but become restricted by wearing shoes later. As in the hand, the interphalangeal joints of the toes move in flexion and extension only.

Muscles moving the foot

The muscles acting on the foot originate in the leg and pass around the ankle to insert into the bones of the foot. Like the hand, the foot also has intrinsic muscles that begin and end in the foot. The arrangement of the intrinsic muscles of the foot is similar to that in the hand. Children with malformation of the upper limb may develop the muscles of the foot to take over the manipulative functions of the hand.

The dorsiflexors and plantar flexors of the ankle have already been described.

Invertors and evertors of the foot

The invertors of the foot are the **tibialis anterior** and **tibialis posterior**. The tibialis anterior is also one of the dorsiflexors already described (see Figure 8.12). The tibialis posterior is the deepest muscle of the calf, originating on the posterior shaft of the tibia and fibula. The tendon of this

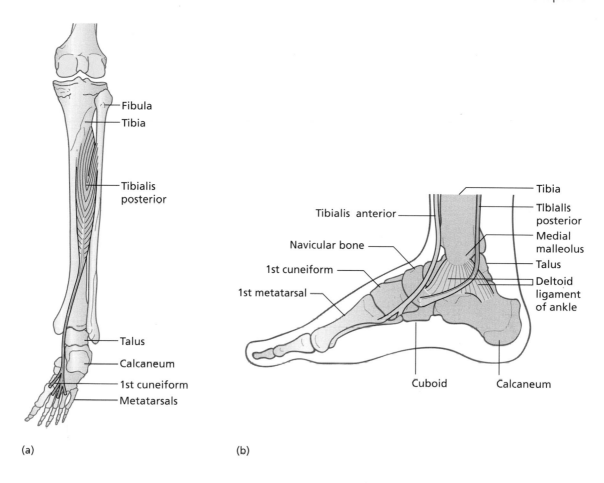

(a)

(b)

Figure 8.18 (a) Tibialis posterior, right leg and foot; (b) tendons of tibialis anterior and posterior, right ankle medial.

muscle passes round the medial side of the ankle and it inserts on the plantar surface of the navicular and adjacent tarsal bones (Figure 8.18a). The relationship between the tendons of the tibialis anterior and posterior on the medial side of the foot can be seen in Figure 8.18b.

The evertors of the foot are the **peroneus longus** and **peroneus brevis**. These two muscles are attached to the lateral shaft of the fibula and their tendons pass round the lateral side of the ankle. The tendon of the peroneus brevis ends at the base of the fifth metatarsal. The peroneus longus turns under at this point and crosses the sole of the foot in a groove on the cuboid bone, to reach the medial cuneiform and the base of the first metatarsal on the medial side of the foot (Figure 8.19).

When the evertors are weak, lateral stability of the ankle is lost and the lateral ligament of the ankle is often torn. When the foot is in contact with an uneven surface, the movements of inversion and eversion, together with the actions of the intrinsic muscles of the foot, allow the foot to adjust to the ground and stabilise the ankle. Shoes reduce the amount of adaptation required, but the foot and the shoe still have to accommodate sloping ground and avoid slipping on wet or icy surfaces.

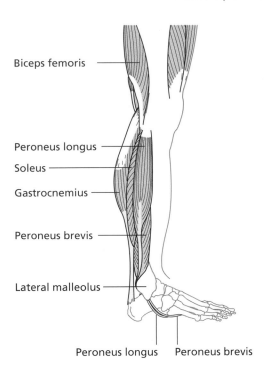

Biceps femoris

Peroneus longus

Soleus

Gastrocnemius

Peroneus brevis

Lateral malleolus

Peroneus longus   Peroneus brevis

Figure 8.19 Peroneus longus and brevis, right leg lateral.

The arches of the foot

The bones of the foot form a complex arched mechanism that combines stability with flexibility.

Reflective task

- Revise the bones of the foot. Place an articulated skeleton of the foot on a flat surface. Note which bones are in contact with the table, and which bones are wholly or partly raised above the surface.
- Stand the feet in a tray of water-soluble paint, then make footprints on a sheet of lining paper laid out on the floor: (i) sitting on a chair, i.e. non-weight bearing; (ii) standing upright; and (iii) walking for several steps. Note the variation in the pattern of footprints in (i), (ii) and (iii). Compare your footprints with those of other students and note any individual differences.

The change seen in the footprints shows an increase in the area of foot in contact with the ground as the force of the body weight on the feet increases in the change from sitting to standing to walking. In all of the prints, the heel and ball of the foot will be seen. The lateral border of the foot will be present when the foot is weight bearing. The medial border of the foot remains absent, except when there is abnormal flattening of the foot.

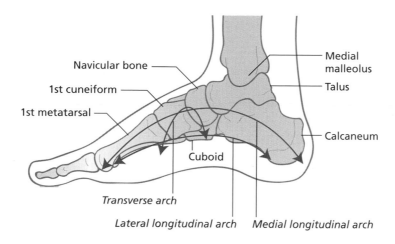

Figure 8.20 Arches of the foot, right medial.

Looking at the bones of the foot and the footprints, it can be seen that the foot is arched in different directions. A longitudinal arch from the heel to the ball of the foot is easy to recognise. The foot is also arched transversely across the distal row of tarsals and the metatarsals (Figure 8.20).

Ligaments bind the bones of the foot together and provide the main factors supporting the arches in standing. During movement, it is the muscles of the leg acting as slings from above, and the intrinsic muscles of the foot acting as bowstrings across the base of the arches, that maintain the arches. The height of the arches varies during different phases of locomotor movements, particularly the medial part of the longitudinal arch.

The bony compartments of the arches are as follows:

- **Medial longitudinal arch**: this arch is formed by the calcaneum, talus, navicular, three cuneiforms and metatarsals 1, 2 and 3. The highest part of the arch is the talus, which sits on the calcaneum supported by a shelf on the medial side known as the sustentaculum tali.
- **Lateral longitudinal arch**: this arch also begins at the calcaneum and extends along the lateral side of the foot to the cuboid and metatarsals 4 and 5. There is considerable stress on this arch during running, when the body weight is transferred along the lateral border of the foot and on to the big toe. The shoes of a marathon runner, which are often worn down on the outer border, show how high this stress can be.
- **Transverse arch**: the foot is most arched in the transverse direction across the distal row of tarsals: the three cuneiforms and the cuboid. The metatarsals are also arched transversely, the region of the heads of the metatarsals is sometimes called the anterior arch. When the foot is stressed from above in standing, the anterior arch is flattened as the weight is taken by the heads of the metatarsals.

Ligaments bonding the arches

- **Spring ligament**: a tough, fibrous band extends from the sustentaculum tali of the calcaneum to the navicular, and supports the head of the talus. This ligament is very elastic and responds to compression of the medial longitudinal arch (Figure 8.21a).

201

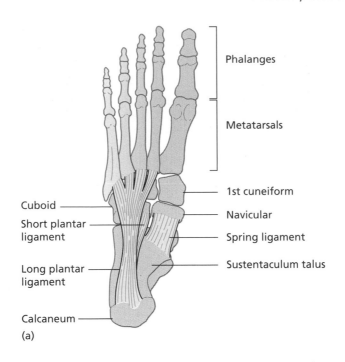

Phalanges

Metatarsals

1st cuneiform

Cuboid

Navicular

Short plantar ligament

Spring ligament

Long plantar ligament

Sustentaculum talus

Calcaneum

(a)

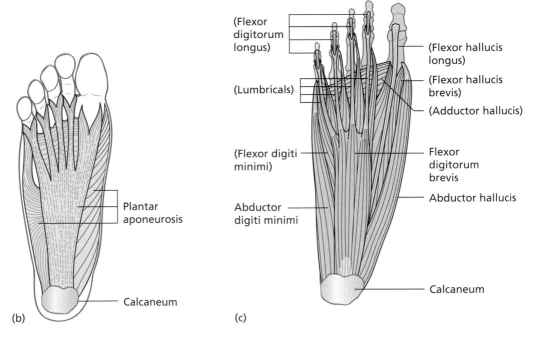

(b)

Plantar aponeurosis

Calcaneum

(c)

(Flexor digitorum longus)

(Flexor hallucis longus)

(Flexor hallucis brevis)

(Lumbricals)

(Adductor hallucis)

(Flexor digiti minimi)

Flexor digitorum brevis

Abductor digiti minimi

Abductor hallucis

Calcaneum

Figure 8.21   Plantar surface, right foot: (a) plantar ligaments; (b) plantar aponeurosis; (c) three muscles of the first layer (second and third layers named in brackets).

- **Long** and **short plantar ligaments**: these two ligaments bind the bones of the lateral longitudinal arch. The long plantar ligament stretches from the calcaneum to the ridge on the cuboid and the bases of the middle metatarsals. Deep to this, the short plantar ligament is attached to the anterior end of the calcaneum and to the cuboid (Figure 8.21a).
- **Plantar aponeurosis**: a thick sheet of dense fibrous tissue is attached to the tuberosities of the calcaneum, and passes forwards over the muscles of the sole, to blend with the ligaments joining the heads of the metatarsals (deep transverse metatarsal ligaments). There are five main bands in the plantar aponeurosis, and each band blends with a fibrous sheath round a flexor tendon to a toe. The plantar aponeurosis joins the two ends of the medial and lateral longitudinal arches (Figure 8.21b).

Muscles supporting the arches

- **Muscles of the leg**: the medial longitudinal arch is supported by the tibialis anterior lifting the middle of the arch and the tendon of the tibialis posterior uniting the medial tarsal bones on the plantar surface. The tendon of the flexor hallucis longus acts as a bowstring for the arch. Further support for the longitudinal arch is provided by the tendons of the flexor digitorum longus lying along the plantar surface of the foot. The chief support for the transverse arch is the peroneus longus, the tendon of which crosses the foot from the lateral border to the medial side.
- **Intrinsic muscles of the foot**: the longitudinal arches are supported by the three muscles of the first layer of the foot that originate on the calcaneum and insert into the toes. Like the plantar aponeurosis, these muscles (abductor hallucis, flexor digitorum brevis and abductor digiti minimi) join the two ends of the longitudinal arches (Figure 8.21c). The transverse arch is supported by the transverse head of the adductor hallucis in the third layer of the foot. This muscle crosses the anterior end of the transverse arch, from the heads of metatarsals 3, 4 and 5 to the proximal phalanx of the big toe. The transverse arch is also supported by activity in the interossei and the flexors that draw the metatarsals towards the axis of the foot, the second metatarsal.

> **Reflective task**
>
> Place the foot flat on the ground while sitting in a chair. Try to pull up the centre of the foot (flexion) with the toes kept flat on the ground. Notice how the foot arches both longitudinally by some flexion at the tarsometatarsal joints, and transversely as the shafts of the metatarsals move towards the axis of the foot.

The maintenance of the flexibility of the foot is important for mobility, especially in dancers and gymnasts who need to balance the body on the whole, or part of, one foot. In the supporting foot in walking and running, the body weight is transmitted from the heel to the big toe at each step. The big toe takes most of the weight in standing, and provides the thrust in driving the body forwards in walking and running. Long-distance runners commonly experience pain in the big toe as a result of the great stress on it.

> **Practice note-pad 8F: flat foot and hallux valgus**
>
> Flat foot is the collapse of the medial arch so that the medial border of the foot almost touches the ground. Predisposing factors are muscle weakness or joint erosion, e.g. rheumatoid arthritis.
>
> Hallux valgus is the most common deformity of the foot. The first metatarsal deviates medially away from the second metatarsal, and the big toe slants laterally towards the second toe. The head of the metatarsal develops a protective bursa where the shoe rubs. There is some evidence for shoes with inadequate support in standing, contributing to the condition. It does not occur in people who have never worn shoes.
>
> In rheumatoid arthritis, pain and swelling occur in the metatarsophalangeal joints of the foot, which gives a feeling of 'walking on stones'.

Summary of the lower limb muscles

- **Muscles of the hip**: gluteus maximus, medius and minimus, tensor fascia lata, iliacus and psoas (ilio-psoas), six lateral rotators.
- **Anterior thigh**: quadriceps femoris (rectus femoris, vastas medialis, intermedius and lateralis) sartorius.
- **Medial thigh**: adductor magnus, longus and brevis, pectineus, gracilis.
- **Posterior thigh**: hamstrings (biceps femoris, semitendinosus, semimembranosus).
- **Anterior leg**: tibialis anterior, extensor hallucis longus, extensor digitorum longus.
- **Posterior leg**: gastrocnemius, soleus, (plantaris and popliteus), tibialis posterior, flexor hallucis longus, flexor digitorum longus.
- **Lateral leg**: peroneus longus and brevis.
- **Sole of the foot**:
  - first layer: abductor hallucis, flexor digitorum brevis, abductor digiti minimi;
  - second layer: lumbricals, flexor digitorum accessorius;
  - third layer: flexor hallucis brevis, flexor digiti minimi brevis, adductor hallucis;
  - fourth layer: plantar interossei, dorsal interossei.

Summary

- The lower limbs form the support for the body in the upright position, with the line of body weight passing from the trunk through the pelvis at the sacroiliac joint and on to the hip joints.
- The pelvic girdle is an irregular ring of bone formed by the sacrum and the two innominate bones bound together by strong ligaments.
- The tilt of the pelvis affects the lumbar curvature and the consequently the upright posture.
- The hip joint is a stable ball and socket joint allowing movements of the thigh in all planes, carrying the foot in all directions around the body.
- The knee joint is a complex synovial joint that moves mainly in flexion and extension. Flexion of the knee shortens the limb so that the foot can clear the ground. Extension of the knee

converts the limb into a pillar of support and also lifts the body in rising from sitting to standing and in walking upstairs.

- The ankle joint moves from the neutral standing position into dorsiflexion and plantar flexion. Dorsiflexion lifts the toes clear of the ground. Plantar flexion gives the 'push-off' in walking and lifts the foot on to the toes.
- The muscles of the lower limb can be divided into groups that are active in support, swing and propulsion.
- In double **support**, the joints of the limb are in close-packed position, supported by strong ligaments and the iliotibial tract on the lateral aspect of the thigh.
- In standing on one leg, the body weight shifts to a position over the supporting foot by the action of the adductors of the hip. The hip abductors in the supporting leg contract to prevent the pelvis dropping on the unsupported side. The knee is stabilised by the extensor muscles.
- In **swing**, the thigh moves forwards and upwards by the action of the hip flexors. The knee flexors and the ankle dorsiflexors lift the foot to clear the ground as the leg swings.
- In **propulsion**, the ankle plantar flexes to raise the heel. This creates a force that moves the body upwards or forwards. Propulsive force is also generated by the extensors of the hip and the knee, particularly in lifting the body upwards.
- The functions of the foot are: to accommodate to the variations in the slope and texture of the ground; to provide spring and lift during movement; and to activate the sensory system from receptors in the skin of the sole of the foot in the maintenance of posture and balance.
- Movements of the foot on the leg occur at the ankle, subtalar and midtarsal joints. Inversion and eversion movements turn the sole of the foot medially and laterally, respectively.
- The bones of the foot are arranged in the form of arches directed longitudinally from the heel to the metatarsal heads, and transversely across the base of the metatarsals. The arches are maintained by strong ligaments on the plantar surface of the foot, and by both extrinsic and intrinsic muscles of the foot, forming a structure that combines stability and flexibility.

9

Nerve supply of the lower limb

Key terms

lumbar plexus (femoral, lateral cutaneous and obturator nerves), sacral plexus (superior and inferior gluteal, sciatic, tibial and common peroneal nerves)

Conceptual overview

Muscle action and sensation in the lower limb as a whole depend on the nerves that originate in the lumbar and sacral spinal segments. This chapter covers the nerve innervation of the lower limb from the spinal nerve root branches which form the plexuses to the terminal branches which form the peripheral nerves of the lower limb.

Tyldesley & Grieve's Muscles, Nerves and Movement in Human Occupation, Fourth Edition. Ian R. McMillan, Gail Carin-Levy.
© 2012 Ian R. McMillan, Gail Carin-Levy, Barbara Tyldesley and June I. Grieve. Published 2012 by Blackwell Publishing Ltd.

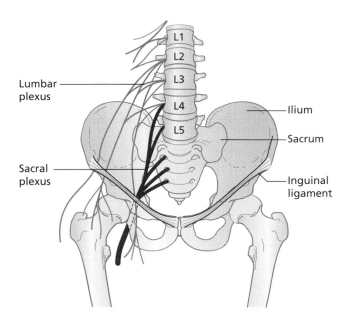

Figure 9.1   Lumbar and sacral plexuses: position and relations.

Introduction

The first four lumbar nerves form the **lumbar plexus**, which lies embedded in the psoas muscle in the posterior abdominal wall. A second **sacral plexus** is formed from the fifth lumbar to the fourth sacral spinal nerves. These spinal nerves of the sacral plexus are part of the cauda equina (see Chapter 4, Figure 4.2) and enter the pelvis through the anterior foramina of the sacrum.

Figure 9.1 shows the position of the lumbar and sacral plexuses in relation to the lumbar spine, the pelvis and the hip. The course of the muscular branches of the lumbar and sacral plexus will be described; the cutaneous branches will be mentioned in outline only.

Lumbar plexus: position and formation

The upper four lumbar nerves (L1–L4) form the lumbar plexus, which lies in the psoas muscle alongside the lumbar vertebrae in the posterior abdominal wall. Branches direct from the plexus supply the hip flexors (psoas and iliacus) and quadratus lumborum (see posterior abdominal wall in Chapter 10). The branches of the plexus emerge from the psoas. Most of the fibres of L4 join the lumbar plexus, but the remainder join L5 to form the lumbosacral trunk, which is part of the sacral plexus. Figure 9.2 shows the roots of the lumbar plexus and the formation of the main terminal branches.

Terminal branches of the lumbar plexus

Three important nerves are formed from the lumbar plexus:

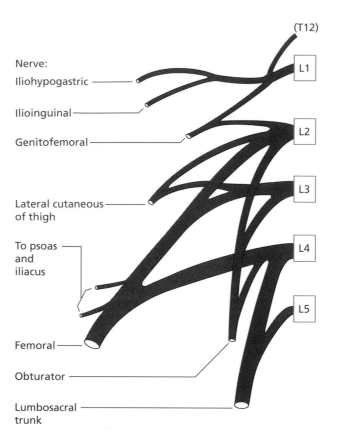

Figure 9.2   Lumbar plexus: roots and main terminal branches.

- the **femoral nerve** supplying the anterior muscles of the thigh;
- the **lateral cutaneous nerve** supplying the skin on the lateral side of the thigh;
- the **obturator nerve** supplying the medial muscles of the thigh.

Figure 9.1 shows the three nerves in relation to the pelvis and the hip.

Femoral nerve

This is the largest nerve of the lumbar plexus. It lies in the psoas muscle in the pelvis, and then emerges from the lateral border of the muscle to lie between the psoas and iliacus, leaving the pelvis anteriorly under the inguinal ligament. In the thigh, the femoral nerve branches to supply the quadriceps group of muscles. The saphenous nerve, a branch of the femoral nerve in the thigh, becomes cutaneous at the medial side of the knee and continues on to the medial side of the ankle (Figure 9.3).

Lateral cutaneous nerve

This nerve emerges from the lateral side of the psoas muscle and crosses the iliacus obliquely to the anterior superior spine of the ilium (Figure 9.4). The nerve passes under the lateral end of

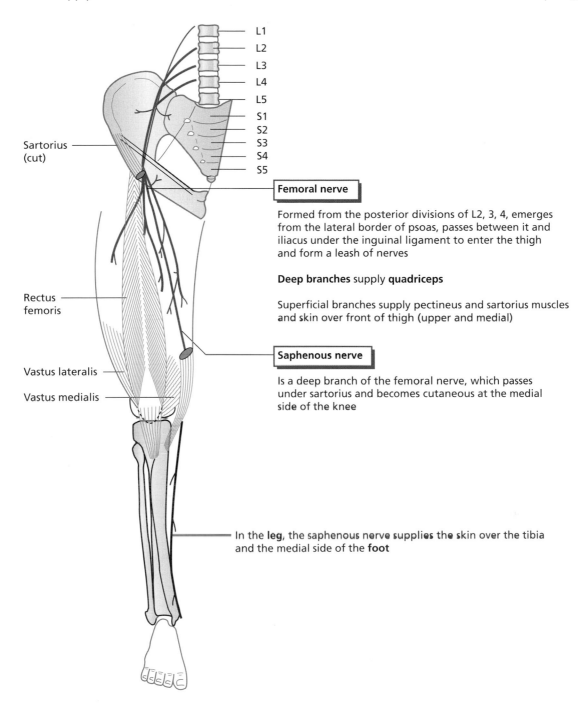

L1
L2
L3
L4
L5
S1
S2
S3
S4
S5

Sartorius
(cut)

Femoral nerve

Formed from the posterior divisions of L2, 3, 4, emerges
from the lateral border of psoas, passes between it and
iliacus under the inguinal ligament to enter the thigh
and form a leash of nerves

Deep branches supply **quadriceps**

Superficial branches supply pectineus and sartorius muscles
and skin over front of thigh (upper and medial)

Rectus
femoris

Saphenous nerve

Is a deep branch of the femoral nerve, which passes
under sartorius and becomes cutaneous at the medial
side of the knee

Vastus lateralis

Vastus medialis

In the **leg**, the saphenous nerve supplies the skin over the tibia
and the medial side of the **foot**

Figure 9.3   Right femoral and saphenous nerve.

209

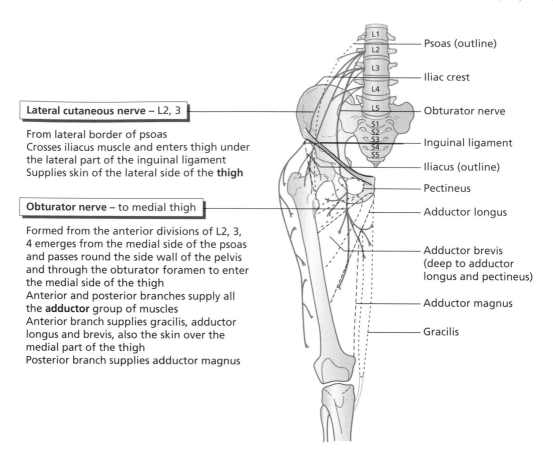

Lateral cutaneous nerve – L2, 3

From lateral border of psoas
Crosses iliacus muscle and enters thigh under
the lateral part of the inguinal ligament
Supplies skin of the lateral side of the **thigh**

Obturator nerve – to medial thigh

Formed from the anterior divisions of L2, 3,
4 emerges from the medial side of the psoas
and passes round the side wall of the pelvis
and through the obturator foramen to enter
the medial side of the thigh
Anterior and posterior branches supply all
the **adductor** group of muscles
Anterior branch supplies gracilis, adductor
longus and brevis, also the skin over the
medial part of the thigh
Posterior branch supplies adductor magnus

Psoas (outline)

Iliac crest

Obturator nerve

Inguinal ligament

Iliacus (outline)

Pectineus

Adductor longus

Adductor brevis
(deep to adductor
longus and pectineus)

Adductor magnus

Gracilis

210

Figure 9.4 Right obturator nerve and lateral cutaneous nerve.

the inguinal ligament and becomes cutaneous in the lateral thigh. Pressure on the nerve in the
area of the iliac spine causes loss of sensation on the lateral side of the thigh.

Obturator nerve

This leaves the medial side of the psoas muscle at the brim of the pelvis and passes through
the obturator foramen of the hip bone to reach the medial side of the thigh (Figure 9.4). In the
medial compartment of the thigh, the obturator nerve supplies all of the adductor group of
muscles.

Reflective task

Look at an articulated skeleton and trace how the three nerves leave the pelvis to enter the
thigh.

Functional importance of the femoral and obturator nerves

The femoral and obturator nerves are both important in walking. The quadriceps, supplied by the femoral nerve, stabilises the knee during support. It propels the body upwards in standing up from sitting. In climbing stairs the quadriceps acts concentrically to lift the body on to the next step, and eccentrically in coming down. The hip adductors, supplied by the obturator nerve, are active to shift the body weight over the supporting foot when the other leg is off the ground. If the adductors are weak owing to damage of the obturator nerve, the leg swings outwards instead of forwards in the swing phase in walking.

Other nerves of the lumbar plexus

Three other cutaneous nerves are formed from the first two nerves of the lumbar plexus. The first lumbar nerve divides into two, the iliohypogastric and the ilioinguinal nerves, which supply the skin of the buttock and groin, respectively. A third cutaneous nerve, the genitofemoral, is formed from L1 and L2, and supplies a small area of skin on the upper front part of the thigh.

Sacral plexus: position and formation

The sacral plexus is formed in the pelvis from the joining of the lumbosacral trunk (L4, L5), the first three and part of the fourth sacral nerves. The landmark to find the position of the sacral plexus in the pelvis is the piriformis muscle, lying across the posterior aspect of the hip joint. The main part of the plexus passes backwards with the piriformis to enter the posterior compartment of the thigh. Figure 9.1 shows the emerging sacral nerves lying on the anterior surface of the sacrum. Figure 9.5 represents the roots of the sacral plexus and the main terminal branches.

Reflective task

- Look at an articulated skeleton and identify the greater sciatic notch of the pelvis, which is converted into the greater sciatic foramen by the sacrospinous ligament joining the sacrum to the ischial spine.
- Look at the anterior surface of the sacrum to see how spinal nerves originating inside the pelvis from the sacral foramina reach the back of the thigh by passing through the greater sciatic foramen. (Remember how the femoral nerve passed anteriorly under the inguinal ligament, and the obturator nerve passed medially through the obturator foramen.)

You should now understand the three directions of exit of nerves from the pelvis to the thigh.

Terminal branches of the sacral plexus

Three main nerves are formed from the sacral plexus: the superior and inferor gluteal nerves and the sciatic nerve. Figure 9.6 shows the three nerves emerging posteriorly through the greater sciatic notch of the pelvis.

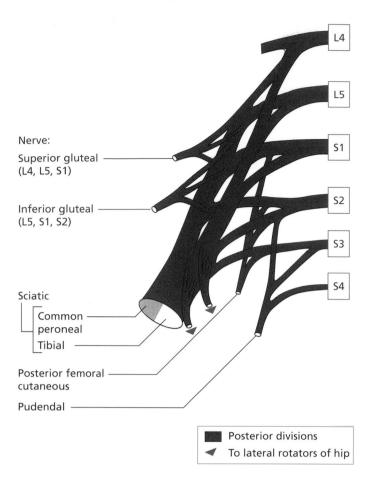

Figure 9.5   Sacral plexus: roots and main terminal branches.

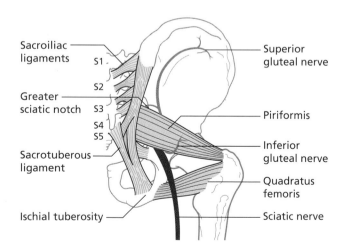

Figure 9.6   Right pelvis and hip, posterior; sciatic nerve and the gluteal nerves emerging through the greater sciatic foramen.

The **superior gluteal nerve** supplies the abductors of the hip: the gluteus medius and minimus and the tensor fascia lata. The **inferior gluteal nerve** supplies the gluteus maximus. These two nerves are found in relation to the piriformis muscles, one of the lateral rotators of the hip. The piriformis is attached to the anterior aspect of the second, third and fourth segments of the sacrum, and passes out of the pelvis into the thigh through the greater sciatic notch of the pelvis to attach to the apex of the greater trochanter of the femur. The two nerves leave the pelvis either above (superior) or below (inferior) the piriformis muscle. Figure 9.6 shows a posterior view of the piriformis muscle with the nerves emerging posteriorly through the greater sciatic notch.

Sciatic nerve

This is the largest nerve in the body, about the same size as the thumb or 2 cm in diameter. The nerve has extensive roots of origin in the spinal cord, L4, L5 and S1–3, and a wide distribution to the posterior muscles of the thigh and all the muscles below the knee (Figure 9.7). This means that pressure on the roots of the sciatic nerve, usually L4 and L5, can have widespread effects in the lower limb.

There are two divisions of the sciatic nerve that lie together as one nerve, deep to the hamstrings in the posterior thigh. The nerve divides into its two components above the knee (Figure 9.7a). Branches of the sciatic nerve high in the thigh supply the hamstring group of muscles. The sciatic nerve also supplies the fibres of the adductor magnus that originate from the ischium. Trauma to the sciatic nerve in the middle of the thigh does not usually affect the hamstrings since the branches to these muscles begin high in the thigh.

The **branches of the sciatic nerve** are the **tibial nerve** and the **common peroneal nerve**.

The **tibial nerve** lies in the popliteal fossa at the back of the knee and continues down the posterior leg between the muscles of the calf. This is the nerve of the posterior muscles of the calf, supplying all of the plantar flexors: the gastrocnemius, soleus, flexor hallucis longus, flexor digitorum longus and tibialis posterior (Figure 9.7a). The **sural nerve** is a cutaneous branch of the tibial nerve in the calf that supplies the skin on the lateral side of the lower calf and the lateral side of the foot (Figure 9.8). A branch of the tibial nerve at the ankle supplies the skin of the heel.

The **common peroneal nerve** (Figure 9.7b) is the lateral part of the sciatic nerve that forms in the upper part of the popliteal fossa. It travels with the biceps femoris of the hamstring group to the lateral side of the knee, where it passes around the neck of the fibula and into the peroneus longus. There it divides into the superficial and deep peroneal nerves.

The **superficial peroneal nerve** lies on the lateral side of the leg, deep to the peroneus longus, and continues over the front of the ankle to supply the skin of the dorsum of the foot. This nerve supplies the evertors, the peroneus longus and brevis.

The **deep peroneal nerve** passes forwards to the anterior compartment of the leg lying on the interosseous membrane between the tibia and fibula. This nerve supplies the dorsiflexors, the tibialis anterior, extensor hallucis longus, extensor digitorum longus and peroneus tertius. The nerve ends on the dorsum of the foot, where it supplies the extensor digitorum brevis and the skin over the first and second toes.

Functional importance of the tibial and the peroneal nerves

The tibial nerve is important for movements that lift the heel to propel the body forwards and upwards in walking, running and jumping. The deep peroneal nerve activates the dorsiflexors of

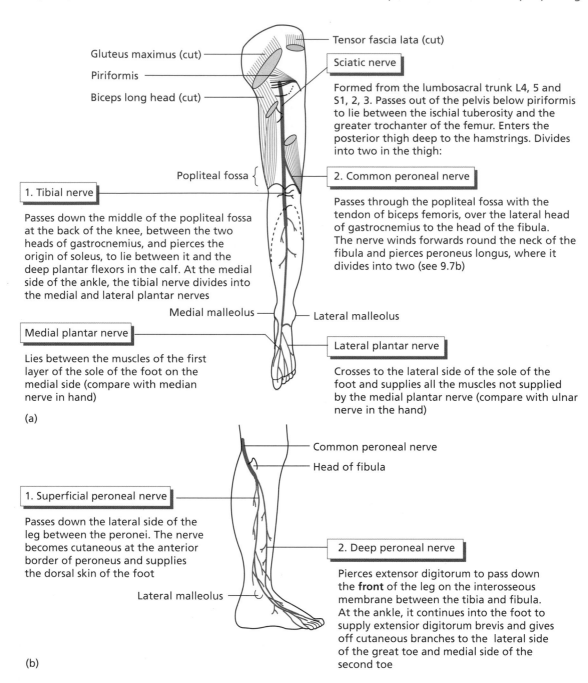

Figure 9.7 Right sciatic nerve and branches; course and distribution: (a) posterior view; (b) lateral view.

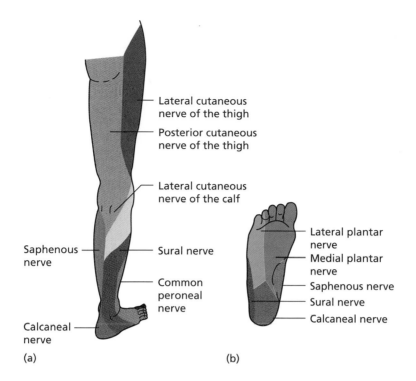

215

Figure 9.8   Cutaneous nerve supply to the right lower limb: (a) posterior view; (b) sole of foot.

the ankle, which lift the toes clear of the ground when the leg swings forwards in locomotion or when kicking a ball. The superficial peroneal nerve stabilises the ankle joint by counteracting the tendency to twist and turn the foot inwards.

Practice note-pad 9A: peroneal nerve lesion

The common peroneal nerve is vulnerable to damage at the lateral side of the knee, at this point it is subcutaneous as it winds round the neck of the fibula. The result of this damage is loss of dorsiflexion and eversion of the ankle, producing 'foot drop' when the leg is lifted off the ground.

Fracture of the shaft of the fibula, common in skiing falls, may injure the superficial peroneal nerve. The foot then tends to go into inversion and the ankle loses stability.

The muscles of the pelvic floor are supplied by the **pudendal nerve** (S2–4), which passes out of the greater sciatic foramen with the sciatic nerve and then turns below the ischial spine to supply the levator ani and coccygeus.

Nerve supply to the foot

The nerves of the plantar surface of the **foot** originate from the tibial nerve at the medial side of the ankle (Figure 9.7a). There are two plantar nerves, which are comparable to the median and ulnar nerves of the hand.

The **medial plantar nerve** supplies the abductor hallucis, flexor hallucis brevis, flexor digitorum brevis and the first lumbrical.

The **lateral plantar nerve** supplies the lateral three lumbricals, all of the interossei, the abductor digiti minimi, flexor digiti minimi and adductor hallucis.

Summary of the cutaneous supply in the foot

The nerve supply to the skin of the sole of the foot is important for sensory information about the contact of the foot with the ground during standing and walking, and the distribution of the body weight over the feet. The major part of the skin of the sole of the foot is supplied by the medial and lateral plantar nerves (Figure 9.8b). The heel receives a branch of the tibial nerve, and the lateral border of the foot receives branches of the sural nerve.

The dorsal surface of the foot is largely supplied by branches of the superficial peroneal nerve, except for a triangular area over the first and second toes which receives branches of the deep peroneal nerve. The saphenous nerve, a branch of the femoral nerve in the thigh, becomes the cutaneous nerve to the medial side of the lower leg and continues to the medial dorsal surface of the foot.

Spinal segmental innervation of the lower limb

In development, the lower limb bud grows out from the side of the embryo. The nerve from the central segment, S1, grows down the limb to end along the outer side of the foot, in the same way that the middle segments of the brachial plexus supply the hand. The later stage of development differs from the upper limb, when the lower limb rotates medially. This means that the dermatomes and myotomes lie in order down the front, and up the back, of the lower limb. Look at Chapter 4, Figure 4.4, to see how the dermatomes of the upper segments L1–5 are in the anterior thigh, knee and leg, while S1–5 are posterior.

The upper lumbar spinal segments supply anterior (quadriceps) and medial (adductors) muscles of the thigh. The lower lumbar spinal segments supply the muscles of the buttock (glutei) and the posterior thigh (hamstrings). All muscles of the leg and foot below the knee are supplied by the fourth and fifth lumbar and the sacral spinal segments. (See Appendix II, Tables A2.3 and A2.4.)

Summary

- The nerve supply of the whole of the lower limb is derived from segments L1–5 and S1–4 of the spinal cord.
- The roots of the spinal nerves emerging from these segments form the lumbar plexus (L1–4) and the sacral plexus (L4, L5, S1–4).
- The femoral, obturator and lateral cutaneous nerves are formed from the lumbar plexus. Direct branches of the lumbar plexus supply the hip flexors, which swing the thigh forwards

in the unsupported limb or move the trunk forwards in preparation for standing up from sitting.

- The functional importance of the femoral and obturator nerves is in stabilising the hip and the knee in standing and walking.
- The sacral plexus forms the superior and inferior gluteal nerves and the sciatic nerve. The superior gluteal nerve supplies the abductors of the hip, which are important in locomotion to prevent the pelvis from dropping on the unsupported side.
- The inferior gluteal nerve supplies the large extensor of the hip, the gluteus maximus. This muscle provides propulsion upwards to lift the body in standing up from sitting, jumping and climbing stairs.
- The sciatic nerve supplies the posterior muscles of the thigh and all the muscles below the knee. Its branches in the leg and the foot supply the muscles that move the ankle in dorsi-flexion and plantar flexion, and the foot in inversion and eversion.
- The course and distribution of the femoral, obturator and sciatic nerves, together with their branches, are shown in Figures 9.3, 9.4 and 9.7.

10

Upright posture and breathing: the trunk

Key terms

structures in maintaining and supporting upright posture, mechanisms of breathing, muscles of the trunk

Conceptual overview

This chapter outlines the structure, musculature and functions of the vertebral column, trunk and pelvis. The collective movements of the trunk are explained in detail in relation to everyday functions that support movement and the maintenance of upright posture during activities of daily living. This chapter also outlines the physical mechanisms of breathing by detailing the muscles involved in movement of the thoracic cage and the role of the diaphragm in facilitating the expansion of the ribs to facilitate breathing. The chapter ends with a brief description of the nerve supply to the muscles of the trunk and neck.

Tyldesley & Grieve's Muscles, Nerves and Movement in Human Occupation, Fourth Edition. Ian R. McMillan, Gail Carin-Levy.
© 2012 Ian R. McMillan, Gail Carin-Levy, Barbara Tyldesley and June I. Grieve. Published 2012 by Blackwell Publishing Ltd.

Introduction

The trunk is the central axis of the body. The limbs use the trunk as the base on which to move. When the body is upright, the trunk supports the head and maintains the erect posture with minimal effort.

The trunk consists of the thorax, abdomen and pelvis, stacked one above the other (Figure 10.1). These three areas form two enclosed cavities, with bony and muscular walls, separated by the muscular diaphragm. Any change in the pressure inside one of the cavities affects the other. The vertebral column links the two cavities posteriorly.

- The **thoracic cavity** extends from the clavicle and first rib above to the muscular diaphragm below. Its walls are formed by the thoracic vertebrae, the ribs and the intercostal muscles in between.
- The **abdominopelvic cavity** has the dome of the diaphragm as the roof and the muscular pelvic floor below. The posterior wall contains the lumbar vertebrae, with muscle on either side of it. The anterolateral wall is formed by the abdominal muscles. The blade of the iliac bone of the pelvis lies in the abdomen. The pelvic part of the cavity is a bowl formed by the sacrum and the two innominate bones, with a muscular floor.

The joints and muscles of the trunk combine to form a stable system when standing upright. The muscles act like guy-ropes keeping the balance when external forces act on the trunk. If a group of muscles becomes weak, the trunk changes its position, in the same way that a tent will lean to one side if a guy-rope is loosened.

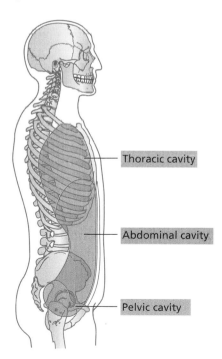

Thoracic cavity

Abdominal cavity

Pelvic cavity

Figure 10.1 Side view of the trunk: outlines of the thoracic and abdominopelvic cavities.

The trunk has a protective function for the lungs, heart, digestive tract, kidneys and pelvic organs (bladder, rectum and reproductive organs). The spinal cord is also protected by being enclosed by the bones of the vertebral column, with pairs of spinal nerves emerging between adjacent vertebrae to be distributed to all parts of the body.

Ventilation of the lungs is the result of changes in the size of the thoracic cavity. Breathing also involves the anterior abdominal wall. Increased abdominal pressure pushes the diaphragm upwards and expels air from the lungs. Changes in the pressure in the abdominopelvic cavity are used to expel urine or faeces and in childbirth.

Lifting, carrying, pushing and pulling heavy loads all involve the trunk. The muscles of the trunk counteract the forces on the limbs, and adjust the line of gravity over the foot base. Carrying a heavy load of shopping in one hand requires muscle activity on the opposite side of the trunk to balance the weight. Increase in pressure in the abdominopelvic cavity, by tensing the anterior abdominal muscles, reduces the stress on the back in lifting loads from the front.

In summary, the trunk:

- maintains the upright posture;
- protects the organs of the thorax, abdomen and pelvis;
- ventilates the lungs in breathing;
- expels urine, faeces, and also the baby at birth;
- adapts to changes in the line of gravity as the body moves;
- releases pressure on the spine when lifting loads.

Most of the movements of the trunk are performed by large muscles arranged in sheets around the axial skeleton. The position of the muscles and direction of the fibres determine the ways in which each contributes to trunk movement.

Upright posture

The bones and ligaments of the vertebral column form a stable balanced support that requires little muscle activity when standing still. Any slight sway is counteracted by the tension in the strong longitudinal ligaments joining the individual vertebrae.

The **vertebral column** contains 33 bony segments. An individual vertebra articulates with the one above and the one below by a cartilaginous joint (intervertebral disc) between the bodies, and by four synovial joints between the articular processes. The position of the articular processes in a thoracic vertebra is shown in Appendix I.

At birth, the vertebral column has a primary curve, concave forwards. As the baby learns to support the weight of the head and trunk in sitting and then standing, two secondary curves develop in the neck and lower back. From 2 years onwards, the vertebral column has four curves as follows: seven cervical vertebrae, convex forwards, secondary; 12 thoracic vertebrae, concave forwards, primary; five lumbar vertebrae, convex forwards, secondary; five sacral vertebrae (fused), concave forwards, primary; and three coccygeal vertebrae.

The four curves provide an efficient way of combining support with flexibility and resilience (Figure 10.2).

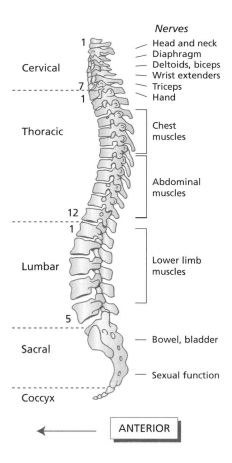

Nerves
- Head and neck
- Diaphragm
- Deltoids, biceps
- Wrist extenders
- Triceps
- Hand

Chest muscles

Abdominal muscles

Lower limb muscles

Bowel, bladder

Sexual function

Cervical
1
7

Thoracic
1
12

Lumbar
1
5

Sacral

Coccyx

ANTERIOR

221

Figure 10.2 Side view of the vertebral column: cervical, thoracic, lumbar and sacral curves.

Reflective task

- Observe a partner standing upright. Look first from the side to imagine a line from the ear through the vertebral column to the hip and knee, ending just in front of the ankle. Move the trunk until the position looks balanced. Notice the curves of the back. Refer to an articulated skeleton to see the curves more easily. Next, look at your partner from the front to see whether the shoulders and hips are level, i.e. no lateral curves.
- Watch a person sitting at a keyboard and notice the shape of the back in relation to the shape of the back of the chair. Try raising and lowering the keyboard to see the effect on the working posture.
- Look at elderly people sitting in easy chairs. Think where a cushion should be placed to support the lumbar curve of the back.

If an abnormal posture is adopted over long periods, the normal relaxed position is progressively lost and muscle activity must be used to a greater extent. Examples of abnormal posture are: **kyphosis**, standing with rounded shoulders; **lordosis**, standing with a hollow back; and **scoliosis**, lateral curvature to the spine, and tilting of the shoulders.

Shoes with high heels throw the body weight forwards and the vertebral column adapts by increasing the lumbar curvature (lordosis). Problems with breathing may develop in scoliosis owing to the effect on the shape of the thorax. Poor working posture increases the possibility of lower back pain, even in the young. In the elderly, degenerative changes in the vertebrae and discs due to disease or ageing, coupled with the loss of the need and motivation to move about during the day, give general loss of mobility, and deformity develops which may become permanent.

Joints and movements of the vertebral column

When the trunk moves in different directions, the movement between adjacent vertebrae is small, but the result of combined movement of vertebrae at all levels results in a considerable range of movement.

Joints of the vertebral column

> **Reflective task**
>
> Look at the structure of a vertebra, seen from above and from the side, in Appendix I and in an articulated skeleton.

There are two series of joints between adjacent vertebrae in the column: anterior and posterior.

The **anterior joints** are between the bodies of the vertebrae: these articulations are secondary cartilaginous joints, the intervertebral discs. They increase in thickness from the upper cervical vertebrae down to the lumbar vertebrae. In the fibrocartilaginous discs, which form about a quarter of the total length of the vertebral column, the collagen fibres are arranged in concentric layers, the annulus fibrosus. The semifluid central mass of the disc is the nucleus pulposus. During movements of the trunk, the cartilaginous discs are compressed on one side (see Chapter 1, Figure 1.6b).

The **posterior joints** are between the articular processes on the vertebral arch of bone which surrounds the spinal cord: these are synovial plane joints. A thin capsule surrounds the adjacent articular surfaces and allows gliding movements between adjacent vertebrae.

All of the vertebrae are joined together by anterior and posterior longitudinal ligaments that extend along the whole length of the vertebral column joining the respective surfaces of the vertebral bodies. Other ligaments join all of the spines and transverse processes of the vertebrae.

> **Practice note-pad 10A: prolapsed intervertebral disc**
>
> Sudden movement that involves compression of the intervertebral disc may result in tearing of the annulus fibrosus (outer coating), and this allows the nucleus pulposus to protrude and press on the spinal cord or the roots of a spinal nerve. Severe pain then radiates down the path of the affected nerve, for example in the lower limb this may be experienced as sciatica.

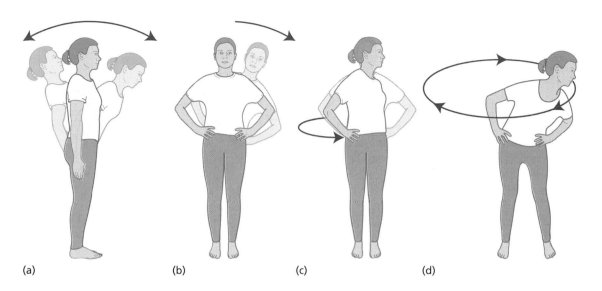

(a)   (b)   (c)   (d)

Figure 10.3   Movements of the trunk: (a) flexion (forwards) and extension (backwards); (b) lateral flexion; (c) rotation; (d) circumduction.

The **movements of the trunk**, shown in Figure 10.3, are described as follows:

*   **Flexion** occurs in bending forwards, or sitting up from lying. The thorax moves towards the pelvis.
*   **Extension** straightens the trunk from flexion and the trunk can bend backwards from the upright position. The thorax moves away from the pelvis.
*   **Lateral flexion** bends the trunk to the side. The ribs move towards the pelvis on one side only.
*   **Rotation** twists the trunk to the right or the left. The head and shoulders are turned so that the eyes can look to the side or behind, either to the right or left.

The trunk-rolling exercise shown in Figure 10.3d is a combination of all of these movements.

The range of the individual movements varies in different parts of the vertebral column, depending on the thickness of the intervertebral discs, the direction of the articular facets of the synovial joints, and the length and angulation of the spines. The regions with secondary curves have the greatest mobility. Movements of the cervical region are important for the eyes to scan a large area. Reversing a car becomes difficult when there is loss of mobility in the neck. The lumbar region has the greatest range for flexion and extension movements. The extreme bending movements of the acrobat and gymnast are achieved by continual exercises to stretch the intervertebral ligaments and increase the separation of the lumbar vertebrae. Conversely, the fusion of the lumbar vertebrae in some pathological changes of the spine will reduce the overall mobility of the trunk by a significant amount.

Muscles moving the trunk

Two systems of muscles collectively perform all movements of the trunk: the deep posterior muscles of the back and the abdominal muscles.

223

Deep posterior muscles of the back

The posterior aspect of the vertebral column, from the sacrum to the skull, provides a long line of bony processes for the attachment of muscle fibres. Some of these muscles fibres are long, extending from the sacrum to the thorax, while others are short and only span one, two or three vertebrae. The vertical fibres pull the column into extension, those arranged obliquely can rotate one vertebra on the next, and the lateral fibres which are attached to the angles of the ribs can assist lateral flexion.

The largest muscle in this group of deep back muscles is the **erector spinae** (also known as the sacrospinalis), which originates from the sacrum by a thick broad tendon. In the lumbar region, this muscle is thick and can be palpated in the lower back. Continuing upwards, the muscle is in three bands in the thoracic region, attached to the spines of the vertebrae, the transverse processes and the ribs. The uppermost fibres in the cervical region end on the base of the skull.

The muscles connecting the trunk to the upper limb, for example the latissimus dorsi and trapezius (described in Chapter 5), are separated from the deep muscles of the back by a layer of deep fascia.

Figure 10.4 follows the line of erector spinae on the right-hand side of the vertebral column. Note how the muscle starts at the sacrum and climbs up the back to the head. Deep to the erector spinae another group of muscles is found (Figure 10.4, left-hand side of the vertebral column). Most of the fibres in this deeper group lie obliquely from the transverse process of one vertebra to the spine of the vertebra above, or they may span three or four vertebrae. The parts found in the thorax and neck are known as **semispinalis**.

In movements of the trunk, the erector spinae acts strongly to raise the body from forward flexion to an upright position. The erector spinae counteracts both the tendency to sway forwards in standing and the force of loads carried in front of the body.

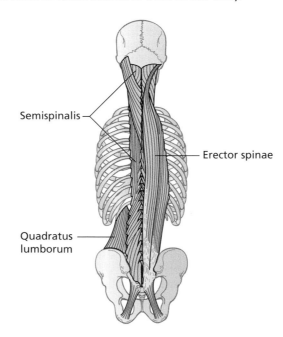

Figure 10.4   Erector spinae (right); semispinalis and quadratus lumborum (left), posterior view of the trunk.

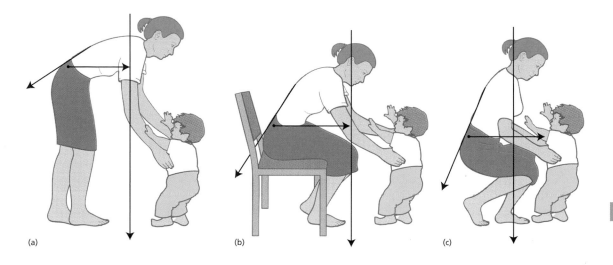

Figure 10.5   Lifting: (a) straight legs; (b) sitting; (c) knees bent. 1 = line of gravity, 2 = load arm; 3 = effort force.

Lifting loads placed in front of the body may cause considerable stress on the lower back. In raising the trunk and the load, the pull of the erector spinae muscle compresses the lumbar intervertebral discs, which may prolapse (see Practice note-pad 10A). The aim of good lifting practice is to reduce the compression force on the lumbar discs. Figure 10.5 shows the application of the principle of levers (see Chapter 2) in three positions for lifting a child.

In lifting with straight legs, the starting position is forward flexion (Figure 10.5a). From this position, the line of weight of the trunk plus the child (1) is some distance from the fulcrum in the lower back, so that the load arm (2) is long. The erector spinae, acting on a short lever arm, must develop considerable effort force (3) to overcome the moment of force of the trunk.

In lifting from the sitting position (Figure 10.5b), the line of weight (1) is even further from the fulcrum and the load arm (2) is longer. The compression load on the discs is therefore much greater as the erector spinae extends the spine. People in wheelchairs should avoid lifting heavy loads, since the stress on the back will be greater than the same load lifted by someone who can stand close to the load.

In lifting with the knees bent and with the load as close to the body as possible, the line of weight (1) is moved nearer to the body, and the load arm of the trunk plus the child (2) is short. This means that the effort force (3) exerted by erector spinae to counteract the load is reduced. In addition, it allows the extensors of the hip and the knee to contribute most of the effort force for the lift. This explains how bending the knees and keeping the trunk as upright as possible puts less stress on the back in lifting.

Anterior abdominal wall

The anterior abdominal wall consists of flat sheets of muscle forming a four-way corset or girdle between the ribs and the pelvis. The position of the individual muscles is as follows. The rectus abdominis lies down the centre of the abdomen, one on either side of the midline. The muscle fibres are in the vertical direction. The external and internal oblique abdominal muscles are two sheets of muscle around the anterior and lateral walls of the abdomen. The muscle fibres are arranged diagonally. The transversus abdominis is a muscle lying deep to the obliques which has horizontal fibres forming a band wrapping round the abdomen.

Figure 10.6a shows the direction of the fibres of the abdominal muscles seen from the side. The fibres of the two oblique muscles and transversus abdominis blend into an aponeurosis (dense fibrous tissue) towards the midline, connecting with those from the opposite side to form a sheath around the rectus abdominis.

The **rectus abdominis** (Figure 10.6b) is a strap-like muscle extending from the lower end of the sternum and the costal cartilages of the fifth, sixth and seventh ribs to the pubis below. The muscle fibres are usually interrupted at three intervals by transverse bands of fibrous tissue, known as tendinous intersections. The four bulges of muscle fibres in between can be seen clearly in men who have done weight training. The rectus abdominis flexes the trunk by pulling the sternum towards the pelvis, so acting strongly in sitting up from lying. When the body is lifted off the ground, as in running and jumping, the rectus abdominis supports the front of the pelvis.

The **external oblique** abdominal muscle is attached to the outer surfaces of the lower eight ribs. The posterior fibres pass vertically to insert on the anterior part of the iliac crest of the pelvis. All of the other fibres lie in a direction downwards and forwards, i.e. like hands in a side-pocket, to attach to the wide central aponeurosis (Figure 10.6c). The lower margin of the muscle and aponeurosis is thickened to form the inguinal ligament, which extends from the anterior superior iliac spine to the pubic crest (see Chapter 8, Figure 8.10). The inguinal ligament acts as a retinaculum forming the division between the trunk and the thigh.

The **internal oblique** abdominal muscle is attached to the fascia of the lower back (thoracolumbar fascia), the anterior iliac crest (deep to the external oblique) and the inguinal ligament. The muscle fibres pass upwards and inwards, to attach to the lower ribs, and become a wide aponeurosis as far as the midline (Figure 10.6d). The aponeuroses of the right and left obliques meet in the midline at the linea alba, a strip of fascia from the lower end of the sternum to the pubic symphysis.

The muscle fibres of the two oblique abdominal muscles lie at right angles to each other. The ways in which the two layers of oblique abdominal muscles work in combination to produce movements of the trunk will now be considered.

- **Flexion** of the trunk involves the external and internal obliques on both sides together.
- **Lateral flexion** involves the external and internal oblique on one side only.
- **Rotation** of the trunk involves the external oblique on one side working with the internal oblique on the opposite side. The trunk then rotates towards the side of the internal oblique (Figure 10.6e).

In standing and sitting, the oblique abdominals work with the neck muscles in turning to look to the side and behind. In walking, the pelvis is carried forwards on the side of the leading leg and the trunk rotates to keep the eyes looking forwards.

Reflective task

Lie down supine and feel the abdominal muscles working in:

(1) sitting up from lying;
(2) lifting the head from lying. Feel the rectus abdominis working statically to fix the thorax so that the neck muscles can act on the head;
(3) sitting up from lying while turning the trunk to the left at the same time. Think which abdominal muscles are working.

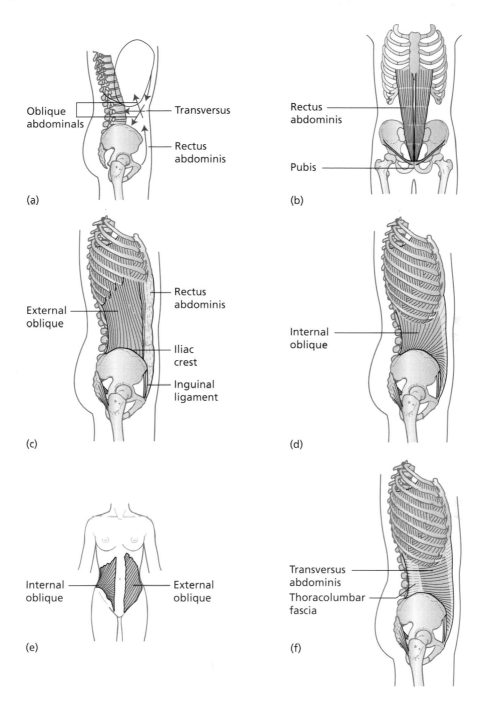

Figure 10.6 Muscles of the anterior abdominal wall: (a) direction of the muscle fibres; (b) rectus abdominis, anterior view; (c) right external oblique abdominal, side view; (d) right internal oblique abdominal, side view; (e) oblique abdominals working togerher; (f) right transversus abdominis, side view.

It should now be clear why it is difficult to sit up from lying if the abdominal muscles are weak, for example after abdominal surgery, with fractured ribs or in the late stages of pregnancy. In these instances sitting up can be performed by turning on to one side and pushing up with the opposite arm to raise the trunk. The legs can then be swung round to the sitting position (see Chapter 13).

The **transversus abdominis** is the deepest abdominal muscle, originating from the inner aspect of the costal margin, the thoracolumbar fascia, iliac crest and inguinal ligament. From this extensive posterior origin, the fibres pass transversely round the abdomen to form a central aponeurosis anteriorly. The muscles from each side meet in the midline at the linea alba. Figure 10.6f shows the right transversus viewed from the side. The transversus has no action in moving the trunk. The tension in the transversus supports the abdominal organs and contraction increases the pressure inside the abdomen. This rise in pressure aids the expulsion of air from the lungs in breathing.

The **functions of the anterior abdominal wall** are: support and protection of the abdominal organs; expulsion of the contents of the pelvic organs in micturition, defecation and parturition; increase in the depth of expiration in breathing; and relief of pressure on the lower back in lifting.

The organs of the digestive system lie in the abdomen. Contraction of the muscles of the anterior abdominal wall improves the circulation of blood and aids digestion. The pelvic organs (the bladder, rectum and uterus) are protected by the bony pelvis. In straining movements, the muscles of the anterior abdominal wall contract and raise the pressure inside the abdomen to expel the urine and faeces. When lifting loads with the back, contraction of the abdominal muscles raises the intra-abdominal pressure. This pressure is distributed upwards and downwards, and reduces the pressure on the intervertebral discs of the lumbar region set up by the back muscles. Weightlifters learn to use the abdominal muscles to reduce the stress on the back. A sudden or unexpected demand for lifting can produce back strain. Even simple everyday tasks, such as making a bed, can cause back injury. Some of the lifting tasks used in the care of the disabled have been replaced by the use of hoists, but it is still important to be aware that contraction of the abdominal muscles can relieve stress on the back when lifting a patient.

The function of the anterior abdominal muscles in breathing will be described later in this chapter with the action of the diaphragm.

The **posterior abdominal wall** between the 12th rib and the posterior part of the iliac crest is formed by the **quadratus lumborum**. This muscle lies lateral to the psoas and deep to the origin of the transversus abdominis (Figure 10.4). Contraction of the quadratus lumborum on one side only assists lateral flexion of the trunk. Acting in reverse, the muscle can lift the pelvic brim on the same side, which prevents the pelvis dropping down on the unsupported side in standing on one leg. The quadratus lumborum on both sides together stabilise the lumbar vertebrae and the pelvis during movements of the upper trunk and upper limb.

Muscles moving the head and neck

The two main functions of the muscles of the head and neck are to hold the head upright on the trunk, and to allow the eyes to focus over a wide field of vision by turning the head.

Two of the muscles supporting the head on the trunk are the upper fibres of the trapezius (described in Chapter 5) and the upper part of the erector spinae. Lying in between these two muscles at the back of the neck is another pair of muscles, the **splenius capitis** and **splenius cervicis** (Figure 10.7). Holding down the deep muscles of the neck in this region, the splenius capitis

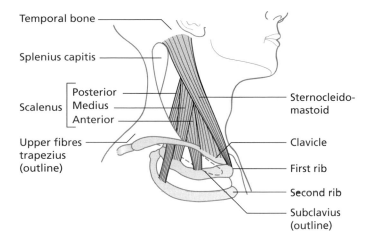

Temporal bone
Splenius capitis
Scalenus [Posterior, Medius, Anterior]
Upper fibres trapezius (outline)
Sternocleido-mastoid
Clavicle
First rib
Second rib
Subclavius (outline)

Figure 10.7   Sternomastoid: scalenus anterior, medius and posterior; right side view of the neck.

has been called the 'bandage muscle'. The splenius muscles are attached to the lower part of the ligament in the midline of the neck (ligamentum nuchae) and to the spines of the upper four thoracic vertebrae. Passing upwards and laterally, the capitis is inserted on the base of the skull, to the mastoid process of the temporal bone and adjacent occipital bone. The splenius cervicis inserts on to the transverse processes of cervical vertebrae 1–4. Working statically, the splenius muscles prevent the head from falling forwards. Both sides working together pull the head backwards in extension. If one side only contracts, the head is rotated to turn the face to the same side.

The most superficial muscle on the front of the neck, clearly visible in action, is the **sterno-cleidomatoid**, often shortened to sternomastoid (Figure 10.7). This strap-like muscle crosses the neck diagonally, and combines with other muscles to perform all of the movements of the head. Its name indicates the attachments of this muscle. From the upper end of the sternum and the medial end of the clavicle, the sternocleidomastoid crosses upwards and outwards to end on the mastoid process of the temporal bone of the skull, extending medially to meet the upper fibres of the trapezius. Both sides of the sternomastoid working together draw the head forwards and act strongly to lift the head up when lying supine. One side contracting produces lateral flexion and rotation to the opposite side. These movements are important in looking from side to side to scan the visual field. The sternomastoid and the splenius muscles combine to produce most of the turning movements of the head. When the head is tilted backwards beyond the vertical, the sternomastoid can act as a neck extensor.

A group of three muscles in the lateral part of the neck comprises the **scalenes**: scalenus anterior, medius and posterior (Figure 10.7). Attached centrally to the transverse processes of the cervical vertebrae, the scalenes pass downwards and laterally to the first and second ribs. These muscles are an important landmark in the location of the brachial plexus, which passes between the scalenus anterior and scalenus medius in its course towards the first rib. The scalenes flex the cervical spine if both sides contract, or produce lateral flexion if one side only is active. The muscles are also used to fix the first two ribs in deep inspiration before a powerful or long exhalation as when singing or playing a wind instrument.

> **Reflective task**
>
> Lie supine and lift the head. Feel the sternomastoid and scalenes in action. Turn the head to the right and feel the left sternomastoid in action.

Breathing

The action of the muscles moving the ribs, and the muscle dividing the thorax and abdomen (the diaphragm), combine to change the size of the thoracic cavity and to ventilate the lungs. The abdominal muscles are also involved in breathing, since their activity affects the position of the diaphragm.

The two lungs fill the thoracic cavity, apart from the space occupied by the heart and major blood vessels. Shaped like two cones, the base of each lung sits on the diaphragm and the apex of each lies above the clavicle. Each lung is surrounded by a narrow, airtight space called the pleural cavity. The pleural membranes which form this cavity are attached to the outer surface of the lungs and the inner wall of the thorax. The cavity between the membranes is a completely enclosed space in which the pressure is lower than the pressure of the air outside the thorax. As the thorax expands as a result of muscle contraction, the lowered pressure in the pleural cavity causes the lungs to be expanded also. The two layers of pleura remain in contact like the sides of a new plastic bag when one tries to separate them.

When the lungs expand, the air pressure within the air sacs is reduced and atmospheric air is drawn in through the nose and trachea to equalise the pressure inside the lungs. Relaxation of the muscles reduces the size of the thorax to the resting volume and the pressure in the air sacs rises, therefore air passes out into the atmosphere.

The exact amount of air entering and leaving the lungs at any one time depends on the amount of movement of the thorax. Other factors that influence the volume of air breathed are the elasticity and inertia of the lung tissue, and the resistance offered by the airways in the lungs.

In quiet breathing, active expansion of the thorax occurs in inspiration, while expiration is passive. Additional muscle activity is recruited during deep inspiration, and expiration becomes active.

> **Practice note-pad 10B: pneumothorax**
>
> In relation to the chest, If the pleural membranes are punctured by a stab wound, or as a result of infection, then air can enter the pleural cavity and the pressure rises. This reduces tension on the elasticity of the lung and it may collapse. Once the pleural membrane heals, the excess air is slowly absorbed into the bloodstream and the lung reinflates.

Joints and movements of the thoracic cage

Articulations

Posteriorly, the 12 ribs articulate with the thoracic vertebrae at the **costovertebral joints**. These are formed between facets on the head of the rib and those on the sides of the bodies of two adjacent vertebrae and the transverse process of the corresponding vertebra. The costovertebral joints are synovial of the plane type.

Anteriorly, the **sternocostal joints** are formed by the costal cartilages of the second to the seventh ribs articulating directly with the sternum by synovial joints, each with a capsule and ligaments. The first sternocostal joint is a primary cartilaginous joint. The eigth, ninth and tenth ribs link indirectly to the sternum by their costal cartilages. The 11th and 12th ribs, which are small and free anteriorly, play little part in breathing.

Reflective task

Look at the position of the ribs on an articulated skeleton. Posteriorly, identify the position of two synovial joints, one between the head of the rib and the body of the vertebra, one between the tubercle of the rib and the transverse process. Anteriorly, the first to seventh ribs join with the sternum by the costal cartilages.

Note two things about the general direction of ribs 2–7: (i) the anterior end is lower than the vertebral articulations; and (ii) when viewed from the side, the central part of each rib is lower than both the anterior and the posterior ends.

Movements at all of the joints provides the mobility of the ribs required to ventilate the lungs. Ribs 2–7 move about two axes simultaneously (Figure 10.8):

- axis A–A′ passes through the neck of each rib. When the rib moves about this axis, the sternum is raised upwards and forwards to increase the anterior to posterior diameter of the thorax;
- axls B–B′ passes through the angle of the ribs posteriorly and the sternocostal joints anteriorly. Movement about this axis lifts the middle of the rib upwards and outwards to increase the transverse diameter of the thorax.

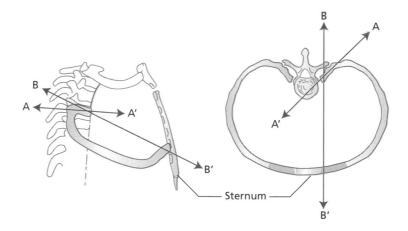

Sternum

Figure 10.8 Movement of a rib in side view and plan view: A–A′ axis through the neck of the rib; B–B′ axis through the vertebral and sternal ends of the rib.

The eight, ninth and tenth ribs have no sternocostal joints and therefore only move about one axis (A–A′).

> **Reflective task**
>
> - Place your hands on the thorax of a partner, first at the sides over the lower rib cage. Ask your partner to breathe in deeply and watch how your hands move further apart, i.e. the thorax becomes wider.
> - Next, stand at the side and place one hand flat on the sternum, the other hand flat on the thoracic vertebrae. Again ask your partner to breathe in deeply, and notice how the hand on the sternum moves forwards and upwards.
>   These two movements occur together each time the ribs move.

Muscles moving the ribs

The external and internal intercostal muscles, which form two layers in the space between adjacent ribs, move the ribs in quiet breathing.

The fibres of the **external intercostal muscles** pass obliquely from the lower border of one rib to the upper border of the rib below. At the anterior end of each intercostal space, the muscle is replaced by membrane. The posterior fibres pass downwards and laterally, and the more anterior fibres lie downwards and medially, i.e. in the same direction as the external oblique abdominal muscles. The first rib does not move in quiet breathing. Figure 10.9 shows the position of the external intercostal muscles in the spaces between ribs 1–6. Contraction of the external intercostals lifts the ribs about the two axes described. The thorax increases in size by expanding in a forwards and sideways direction, and air is drawn into the lungs.

The **internal intercostal muscles** lie deep to the external intercostals, and their fibres are at right angles, downwards and backwards from one rib to the one below. The muscle fibres are

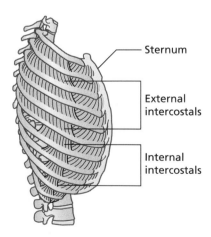

Figure 10.9   Intercostal muscles: external intercostals shown in the upper five intercostal spaces; internal intercostals (deep to the external) shown in the lower six spaces.

replaced by membrane at the posterior end of the intercostal space, between the angle and head of each rib. Figure 10.9 shows the position of the internal intercostal muscles in the spaces between ribs 6–10. There is conflicting evidence about the action of the internal intercostals. It has been shown that the anterior fibres between the costal cartilages are active in inspiration. Other studies have shown activity during speech, which is expiratory. The contribution of the internal intercostals to rib movements probably depends on which fibres are active, and on the level of inflation of the lungs.

Relaxation of the intercostal muscles lowers the ribs to their resting position, and air leaves the lungs. Expiration in quiet breathing is therefore passive.

In **deep breathing**, the muscles in the neck that elevate the shoulder girdle and upper ribs allow the thorax to expand further in inspiration. The main muscles that are recruited to increase the depth of inspiration are the sternomastoid, the scalenes (Figure 10.7) and the pectoralis minor (see Chapter 5, Figure 5.6). These muscles pull the clavicle and first two ribs upwards when their upper attachments are fixed. The result is that the other ribs can move up further.

Reflective task

Watch the neck of a person breathing deeply to see the activity in neck muscles.

In deep expiration, the latissimus dorsi (see Chapter 5, Figure 5.11a), which wraps round the rib cage from the lower back to the shoulder, can compress the ribs further if the humerus is fixed. The abdominal muscles are also involved in deep expiration, see later in this chapter.

Practice note-pad 10C: asthma and chronic obstructive airways disease (COAD)

Asthma can occur in children and adults. Attacks of breathing difficulty occur in response to certain protein substances, such as pollen or animal protein, which release allergens within the body. The muscular walls of the narrow airways in the lungs constrict. Inspiration that is initiated by muscle activity can take place, but passive expiration becomes difficult. Expiratory muscles have to be used to try to force the air out of the lungs.

COAD can be seen in older people. There is a chronic inflammation of the lining of the airways (chronic bronchitis) and the air sacs become distended (emphysema). The thorax and the lungs become less elastic. The muscles of the neck and shoulders, normally used in deep inspiration, are used for quiet breathing, and diaphragmatic breathing becomes more important.

The diaphragm

The diaphragm is a dome-shaped muscle that forms the floor of the thoracic cavity. At rest, the fibres of the peripheral part of the dome are almost vertical. Converging inwards, the muscle fibres end in a central tendon, a strong flat aponeurosis shaped like a trefoil or clover leaf. The central tendon is nearer to the front of the thorax than the back, so that the posterior fibres are longer. The heart lies immediately above the central tendon with the pericardium, the membrane round the heart, attached to it.

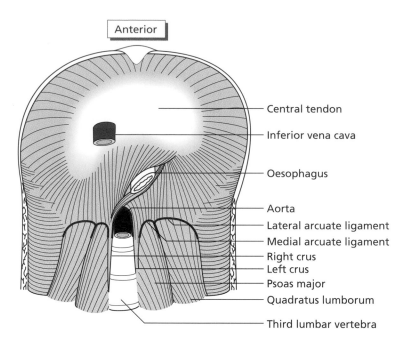

Anterior

— Central tendon

— Inferior vena cava

— Oesophagus

— Aorta
— Lateral arcuate ligament
— Medial arcuate ligament
— Right crus
— Left crus
— Psoas major
— Quadratus lumborum
— Third lumbar vertebra

234

Figure 10.10   Diaphragm viewed from below.

Reflective task

Look at an umbrella (with a very curved shape if possible). The ribs of the umbrella are in the direction of the muscles fibres of the dome of the diaphragm. Imagine the point of the umbrella compressed into a flat trefoil shape to understand the position of the central tendon.

Figure 10.10 is a view of the diaphragm from below (i.e. in the abdomen looking up to the undersurface of the muscle). The muscle fibres of the diaphragm originate all round the lower margin of the thorax. Beginning anteriorly, fibres originate from the xiphoid process of the sternum. Next, ribs 7–12 and their costal cartilages form the largest surface for the attachment of fibres. Posteriorly, the origin from the 12th rib is interrupted by the muscles of the posterior abdominal wall, the quadratus lumborum and psoas. These two muscles are bridged by fibrous bands, known as the lateral and medial arcuate ligaments, which provide a base for the attachment of the diaphragm. The most posterior fibres originate from the sides of the lumbar vertebrae by two bands, the right crus (from L1, L2 and L3) and the left crus (from L1 and L2), which arch over the aorta in the midline. The right crus is longer to overcome the resistance of the larger liver lying below the diaphragm on the right side.

Figure 10.10 follows the complete circle that forms the origin of the diaphragm, which can be summarised as follows: sternal fibres from the xiphoid process of the sternum; costal fibres from the inner surfaces of ribs 7–12; lumbar fibres from the arcuate ligaments over the muscles of the posterior abdominal wall, and from lumbar vertebrae by two crura.

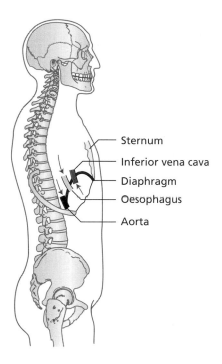

Sternum

Inferior vena cava

Diaphragm

Oesophagus

Aorta

Figure 10.11   Diaphragm viewed from the side.

Figure 10.11 shows how the sternal origin is higher than the lumbar origin. The inferior vena cava passes through the central tendon and the oesophagus passes through the muscular part just towards the left of the midline. The aorta lies posteriorly against the vertebral column.

The **action of the diaphragm** can be understood by focusing on the shape of the dome. When the diaphragm is active, the contractile muscle fibres pull the central tendon downwards and the dome becomes flatter. When the diaphragm relaxes, the muscle fibres return to their resting length and the central tendon moves upwards. Remember: contract – down; relax – up.

The muscles of the anterior abdominal wall can actively participate in breathing out. Contraction of the abdominal muscles raises the pressure inside the abdomen and the diaphragm is pushed upwards. The vertical diameter of the thorax is decreased and air is expelled from the lungs in expiration. The diaphragm and abdominal muscles co-operate in breathing movements.

> **Reflective task**
>
> Place your hands on your anterior abdominal wall. Breathe in deeply, lifting the ribs, and feel the abdominals relax as the diaphragm moves down. Breathe out deeply, contracting the abdominals to expel as much air as possible.

During quiet breathing, the contribution of the abdominal muscles to the ventilation of the lungs varies in different individuals. In deep breathing, the contraction of the abdominal muscles increases the depth of expiration. The ability to control the muscle work of the abdominals is important in singing and in some relaxation techniques.

Pelvic tilt and the pelvic floor

The pelvis is a staging post for muscles passing upwards to the trunk or downwards to the lower limbs. Muscles of the trunk that are attached to the pelvis are the rectus abdominis, oblique abdominals, erector spinae and quadratus lumborum. Muscles of the lower limb attached to the pelvis are the iliopsoas, gluteus maximus, medius and minimus, hamstrings, hip adductors, rectus femoris, tensor fascia lata and sartorius (see Chapter 8).

The **tilt** of the pelvis in relaxed standing largely depends on the weight of the trunk above, that tends to tilt the upper end of the sacrum forwards and the lower end backwards. This tendency for rotation of the sacrum is prevented by the sacrospinous and sacrotuberous ligaments, two strong bands that bind the sacrum to the hip bone (Figure 10.12). Pelvic tilt is affected by the opposing tension in the rectus abdominis pulling the pubis up towards the ribs, and the gluteus maximus pulling on the posterior surface of the sacrum in the opposite direction. Wearing shoes with high heels tilts the pelvis anteriorly and the lumbar lordosis increases to compensate. Posterior or backward tilting occurs when sitting in low chairs with poor back support. In this sitting position the lumbar curvature of the spine is lost.

Lateral tilting of the pelvis when one leg is lifted off the ground is counteracted by contraction of the gluteus medius and minimus on the supported side (see Chapter 8). When the glutei and the knee flexors are weak, the toes of the swinging leg in walking drag on the ground. In this case,

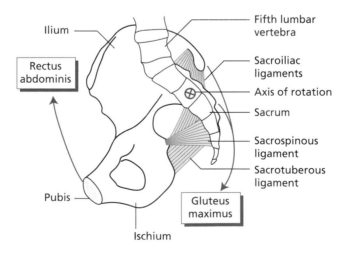

Figure 10.12   Pelvic tilting. Arrows indicate the direction of pull of the rectus abdominis and gluteus maximus. Right innominate bone and sacrum viewed from the inside of the pelvis.

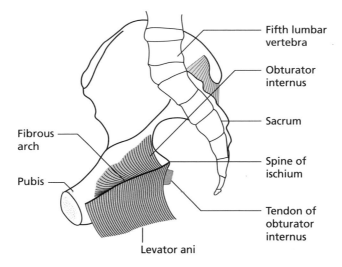

Fifth lumbar vertebra

Obturator internus

Sacrum

Fibrous arch

Spine of ischium

Pubis

Tendon of obturator internus

Levator ani

Figure 10.13   Levator ani of the pelvic floor. Right innominate bone viewed from the inside of the pelvis.

the dropping of the pelvis to the unsupported side can be conteracted by the contraction of the quadratus lumborum and the latissimus dorsi on that side; this is known as 'hip hitching'.

Pelvic floor

The muscles of the floor of the pelvis are suspended from the bony walls of the pelvis, and from a fibrous arch, a thickened band in the pelvic fascia. This fibrous arch extends from the pubis anteriorly to the spine of the ischium posteriorly. The main muscle of the pelvic floor, the levator ani, is attached to this band of fascia (Figure 10.13). The fibres of the levator ani descend and then turn inwards to meet those from the opposite side in the midline. Posteriorly to the levator ani, the pelvic floor is completed by the coccygeus muscle, which extends from the spine of the ischium to the lower part of the sacrum and the coccyx.

The functions of the pelvic floor are to support the pelvic organs, and to withstand any increase in pressure in the abdominopelvic cavity, for example in lifting, coughing and sneezing. In women, the levator ani surrounds the vagina and supports the uterus.

Practice note-pad 10D: stress incontinence

Stretching of the muscles of the pelvic floor in childbirth may affect the action of the levator ani on the control of the bladder and the rectum. This leads to incontinence, particularly at times when there is a sharp rise in intra-abdominal pressure such as coughing, sneezing and laughing.

Nerve supply of the muscles of the neck and trunk

The muscles of the trunk are supplied by branches of spinal nerves at the cervical, thoracic and sacral levels.

In the **neck**, the spinal accessory (cranial) nerve, together with branches of C2 and C3, supply the sternomastoid muscles. Branches of C6, C7 and C8 supply the scalene muscles.

In the **thorax**, the **phrenic nerves** supply the two sides of the diaphragm. They are formed from branches of the third, fourth and fifth cervical nerves in the neck. Each nerve passes down the neck deep to the sternomastoid and enters the thorax. The right phrenic nerve lies on the pericardium covering the right atrium and pierces the central tendon of the diaphragm with the inferior vena cava. The left phrenic nerve lies on the pericardium over the left ventricle and pierces the diaphragm in front of the central tendon (Figure 10.14). Each phrenic nerve is the motor and sensory supply to the corresponding side of the diaphragm.

Practice note-pad 10E: cervical spine injuries

Injuries to the neck may occur by falls from a height, a blow on the head, or violent free movements of the neck, for example in a road traffic accident. If there is damage to the roots of the phrenic nerves (C3–5), a loss of the action of the diaphragm in breathing occurs and a ventilator must be used.

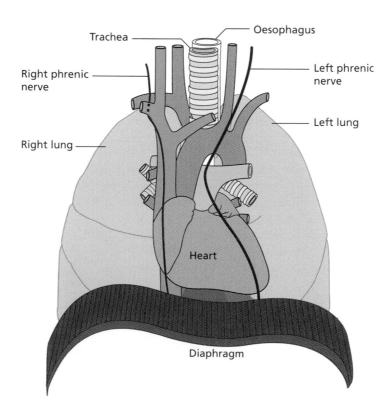

Figure 10.14   Phrenic nerve: position and relations in the thorax.

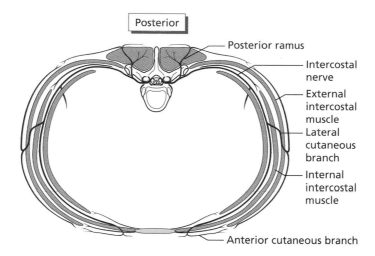

Figure 10.15 Transverse section of the thorax through an intercostal space showing one pair of intercostal nerves.

The thoracic spinal nerves form the **intercostal nerves**, which supply the intercostal muscles. Intercostal nerves 1–6 run parallel to the corresponding rib and deep to the internal intercostal muscles (Figure 10.15). Branches of the intercostal nerves 7–12 continue forwards from the intercostal spaces to the muscles of the **anterior abdominal wall**. Each layer of the anterior abdominal wall (the rectus abdominis, the oblique abdominals and transversus) receives branches of the thoracic nerves 7–12 from above downwards. Thoracic nerve 12 branches to supply the quadratus lumborum in the posterior abdominal wall.

The muscles of the **pelvic floor** are supplied by branches of the third and fourth sacral spinal nerves.

Summary of the muscles of the trunk

- **Muscles moving the head and neck**: sternocleidomastoid; scalenus anterior, medius and posterior; splenius capitis and cervicis.
- **Muscles moving the thorax in the ventilation of the lungs**: external and internal intercostals; diaphragm.
- **Deep posterior muscles of the back**: erector spinae (sacrospinalis).
- **Abdominal muscles**:
  - anterior abdominal wall: rectus abdominis, external oblique, internal oblique, transversus abdominis;
  - posterior abdominal wall: quadratus lumborum.
- **Pelvic floor**: levator ani and coccygeus.

Summary

- The trunk consists of the thoracic and the abdominopelvic cavities, bounded by bony and muscular walls, and separated by the muscular diaphragm.

- The functions of the trunk can be summarised as: maintenance of the upright posture; protection of the thoracic and abdominal organs; ventilation of the lungs; and expulsion of urine and faeces.
- The trunk supports the head and provides a base for the movements of the limbs.
- The bones of the vertebral column, which supports the trunk and the head, are arranged as four curves, forming a strong and resilient unit of structure.
- Seven cervical vertebrae form a secondary curve that supports the head above. A primary curve, concave forwards, is formed by 12 thoracic vertebrae that articulate with the ribs. The five large lumbar vertebrae combine strength with mobility for the movements of the trunk. The five sacral vertebrae are fused to form the sacrum, which anchors the two innominate bones in the pelvic girdle.

- Movements between adjacent vertebrae occur at anterior secondary cartilaginous joints between the bodies of the vertebrae, and posterior synovial plane joints between the articular processes.
- Movements of the vertebral column as a whole produce flexion, extension, lateral flexion and rotation of the trunk.
- The deep posterior muscle of the back (erector spinae) performs extension movements of the trunk, and counteracts both forward sway in standing and the force exerted by loads carried in front of the body.
- The anterior abdominal wall is composed of four layers of muscles which, combining in different ways, produce flexion, lateral flexion and rotation of the trunk. The anterior abdominal wall supports the digestive organs and assists in expiratory movements in breathing.
- In lifting loads, contraction of the anterior abdominal wall raises the intra-abdominal pressure and relieves the pressure on the lower back. The load force of the body plus a load is counteracted by the effort force exerted by the erector spinae. The effort required is least when the load is placed near to the body.
- Ventilation of the lungs is achieved by movements of the ribs, which change the size of the thoracic cavity.
- In inspiration, the thoracic cage is enlarged by the action of the intercostal muscles and the diaphragm. The action of the muscles of the neck increases the depth of inspiration.
- The depth of expiration is increased by contraction of the anterior abdominal wall which pushes the diaphragm up further.
- The pelvis forms a bowl, with a bony wall and a muscular floor, at the inferior end of the abdominopelvic cavity.
- In upright standing the pelvis can tilt forwards and backwards, and in standing on one leg the pelvis tends to drop on the unsupported side. Forward tilting is resisted by the action of the rectus abdominis and the gluteus maximus. Lateral tilting is counteracted by gluteus medius and minimus on the supported side.
- The muscles of the pelvic floor support the pelvic organs.

Section III

Sensorimotor control of movement

Sensory background to movement and motor control

- Sensory background to movement
- Motor control

11

Sensory background to movement

Key terms

somatosensory system, pain, vestibular system, visual system, regulation of posture

Conceptual overview

All movement starts with a background of sensory information about the surrounding space and about the position of the body entering the central nervous system. As movement proceeds, this sensory activity changes from moment to moment. We are aware of some of the changes, but many of the motor responses to the changing input are entirely automatic. Obstacles in the way can be recognised and avoided by changing direction. In the absence of information from the eyes, there is more reliance on information from the other senses, including sound and smell. The sensory system is composed of subsystems, each transmitting specific information to the central nervous system. Activity in the subsystems is integrated in association with areas of the brain. In this chapter, the three subsystems (somatosensory, vestibular and visual) will be considered, with emphasis on their role in movement. The chapter ends with a summary of the contribution of these three subsystems to the regulation of posture during movement.

Tyldesley & Grieve's Muscles, Nerves and Movement in Human Occupation, Fourth Edition. Ian R. McMillan, Gail Carin-Levy.
© 2012 Ian R. McMillan, Gail Carin-Levy, Barbara Tyldesley and June I. Grieve. Published 2012 by Blackwell Publishing Ltd.

Somatosensory system

The functions of the somatosensory system are:

● to monitor the contact of objects and surfaces with the skin, particularly the hands and feet;
● to report the position of body segments in space and in relation to each other (body scheme);
● to initiate sensory activity for the interpretation of harmful stimuli.

From this system, one knows where the arms are in space, the pressure of a pencil held in the fingers, and how cold the wind is on the face.

The skin is not only a simple sense organ for touch, but responds to the particular pressure and temperature of surfaces. In gripping, the feedback from all the receptors of the skin in contact with the object guides the muscle force that is required. Pressure receptors in the skin of the soles of the feet monitor the distribution of body weight over the feet, and therefore assist balance reactions.

In reaching out to grasp an object, the proprioceptors in the upper limb monitor the changing angulation of the joints as the movement proceeds. We can judge the weight of an object held in the hand from activity in the proprioceptors of the elbow flexors and the mechanoreceptors in the skin of the palm of the hand.

The sensory information from the somatosensory system forms the body scheme and regulates posture during movement. We are unaware of a large amount of the activity of the somatosensory system and its role in movement is often underestimated.

Somatosensory information is transmitted in two main ascending pathways in the spinal cord and the brain, known as the **posterior (dorsal) column pathway** and the **anterolateral pathway**. Alternative names are the medial lemniscus pathway and the spinothalamic tracts, respectively. Both systems link the receptors on one side of the body with the somatosensory area in the opposite parietal lobe. The anterolateral pathway crosses at the spinal level, while the posterior column crosses in the sensory decussation in the medulla of the brain. The pathways converge in the brain stem, and both synapse in the thalamus. All fibres from both the anterolateral and posterior column pathways pass through the internal capsule to end in the somatosensory area of the parietal lobe, where the body parts are represented in a particular topographical arrangement (see Chapter 3).

Reflective task

● Revise the composition of a spinal nerve from Chapter 4, and the position of ascending tracts of the spinal cord described in Chapter 3.
● Look at Figure 11.1 to follow the general plan of these two pathways.

The function of each of the two sensory pathways is different, even though some of the sensation transmitted appears to be the same. The posterior column pathway is concerned with fast-acting information that has a high degree of discrimination. For example, changes in joint position occur rapidly during movement. The changing activity in the joint proprioceptors is conducted via this route. The anterolateral pathway conducts the reponses from stimuli, such as temperature, that are neither urgent nor require precise location.

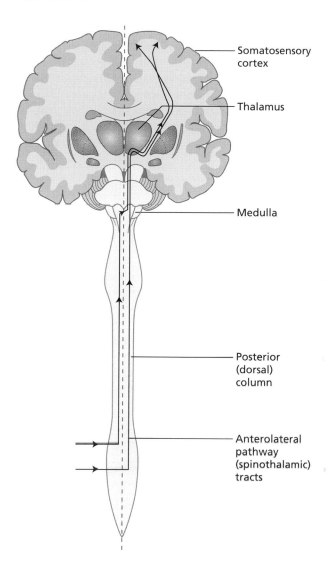

Figure 11.1 Ascending pathways to the somatosensory cortex, general plan. Frontal section of the brain with spinal cord.

Posterior (dorsal) column

The posterior column pathway provides the route for touch and proprioception. This ascending route also plays a part in the interpretation of pain. The important role of this ascending system is in the combination of input from more than one modality to interpret complex sensations. For example, both touch and proprioception are involved in the ability to distinguish the size and the shape of an object without vision.

The activity in the posterior column route is initiated by receptors that are fast adapting with large-diameter axons. These receptors are found in the skin and also lying in muscles, tendons and joints (proprioceptors). The sensory neurones enter the posterior horn of the spinal cord, and then pass into the posterior (dorsal) column of white matter of the same side. Many of the first-order neurones branch to synapse with interneurones in the posterior horn at the spinal level of entry. The posterior column of white matter, lying underneath the lamina of each vertebra, becomes larger as it ascends the spinal cord, collecting sensory fibres from each spinal nerve. In the medulla of the brain, the neurones end in the gracile and cuneate nuclei. At this level, the second-order neurones cross to the opposite side and pass through the brain stem in the medial lemniscus to the thalamus. The third-order neurones project to the somatosensory cortex.

> **Reflective task**
>
> Look at Figure 11.2 to trace the route followed by the posterior column pathway in the central nervous system. Identify the three orders of neurone.

The fibres in the posterior columns are ipsilateral, i.e. they carry sensation from the same side of the body. Fibres from the lower limbs are most medial and form the fasciculus gracilis. As more fibres enter the spinal cord from sacral to cervical segments they are added laterally. In this way, the fibres from the upper limb form the fasciculus cuneatus.

Figure 11.3 shows the position of the main ascending tracts in position in the spinal cord at the level of the cervical segments. A similar section at the level of the lumbar segments would have a smaller posterior column with no fasciculus cuneatus. The posterior spinocerebellar tract is formed by some of the fibres from proprioceptors that enter the lateral white matter and reach the ipsilateral cerebellum.

Anterolateral pathway (spinothalamic tract)

This pathway is primarily concerned with temperature and nociceptive sensations. The spinothalamic tracts play a supplementary role for touch sensation, but probably only become important when the posterior column is damaged.

Activity in the anterolateral pathway originates in sensory neurones with slowly adapting receptors in the skin. The sensory neurones have small-diameter axons with slow conduction velocity. These sensory neurones enter the spinal cord and synapse in the posterior horn before crossing to the opposite side to enter the spinothalamic tract. The fibres of the spinothalamic tract lie in the anterolateral white matter of the spinal cord. This route has been divided into anterior and lateral spinothalamic tracts, but more recent work has shown no difference in the spread of fibre types across the pathway. There is a topographical arrangement of the fibres in the anterolateral pathway, with those from distal body segments more lateral, and proximal areas more medial.

The anterolateral route continues in the brain stem, to end in the thalamus. The third-order neurones project from the thalamus to the somatosensory area in the parietal lobe.

> **Reflective task**
>
> Look at Figure 11.4 to trace the route followed by the anterolateral pathway in the central nervous system. Identify the three orders of neurone in the pathway. Return to Figure 11.1 to find the fibres from both the ascending pathways lying in parallel in the brain stem.

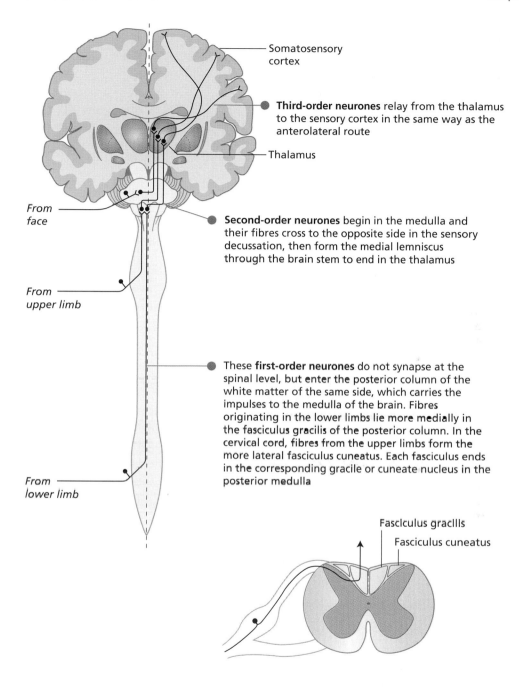

Somatosensory cortex

Third-order neurones relay from the thalamus to the sensory cortex in the same way as the anterolateral route

Thalamus

From face

Second-order neurones begin in the medulla and their fibres cross to the opposite side in the sensory decussation, then form the medial lemniscus through the brain stem to end in the thalamus

From upper limb

These **first-order neurones** do not synapse at the spinal level, but enter the posterior column of the white matter of the same side, which carries the impulses to the medulla of the brain. Fibres originating in the lower limbs lie more medially in the fasciculus gracilis of the posterior column. In the cervical cord, fibres from the upper limbs form the more lateral fasciculus cuneatus. Each fasciculus ends in the corresponding gracile or cuneate nucleus in the posterior medulla

From lower limb

Fasciculus gracilis

Fasciculus cuneatus

Figure 11.2 Posterior (dorsal) column pathway seen in a frontal section of the brain with spinal cord, and its position in a transverse section of the spinal cord.

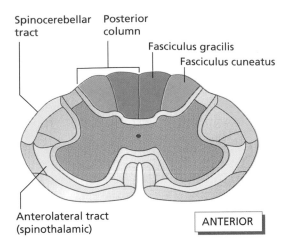

Spinocerebellar tract

Posterior column

Fasciculus gracilis
Fasciculus cuneatus

Anterolateral tract
(spinothalamic)

ANTERIOR

Figure 11.3   Position of the ascending tracts at the cervical level.

In the brain stem, some of the second-order neurones branch to link with the reticular formation.

Sensory information from the face

Receptors in the skin and the muscles of the face and in the mouth enter the brain stem mainly in the trigeminal (fifth cranial) nerve and synapse in the sensory nuclei of this nerve. Second-order neurones cross to the opposite side and lie alongside the medial lemniscus to reach the thalamus. Third-order fibres end in the region representing the face in the somatosensory cortex in the parietal lobe. Input from this trigeminal system is important for the sensory background to the movements of facial expression, swallowing and speaking.

> **Practice note-pad 11A: sensory loss in spinal cord damage**
>
> Sensory loss occurs when the posterior roots of the spinal nerves and/or the posterior column of white matter are damaged in the following ways:
>
> - degeneration of myelin in the spinal cord in multiple sclerosis;
> - infection, e.g. acquired immunodeficiency syndrome (AIDS);
> - diseases involving the vertebral column and/or intervertebral discs, e.g. ankylosing spondylitis and prolapsed intervertebral discs.
>
> The outcome depends on the segmental level and the extent of the spinal cord damage. Sensory loss occurs on the same side of the body below the spinal level affected, so that cervical damage affects upper and lower limb function. Loss of position and movement sense in the lower limbs infers walking may be diffcult. The overall sensory loss is severe in a bilateral lesion of the posterior columns.

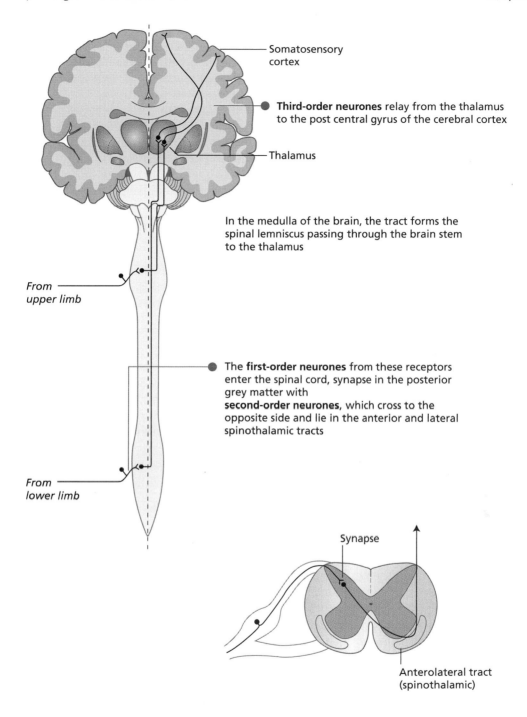

Figure 11.4 Anterolateral (spinothalamic) pathway seen in a frontal section of the brain with spinal cord, and its position in the transverse section of the spinal cord.

Interpretation of pain

In the past, pain was thought to be a unidimensional sensory experience. There was a belief that neural mechanisms responsible for the transmission of pain were solely 'hard-wired', and sensory nerves carried 'damage information' to a single pain centre in the brain. This single pathway reproduced a pain sensation in proportion to the original damage. In other words, the more damage done, the more pain was felt, and when the damage 'healed', the pain would stop. The return of function would automatically follow. This account of the experience of pain leads to frustration when individuals still report pain, in the absence of ongoing tissue damage, and it is inferred that the pain the person reports is imaginary.

It is now well recognised, especially by people who experience pain, that tissue healing after damage does not always stop pain. The current view of neural mechanisms responsible for the transmission of pain is that they have a dynamic/plastic nature with the capacity to change. The formulation and continuation of pain is a multidimensional experience that incorporates sensory, emotional, affective, cognitive and behavioural elements. The interaction between people and the environment is also affected. Individuals may report spontaneous ongoing pain, pain during occupations that would not be expected to provoke it, and chronic pain over many years despite the absence of tissue damage. In other words, the extent and severity of pain appear to be disproportionate to the original damaging stimulus. This is because pain is a perception that is the sum of many individual mechanisms occurring in the central nervous system and therefore is reported to be multidimensional in nature.

In summary, there is no single route from nociceptors to the somatosensory cortex or other areas of the brain that can explain how pain is experienced at any one time. Pain is a subjective perception and different individuals may interpret the same damaging (noxious) stimulus in different ways at different times.

In order to understand more fully why this is the case, the different types of pain that individuals can perceive must be appreciated.

Transient pain is usually brief in duration and is of little consequence, because tissue damage is minimal. Accidentally sticking a pin into the finger, would be an example of this type of pain. The sensation is usually sharp and then a dull sensation is experienced, which usually subsides quickly. A function of this type of pain is to prevent further damage by initiating escape from the stimulus and protection of the body.

Acute pain describes pain of recent onset and is probably time limited. It is usually associated with disease or injury that takes longer for the body to repair than transient pain. Acute pain that lasts for more than 3 months may be classified as chronic.

Chronic pain lasts for long periods, for example years, and persists beyond tissue healing. This may occur in chronic conditions such as joint disease, nerve damage or cancer. However, chronic pain may also be experienced in the absence of tissue damage. It is now thought that pain mechanisms and neural pathways can become dysfunctional and undergo plastic changes leading to maladaptive responses. Chronic pain by definition is more than a sensation and is multidimensional in nature.

Neural mechanisms of transient and acute pain

Peripheral and central mechanisms have been studied to understand the perception of pain. Once understood, the plastic changes that can take place in the nervous system contributing to the perception of chronic pain can be appreciated.

The mechanisms in the 'normal state' of transient and acute pain are presented as **transduction**, **transmission**, **perception** and **modulation**.

Transduction: this is the process of converting the energy content of a stimulus applied to a receptor into action potentials in sensory nerve fibres. Nociceptors are activated by noxious stimuli, which may be mechanical, thermal or chemical (released from damaged tissues), or any combination. The energy of the stimulus is converted into electrochemical impulses in the sensory neurones with **small-diameter nerve fibres** transmitting noxious information from the periphery to the spinal cord (see Chapter 1). Nociceptors are normally only activated transiently by intense levels of stimulation. Long-term stimulation by locally released endogenous pain-producing chemicals associated with tissue damage can result in changes in receptor sensitivity. If the receptors become more sensitive (hyperalgesia), the experience of pain is exaggerated. Pain may also be felt from a stimulus that would not normally cause pain (allodynia).

Remember there are other types of receptor in the skin, joints and muscles responding to non-noxious tactile and proprioceptive stimuli. When activated, this information is transmitted towards the spinal cord in **large-diameter fibres**.

Transmission: noxious information in small-diameter fibres and non-noxious information in large-diameter fibres is transmitted to the spinal cord and directed to the posterior horns. In the posterior horn there is a layer known as the substantia gelatinosa (SG cells), owing to its appearance, composed of interneurones with short axons. The sensory neurones synapse with the SG cells and in turn with the transmission (T) cells, the fibres of which link with the ascending pathways to the brain. This pain gate mechanism in the spinal cord integrates the incoming information so that onward transmission of information towards the cortex depends on the balance between noxious and non-noxious input. Figure 11.5 shows the SG and T cells in the gate control system, which will be considered further under modulation.

The ascending pathways include the spinothalamic tract (STT) and the spinoreticular tract (SRT).

- The STT is a direct nociceptive pathway that ascends in the cord, synapses in the thalamus and then goes on to the somatosensory strip of the cortex (see Figure 11.4).
- The SRT is a less direct nociceptive, multiple pathway that ascends the cord and synapses in the medial aspect of the thalamus and then to multiple regions of the brain.

Perception: pain is not perceived as 'pain' until it is interpreted within various structures and areas of the cerebral cortex. This implies that pain is not merely a sensation but a perceptual experience. Nociceptive information via the STT is projected from the thalamus to the primary somatosensory cortex, where the pure sensory component of pain is registered and discriminated in terms of quality, intensity, localisation and duration. The STT is responsible for the primary processing of pain, which centres on identification of stimuli. Some information is also transmitted to the brain stem, where the reticular formation influences the state of arousal of the cortex.

Nociceptive information via the SRT is projected diffusely and bilaterally to many other areas of the brain. This secondary processing of pain, related to recognition and meaning, is dependent on the association areas of the brain that form part of the **cognitive control system** (Figure 11.5). The prefrontal lobe initiates the cognitive evaluation of pain and the development of coping strategies. The hypothalamus and the limbic system are involved in the development of pain behaviours. The hypothalamus regulates autonomic responses, e.g. blood pressure and breathing; and the limbic system is concerned with mood and emotional responses. The individual may exhibit holding and guarding a limb, adopting awkward postures, facial grimacing and wincing, vocalising pain, and feeling nauseous, sweaty and light-headed. The construction of the

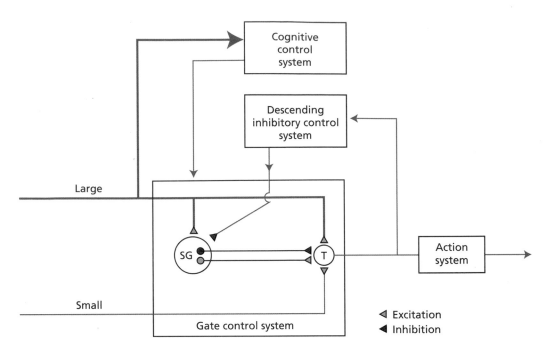

Figure 11.5 Gate control theory based on Melzack & Wall (1983). SG = cells in substantia gelatinosa; T = transmission cells. (Redrawn from Main C.J. & Spanswick C.C. (2000) *Pain Management – An Interdisciplinary Approach*, Churchill Livingstone, Edinburgh, with kind permission.)

perception of pain relates both to volition and mood (motivational–affective components) and to the future implications of pain in the individual's life (cognitive–evaluative components).

Modulation: this is the process by which the level of excitability of a group of neurones is altered. Modulatory influences can raise the base level of excitability or lower it. In the interpretation of pain, modulation balances noxious and non-noxious information within the nervous system. This ultimately defines the quality of the perception of pain at the cortical level.

Two control systems of neural mechanisms that are linked together are implicated in the modulation of pain. These are the pain gate system and the descending inhibitory system.

The **pain gate control system** (see Figure 11.5) is explained as follows.

- Activity in the **small**-diameter fibres, originating in nociceptors, stimulates the transmission cells in the posterior horn. Impulses then enter the anterolateral system ascending to the somatosensory cortex and pain is perceived. The pain gate is **open**, and increased noxious traffic is ascending to the cortex.
- Activity in the **large**-diameter fibres stimulates the interneurones of the SG cells and these, in turn, inhibit the transmission cells. This prevents information from entering the anterolateral pathway and no pain is perceived. The gate is **closed**, and less noxious traffic is ascending to the cortex.

The prediction from the pain gate theory is that large-diameter fibre activity in spinal nerves can block the transmission of noxious information arriving in the small-diameter fibres by the action of interneurones in the substansia gelatinosa in the posterior horn of the grey matter. The ultimate transmission of noxious impulses depends on the balance of activity in the large- and small-diameter sensory neurones entering the spinal cord.

The pain gate theory explains how rubbing the skin over a painful area often reduces the perception of pain. Tactile stimulation increases activity in the large-diameter fibres and helps to close the gate. The effectiveness of acupuncture in the relief of pain may be partly explained by the stimulation of large-diameter fibres. Electrodes implanted in the posterior column of the spinal cord, which can be switched on by the subject, have been used to relieve chronic pain. A less invasive approach for the management of chronic pain is to use transcutaneous electrical neural stimulation (TENS), which activates the large-diameter axons through the skin. Patients can then control the stimulation of large-diameter fibres and close the gate.

The **descending inhibitory control system** originates in the cerebral cortex, the midbrain and medullary reticular formation. The neurones of these descending pathways use endorphins, which are natural painkillers, as a neurotransmitter. They lie in the spinal cord white matter and terminate on the SG cells at all levels (Figure 11.5, descending inhibitory control). Large numbers of corticospinal fibres also terminate in the same area of the posterior horn. The SG cells, in turn, inhibit the transmission cells (T cells) and close the gate, thus reducing noxious activity in the ascending anterolateral pain pathway. In this way, descending inhibitory pathways from the brain stem modulate the activity of the ascending systems.

The descending inhibitory control system may explain how the pain from an injury may not be felt by a footballer or an athlete during the match or race. A high level of activity in this descending pathway may also account for the absence of pain often reported by victims of severe trauma at the time of injury.

The descending pathways are positively or negatively influenced by cortical perceptual mechanisms. This means that the way in which pain is perceived can be changed by focusing on the positive rather than negative emotions and attitudes, and maintaining emotional stability by avoiding excess anger and fear. Engaging in occupations that distract attention from cognitive processing of pain towards attending to external stimuli, for example involvement in leisure activities, may energise the descending system and have an effect on the pain gate.

In conclusion, the interpretation of noxious stimuli depends on activity in three control systems which influence the transduction, transmission, perception and modulation of sensory information.

Practice note-pad 11B: chronic pain

Chronic pain may occur as a result of disease or trauma. Damage to the low back is particularly implicated. The persistence of pain, after tissue healing or outlasting the pathological condition, suggests that structural neuroplastic changes occur that increase the sensitivity of neurones at both the receptor and transmission levels. Action potentials may be evoked by innocuous pressure and temperature changes at the receptor level. Neurones at the spinal level become excitable by low-threshold inputs and the pain gate mechanism is opened. The result is an increase in the noxious information transmitted to the cerebral cortex. Another factor may be a decrease in the modulatory effects of the descending pathway to the spinal cord. These changes in the processing of noxious information result in abnormal postures, and autonomic effects such as sweating and nausea. Negative perceptions continuing after the tissues have healed and cognitive evaluation of the consequences for the future may lead to depression and decreased engagement in occupations.

253

Vestibular system

The functions of the vestibular system are:

- to monitor the position of the head in space;
- to co-ordinate head and body movements to keep the body balanced;
- to stabilise the gaze when the head is moving.

The receptors lie in the vestibule of the inner ear, adjacent to the hearing organ (the cochlea). In the vestibule there are five fluid-filled sacs communicating with each other, arranged in the form of: (i) two oval bulbs, about 5 mm in diameter, known as the utricle and saccule; and (ii) three semicircular canals, about 1 mm in diameter, lying above and behind the utricle and saccule. One canal lies in each of the three planes of the head: superior, posterior and lateral (Figure 11.6).

The proprioceptors found in the walls of these sacs respond to movement of the fluid in the sacs as the head moves in space and in relation to gravity. Each receptor responds to a particular direction and velocity of head movement. People are not generally aware of vestibular activity, so it may be difficult at first to appreciate its importance in everyday movement.

The receptor areas that lie in the walls of the **utricle** and **saccule** are called otoliths or maculae. The receptor cells have projecting cilia embedded in a jelly-like mass, which contains particles of calcium called otoconia. If the head tilts, the fluid in the sacs lags behind the movement of the walls of the utricle and saccule, the cilia are bent and the sensory cells are stimulated. Sideways tilting of the head results in increased firing of impulses from one saccule and less from the opposite saccule. The otoliths on the base of the utricle signal when the head is bent forwards and backwards. In horizontal movement of the head and body, for example when sitting in a car or a train moving forwards, the otoconia lag behind the movement of the wall of the sac, the cilia are again bent and the sensory cells stimulated.

A simple way to try to understand the mechanism of the utricle or saccule is to imagine a football filled with fluid. If the football is tilted or moved steadily in a horizontal direction, there

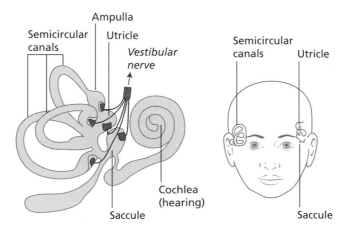

Figure 11.6 The vestibule in the inner ear (utricle, saccule and semicircular canals): position in the head.

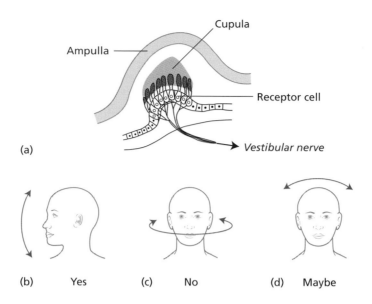

Figure 11.7   Semicircular canals: (a) cupula receptor in the ampulla of a canal; (b–d) stimulation of each canal on the left side of the head.

is always a delay in the movement of the fluid inside the football. This moment of delay would be signalled by flexible pins projecting from the inner side.

Receptor areas in the **semicircular canals** are found in the ampulla, a swelling at the base of each canal. Sensory cells in the ampulla also have cilia embedded in a jelly-like structure called the cupula, but there are no calcium particles (Figure 11.7a). The cupula forms a flap like a swing-door, moving backwards and forwards in response to movement of the fluid along the canal as the head moves. As the cupula bends, the cilia move and the hair cells are stimulated.

Rotation of the head affects the canal lying in the same plane of movement. Figure 11.7 shows the direction of head movement that stimulates each of the canals on the left side of the head.

Although individual receptors may respond to a greater extent in particular movements of the head, it is the combined effect of movement of the fluid in all the cavities that is integrated in the vestibular nucleus.

The output from the vestibular nucleus is to the spinal cord, the cerebellum and to the nuclei of the cranial nerves supplying the muscles that move the eyes. Information about the orientation of the head with respect to gravity is relayed directly to the spinal cord, while changes in the head and body position during movement reach the spinal cord via the cerebellum. The body balance is then maintained by activity in the contralateral muscles of the neck and the ipsilateral extensors of the trunk and lower limbs. The descending spinal pathways, the vestibulospinal tracts, will be described in Chapter 12.

The vestibular system plays a role in the movements of the eyes. The detection of head movements by the vestibule activates the cranial nerve nuclei of the eye muscles via the brain stem. If the head turns to one side, the eyes move in the opposite direction. This means that when the head moves, the visual field remains stable and images are focused on the macula of the retina, which has the greatest visual acuity (see the next section: Visual system).

Visual system

The visual system plays an important role in movement for the:

- detection of the features of the environment, their location and movement;
- maintenance of a stable gaze when the head moves;
- recognition of the objects used in task performance;
- maintenance of the balance of the body.

Light entering the eyes passes through several transparent layers of cells and blood vessels to reach the rods and cones, the primary receptor cells. The retina is like a 'mini-brain' and some processing occurs in its layers of cells before transmission along the fibres of the optic nerve to the brain. An area of the retina opposite the pupil and the lens is densely packed with rods and cones. This area is the macula lutea, which is best adapted for the discrimination of form and colour.

The visual pathway extends from the retina to the striate cortex in the occipital lobes of the cerebral hemispheres (Figure 11.8), where the processing for visual identification begins. Further

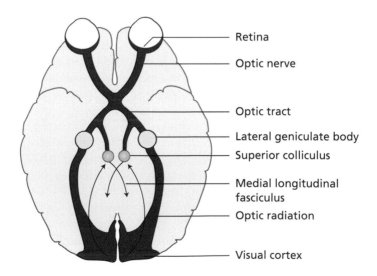

Figure 11.8   The visual system.

processing for meaning occurs in the prestriate cortex, and finally in the temporal and parietal lobes for object and face recognition.

Vision can be divided into central and peripheral, relating to the area of the retina involved.

Central vision is centred on the macula lutea, where visual acuity is greatest. The output from this area is processed in the brain for the perception of the shape, distance and size of objects. Further processing leads to object recognition and to praxis, which is the activation of the movements associated with the functional use of objects. These are essential components for the planning and execution of the movements in task performance.

Vision from the receptors in the **periphery** of the retina detects the features of the environment as an individual moves around. The location, orientation and movement in the environment are signalled by the peripheral receptors. This aspect of vision is important for functional mobility, enabling a person to react to obstacles in the way by changing direction. Peripheral vision is involved in keeping the body balanced by monitoring the verticality of the features of the environment. Vertical and horizontal structures, such as walls, doors and furniture, are used to align the position of the body. When the eyes are closed, postural sway increases. The contribution of vision to our sense of balance can be demonstrated as follows.

257

Reflective task

Stand on one leg with the eyes open, and then with the eyes closed. Notice how much you sway, and you may fall over when the eyes are closed.

The visual system controls the movements of the eyes. The visual pathway branches in the midbrain just before the lateral geniculate nucleus (Figure 11.8). These fibres, which synapse in the superior colliculus of the midbrain, link with the nuclei of the cranial nerves supplying the eye muscles. The position of the eyes keeps the centre of gaze directed on to the central macular area of the retina. When the head turns to one side, the eyes move in the opposite direction to maintain a constant gaze. If the head continues to turn, a rapid eye movement occurs in the same direction as the head to focus on a new fixed point. The rapid eye movements are known as saccades. These eye movements are controlled by co-operation of the vestibular and visual system in the vestibulo-ocular reflex (see Chapter 4, Figure 4.8).

A different type of eye movement occurs when the eyes track a moving object, known as pursuit eye movements. The manipulation of objects in many kitchen tasks involves tracking movements of the eyes. In all reaching and locomotor movements vision becomes more important at the stage when the target is approached. In reaching out to grasp a glass of water, or starting to ascend and descend stairs, visual information is crucial in the stage just before gripping the glass or negotiating the step.

Practice note-pad 11D: visual impairment

The visually impaired person has to rely on alternative input for detecting the presence of obstacles, the nature of supporting surfaces and the form of objects to be manipulated. Touch, pressure, sound, smell and proprioception all help to compensate for loss of vision. Perceptual and cognitive functions such as spatial awareness, visual imagery and memory are also important.

Regulation of posture

The static posture of the body depends on the postural tone in the muscles that support the body against gravity, together with muscle activity required to keep the body balanced over its base of support. As the body segments move from one position to another during movement, the line of gravity of the whole body is constantly shifting. Muscles all over the body can be involved in automatic postural adjustments to maintain balance.

Quiet standing requires remarkably little muscle activity, but the situation changes when there is an added weight. For example, a shopping bag held in the hand moves the centre of gravity horizontally to the side of the body with the extra load. If this movement is great enough, balance will be lost. The postural reflex response moves the centre of gravity back again by contraction of the neck and trunk muscles on the opposite side to the load, which keeps the head and trunk in line over the feet. At the same time postural tone is increased in the muscles of the lower limbs.

The response to postural disturbance depends on the direction of the force causing the imbalance and the strategy adopted by the postural system to maintain balance. For example, the force on the body when standing on a braking train is counteracted by grabbing a handrail. In lifting a heavy load that might topple the body, the position of the feet is changed to increase the base of support.

The postural disturbances are detected by the somatosensory, vestibular and visual systems. The proprioceptors in the somatosensory system are sensitive to changes in the position of the body. The skin is stimulated by a change in the contact of the foot with the ground and by any object interacting with the body. The visual system detects changes in the orientation of the environment. The vestibular system responds to any movements of the head that have occurred. The same postural reflex response can be produced by changes in any one of the three sensory systems.

The relative contribution of each of the three systems has been studied by neurophysiologists. A patient with no vestibular function and with sensory loss below the knees was reported. He relied on visual information to maintain balance and he could only stand for one second if he closed his eyes. With his eyes open he could walk but he required great concentration. Removal of all three inputs makes it impossible to stand unaided. The contribution of the somatosensory and visual inputs can be experienced as follows.

Reflective task

Stand on a piece of foam rubber with your eyes closed and hold the position for a minute or two. Change to eyes open and hold that position. Note whether you feel any difference with respect to balance in the two conditions.

The foam-rubber mat reduces the somatosensory input from the feet. In the first condition, you were relying on vestibular input for balance. Patients with no vestibular function would fall over in this situation. Studies of balance have shown that at least one of the three main sources of sensory input is necessary for balance.

Disturbance of balance also occurs during **active movements** of the body, for example when kicking a ball or reaching for an item on a shelf. The movements of the head and the limbs shift the line of weight on the base of support. This recruits the postural support necessary for that

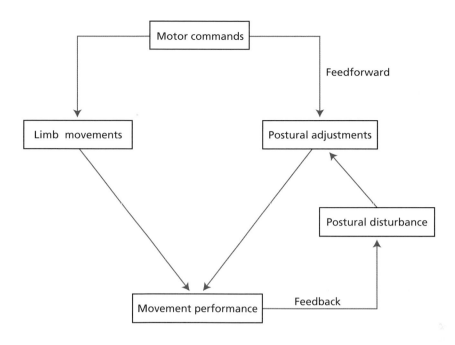

Figure 11.9   Model of the regulation of posture during movement.

movement. It has been proposed that the central motor commands for voluntary movement include output to the postural muscles as well as those to the prime movers. In this way, the disturbances of posture that the prime movers will produce are anticipated and the likelihood of imbalance is reduced to a minimum. This is known as **feedforward**. The anticipatory mechanism improves with practice, so that movements are performed with greater smoothness and stability. This is a major component in the acquisition of motor skills in sport. The loss of anticipatory postural control is one of reasons for instability in patients with neurological impairments such as stroke and Parkinson's disease.

If a postural disturbance occurs during the progress of the movement, due to body sway or changes in external conditions, further adjustments are made in response to **feedback**. A model of postural control during the performance of voluntary movement showing feedback and feed-forward is presented in Figure 11.9.

The overall ability to maintain balance during movement depends on a background of normal muscle tone, anticipatory motor commands to postural muscles and the response to feedback from the sensory systems.

Summary

- The wide variety of sensory information entering the central nervous system during movement can be divided into visual, vestibular and somatosensory.
- The visual system is not only a monitor of visual changes in the external environment, but also reinforces proprioceptive information about the movement of body parts, and co-operates with the vestibular system in maintaining balance.

259

- The somatosensory system is concerned with body sensation. Two ascending pathways in the central nervous system carry information from the skin, muscles and joints to the somato-sensory cortex in the parietal lobe. Tactile and proprioceptive information is transmitted in the posterior (dorsal) column pathway. Sensation from receptors responding to thermal and nociceptive stimuli follows the anterolateral pathway to the cortex.
- The interpretation of pain involves modulation at the spinal level of the activity originating in nociceptors.
- The pain gate theory proposes that large-diameter sensory neurones can block the transmission of nociceptive input from small-diameter axons, via the action of interneurones in the posterior horn of the spinal cord.
- Activity in a descending inhibitory pathway from the cortex to the spinal level provides another modulatory influence. The influence of these two mechanisms together with a cognitive evaluation determine the experience of nociceptive activity in the individual.

- The vestibular system monitors the position of the head in space via receptors in the inner ear. Processing in the brain stem of this information about the orientation and the dynamic movements of the head results in output to the muscles of the neck and the extensors of the trunk and lower limbs.
- The vestibular system also initiates reflex movements of the eyes to keep the image of an object centred on the macula of the retina of the eyes during movements of the head.
- The visual system orientates the upright body in relation to vertical and horizontal lines in the environment.
- During manipulative movements, the visual system is important for the perception of distance and depth in reaching and grasping, and also for the recognition of objects and the tracking of their movements during task performance.
- The regulation of posture involves feedback from the three sensory systems about the position of the body and the features of the environment as the movement proceeds. At the same time, a feedforward system issues motor commands to the postural muscles as well as the prime movers to anticipate any adjustments required.
- The importance of the integration of all of the sensory input entering the nervous system at any one time was identified by Jean Ayres, who observed children with problems in learning movement and behaviour. By facilitating sensory integration she was able to improve their ability to interact with the environment effectively and to experience satisfaction. Like a radio receiver with an infinite number of channels, the integrating centres of the brain are tuned to 'listen' to particular combinations of signals so that they can be recognised and acted on. Other signals may be ignored to reduce irrelevant activity.

12

Motor control

Key terms

motor control, spinal mechanisms, descending motor systems, planning coordination and motor learning and a summary of the three levels of motor control

Conceptual overview

This chapter outlines the interrelated components that control motor activity, from important centres in the brain via descending pathways in the spinal cord to groups of muscles that produce a wide range of activities from walking to facial expression.

Tyldesley & Grieve's Muscles, Nerves and Movement in Human Occupation, Fourth Edition. Ian R. McMillan, Gail Carin-Levy.
© 2012 Ian R. McMillan, Gail Carin-Levy, Barbara Tyldesley and June I. Grieve. Published 2012 by Blackwell Publishing Ltd.

Introduction

The motor system moves the arms in skilful activity and the legs in walking, and at the same time controls the background posture of the whole body. The same system is involved in movements of the tongue, lips and larynx needed for speech. Movements are controlled by motor centres in the brain and activity passes down from these motor centres in descending pathways to the motor neurones of the cranial nerves in the movements of speaking, eating and facial expressions, and to the motor neurones of spinal nerves in the movements of the limbs and trunk.

Movement is executed in response to commands from the motor centres of the brain. The commands have been called **motor programmes**, which specify not only which muscles are activated but also the force, direction and timing of the activity. Motor programmes, developed with practice and stored in the brain, can be activated by internal decision making and/or input from the environment.

In simple ballistic movements, known as open loop, the action is planned and executed over a very short period. Examples of open-loop movements are pressing a key on a keyboard, throwing a ball and chopping vegetables. However, most actions take longer. In these closed-loop movements, the motor commands can be modified during the progress of the movement in response to feedback from the sensory system.

The cortical motor areas, together with the basal ganglia and the cerebellum, form the **higher centres** for the production and regulation of the motor commands to the muscles. Motor nuclei in the **brain stem** control the posture and the balance of the body as the movement proceeds. Motor commands reaching the **spinal level** are fine tuned as a result of a variety of influences from the descending pathways from the brain and from local spinal reflexes.

In this chapter, activity at the spinal level will be considered first, followed by the influence of descending pathways from the brain stem and the higher centres.

Spinal mechanisms

In the spinal cord, the **lower motor neurones** form the final common pathway for activation of the muscles in all movement, both voluntary and reflex. Chapter 1 included a description of how the cell bodies of the lower motor neurones lie in the anterior horn of the spinal cord and in the nuclei of the cranial nerves. The axons of the lower motor neurones lie in the peripheral nerves supplying the muscles (see Chapter 1, Figure 1.15).

The spinal cord also contains **interneurones**, in larger numbers than the motor neurones. An interneurone is a nerve cell found in the central nervous system with no branches in a peripheral nerve. The abundance of interneurones reflects the complex information processing performed by the spinal cord. Interneurones provide an inhibitory influence for the regulation of activity in the lower motor neurones and for the reciprocal inhibition of antagonist muscles. Interneurones are important in all bilateral movements when there is activity on both sides of the spinal cord, and in movement patterns when several adjacent spinal segments are involved. The spread of activity across the spinal cord by interneurones is the basis of associated reactions.

> **Reflective task**
>
> Ask a partner to remove an elastic band placed round the fingers and thumb of one hand without using the other hand. Watch how the complex movements attempting to release the fingers from the band are mirrored in the untied hand.

The associated reaction movements may become exaggerated when the interruption of descending pathways releases spinal reflexes from the control by higher centres.

Lower motor neurone activity controls the changes in the length and tension of all the active muscles as the body moves from one position to another. Two **spinal reflexes** provide the basis for the regulation of these changes to achieve co-ordinated movement. The two reflexes are the muscle stretch reflex and the Golgi tendon reflex.

Muscle stretch reflex

When the body holds a position, muscles are maintained at a constant length by activity in the muscle stretch reflex (see Chapter 1, Muscle tone). During movement, muscles change in length, and the level of stretch reflex activity is then modified by the influence of descending pathways in the spinal cord which change the setting of the spindles in the following way. Fusimotor (gamma) neurones supply the intrafusal muscle fibres of the spindles themselves. When these neurones are excited, the intrafusal fibres of the spindle contract. The spindle then becomes taut and more sensitive to length changes in the muscle (Figure 12.1a). When the influence from the descending tracts inhibits fusimotor neurones, the spindle becomes slack and only responds to marked changes in length of the muscle (Figure 12.1b). In this way, spinal stretch reflex activity is regulated during movement by the higher levels of the central nervous system.

Consider the hand performing fine manipulative movements, such as doing up buttons and tieing shoe laces. Stretch reflex activity must be dampened in the muscles of the hand to allow rapid length changes to occur. At the same time, muscles of the shoulder and arm perform background activity to hold the postion of the limb and allow the fingers to move accurately. The spindles in the supporting muscles are set at a high level, so that any change in length is resisted.

Static and dynamic intrafusal fibres

Looking in more detail at the structure of the muscle spindle, two different types of intrafusal fibre can be identified. Both types have a primary sensory ending wound round the central area, the annulospiral ending. In addition, some of the intrafusal fibres have secondary sensory endings towards the periphery of the fibre, known as flower-spray endings, which respond to the rate of change in length of the muscle during movement. The two types of intrafusal fibre are: (i) nuclear bag fibres with a bulge in the middle where the nuclei are found, and secondary sensory endings are present; and (ii) nuclear chain fibres, which are thinner and their nuclei are lined up in a row.

The nuclear bag (dynamic) fibres respond to rapid changes in length of the muscle, while the nuclear chain (static) fibres respond to prolonged slow stretch. The muscles spindles, therefore, relay detailed information to the spinal cord about both the length, and the rate of change in length, of a muscle during movement.

The muscle stretch reflex provides a feedback mechanism so that muscle groups producing movement change length appropriately and supporting muscles are held at the desired length.

Golgi tendon reflex

Golgi tendon organs are proprioceptors found at the junction between the muscle fibres and the tendon of a muscle. Each consists of a nerve ending embedded in collagen fibrils surrounded by a capsule. Since the Golgi tendon organs lie in series with the muscle fibres, they respond to an increase in tension in the whole muscle. (Remember that muscle spindles lie in parallel and

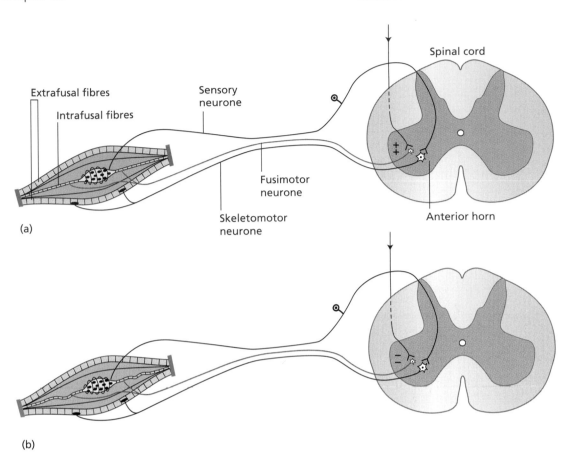

(a)

264

(b)

Figure 12.1 Muscle spindle sensitivity: (a) high – descending pathways stimulate fusimotor neurones, the intrafusal fibres contract and the muscle spindle is very sensitive to distortion; (b) low – descending pathways inhibit fusimotor neurones, intrafusal fibres are slack and the muscle spindle is less sensitive to distortion.

respond to a change in length of a muscle.) When the tension in a muscle rises, the muscle pulls on the tendon and the Golgi tendon organs are stimulated. This activity stimulates sensory neurones, which synapse with interneurones in the spinal cord. The interneurones are inhibitory to the lower motor neurones of the same muscle (Figure 12.2) and also exert an influence on motor neurones supplying other muscles around the same joint. In this way, the Golgi tendon reflex provides a feedback mechanism to regulate muscle tension and to keep it within the limits required for the performance of any task.

It has been suggested that the Golgi tendon reflex can act as a protective mechanism to prevent damage to tendons when a sudden high level of tension develops in a muscle. In these conditions, stimulation of the tendon organs inhibits the lower motor neurones and a loss of muscle tension occurs. An example is a weight-lifter who experiences a sudden loss of power when attempting to lift a load that he cannot move.

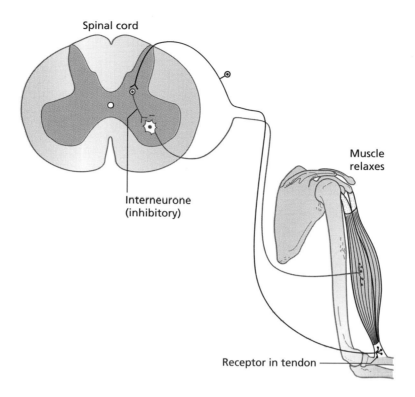

Figure 12.2   Golgi tendon reflex.

The two spinal reflexes described, which are mediated by muscle spindles and Golgi tendon organs, co-operate to control the length and tension in the muscles at the correct levels during normal movement.

Spinal integration and synergy

The motor neurones in the spinal cord are organised systematically. Motor neurones of flexor muscles lie laterally and extensor motor neurones lie medially in each anterior horn of grey matter. Motor neurones of the proximal muscles of a limb lie towards the centre and those of the distal muscles lie towards the periphery in the grey matter. A large number of interneurones link all of these groups of neurones, forming a neural network.

Within a network of neurones, the axon of each neurone branches to synapse with many other neurones (divergence) and each cell body receives branches from many other neurones (convergence) (Figure 12.3). Some of the neurones in a network will exert excitatory influences, while others will inhibit activity.

Inhibition is the term for the changes in the cell membrane of a neurone that make it more difficult for it to respond to activity from another source. The balance of excitatory and inhibitory influences within a network of neurones determines the final output. There are two main types of inhibition in the spinal cord: presynaptic inhibition and recurrent inhibition (Renshaw cells).

265

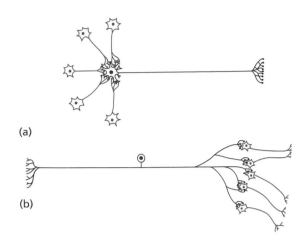

(a)

(b)

Figure 12.3   Neurone circuits: (a) convergence; (b) divergence.

Presynaptic inhibition occurs when the neurotransmitter substance from a terminal bouton of an inhibitory interneurone prevents the release of excitatory neurotransmitter by another neurone at a synapse (Figure 12.4a). An example of presynaptic inhibition is found in the pain gate mechanism that regulates the activity of the pain transmission cells (see Chapter 11). Another example is the suppression of stretch reflex activity by descending pathways from the brain via spinal interneurones.

Recurrent inhibition occurs in the skeletomotor neurones when collaterals or branches of the axons synapse with small inhibitory interneurones called Renshaw cells in the spinal grey matter. The inhibitory neurones, in turn, synapse with the cell bodies of the skeletomotor neurones supplying the same muscle and synergistic muscles (Figure 12.4b). It has been proposed that the Renshaw cells form a closed-loop feedback control system for alpha-motor neurone activity at the spinal level.

Functional movements involve the repetition of particular patterns of muscle activity to perform specific tasks. Reach and grasp movements require simultaneous activity in the flexors of the shoulder, the extensors of the elbow and wrist, and the flexors of the fingers. Walking involves the repetition of alternating flexion and extension movements of the hip, knee and ankle in a particular order. These patterns of movement are called **synergies**. Movement synergies are executed by spinal neural networks, containing motor neurones and interneurones, which generate repeated activity in the same groups of neurones.

> **Practice note-pad 12A: lower motor neurone lesion**
>
> Interruption of lower motor neurones may be due to damage of the cells in the anterior horn of the spinal cord (for example in poliomyelitis) or to the axons in peripheral nerves (for example in peripheral nerve injury). The result is loss of tendon reflexes, and of muscle tone in the absence of stretch reflex activity. The muscles usually feel limp and have no 'life' (hypotonia). Muscle wasting occurs with time and there is a risk of shortening of the muscle tissue.

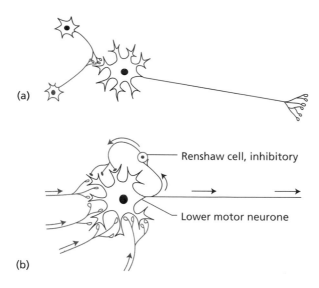

Figure 12.4   Inhibitory neurones: (a) presynaptic inhibition; (b) recurrent inhibition.

Descending motor system

Motor centres in the cerebral cortex plan and initiate motor commands to the brain stem and the spinal cord. In the brain stem, the background posture and balance during movement is regulated by other motor centres that receive background information about the position of the head and body, and about the visual field ahead. The axons of the neurones in all these motor centres in the brain lie in tracts that terminate at all levels in the spinal cord. Together they form the descending motor system. The neurones in this system are known as **upper motor neurones**. The collective output from these upper motor neurones influences the level of activity in the lower motor neurones of the spinal cord which, in turn, controls the active muscles during movement.

Upper motor neurones synapse at all levels in the spinal cord with skeletomotor neurones supplying type I and type II muscle fibres (see Chapter 1), and also with fusimotor neurones innervating the intrafusal fibres of muscle spindles. In this way, the upper motor neurones affect both the recruitment of motor units for different levels of muscle activity, and the level of stretch reflex activity in the muscles for the regulation of postural tone.

Motor commands to the muscles: corticobulbospinal tracts

Upper motor neurones originating in the cortical motor areas form a fast, direct route via the brain stem and the spinal cord to the lower motor neurones. The motor areas contributing to this descending pathway are the primary motor cortex, the premotor cortex and the supplementary motor area (see Chapter 3). The neurones in the primary motor cortex are large pyramidal cells with large-diameter, fast-conducting axons. The individual tracts in this descending system are the lateral and anterior corticospinal tracts, and the corticobulbar (or corticonuclear) tract.

The **corticospinal tracts** descend from the cerebral cortex through the brain stem to the spinal cord. The corticospinal fibres converge as they enter the internal capsule (see Chapter 3, Figure 3.13). Passing into the brain stem, the fibres lie anteriorly in the midbrain and continue down through the pons. At the level of the medulla, 85% of the fibres cross to the opposite side and enter the lateral white matter of the spinal cord to become the lateral corticospinal tract. The other fibres continue anteriorly in the white matter of the spinal cord as the anterior corticospinal tract. The area where the fibres cross in the medulla is known as the decussation of the pyramids (see Chapter 3, Figure 3.16c). The anterior corticospinal fibres cross at the level of the segment that they supply. Fibres of both tracts terminate in the spinal cord, where they synapse with lower motor neurones either directly or via interneurones. Figure 12.5 shows the route followed by the corticospinal tracts.

The **corticobulbar tract** originates in the same cortical areas as the corticospinal pathway. A large part of the corticobulbar tract ends in the brain stem in the motor nuclei of cranial nerves, the red nucleus and the motor nuclei of the reticular formation. The corticobulbar tract activates the muscles involved in eye movements, facial expression and speech via the links with cranial nerves. The influence of the corticobulbar tract also extends to the spinal cord via the links with the brain stem motor centres and their descending tracts.

Together, the corticospinal and corticobulbar tracts represent the cortical descending system for the motor commands to the muscles in movement. In the corticospinal component, muscle action on one side of the body is initiated by the motor areas of the opposite cerebral cortex. Muscle activation by the corticobulbar component is either ipsilateral or contralateral, depending on the target brain stem nucleus involved. The corticospinal system plays a major role in the control of skilled precision movements of the distal muscles of the limbs, while the corticobulbar system controls movements of the eyes and the face.

Postural control: brain stem motor centres

The motor centres in the brain stem are the origin of descending tracts that terminate by synapse with lower motor neurones in the spinal cord. Overall, the fibres of these tracts are excitatory to the skeletomotor neurones of the extensor muscles of the neck and trunk, and the proximal muscles of the limbs. Their effect on the fusimotor neurones is inhibitory, which eliminates unwanted tone, so allowing skilful movement to take place.

Figure 12.6 shows the motor centres in the brain stem and their descending tracts to the spinal cord.

The **tectum** of the midbrain contains two pairs of nuclei, the superior and inferior colliculli. Visual and auditory information is processed in these nuclei. The output from these nuclei is to the cervical segments of the spinal cord via the tectospinal tract and to the muscles of the neck. This pathway initiates changes in the position of the head in response to sound and to changes in the visual field. Examples of this response are experienced when a person turns towards the sound of someone calling their name, or towards a car overtaking them in driving. In group sports, a player responds to the position of other members of the team from the sound and sight of their changing positions.

The **red nucleus** in the midbrain (sometimes included with the basal ganglia) is a motor nucleus that receives input from the cerebellum and the primary motor area. The descending pathway from the red nucleus to the lower motor neurones of the spinal cord is the rubrospinal tract. This is an important route from the cerebellum, which has no direct descending pathway to the spinal cord. The rubrospinal tract is closely linked with the corticospinal tract for the activation of the proximal flexor muscles of the limbs, which provide support during movement.

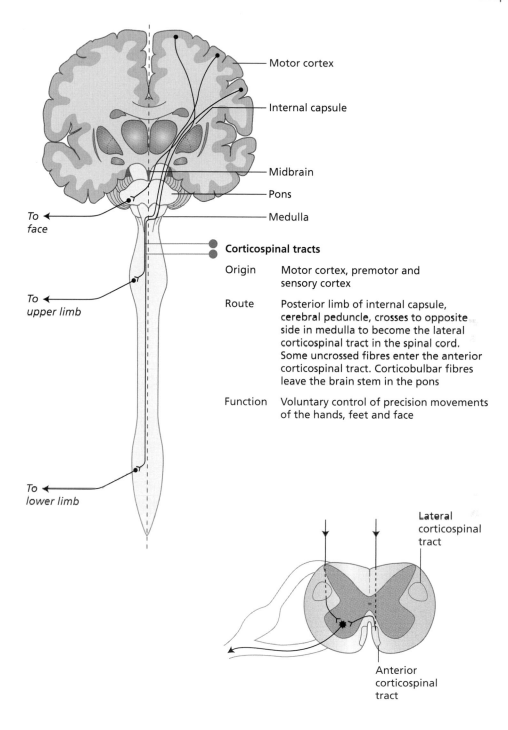

Figure 12.5 Corticospinal tracts seen in frontal section of the brain with the spinal cord. Position of the tracts in a transverse section of the spinal cord.

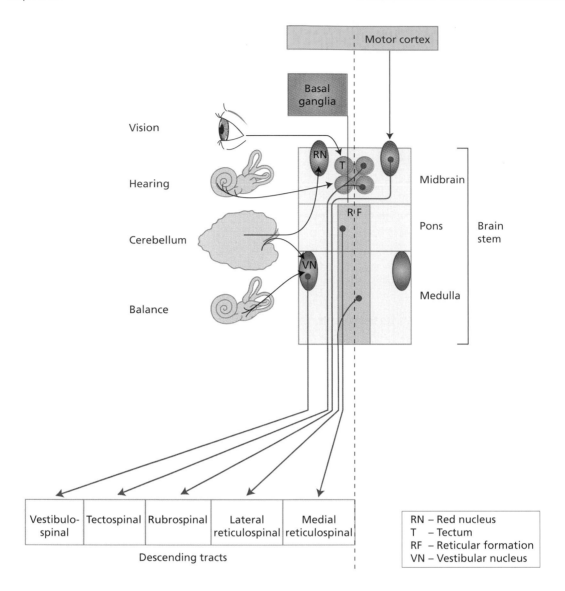

Figure 12.6   Motor centres in the brain stem (diagrammatic). Origin of the descending tracts from the brain stem.

The **vestibular nucleus** in the medulla receives input from the vestibule of the ear (see Chapter 11). The descending tracts from the vestibular nucleus activate the muscles of the neck, which stabilise the position of the head. Some fibres of the vestibulospinal tract continue to all levels of the spinal cord, innervating predominantly extensor motor neurones for postural control. The vestibular nucleus is part of the vestibulo-ocular reflex, which controls eye movements when the head turns (see Chapter 11, Visual system).

The **reticular formation**, which extends along the core of the brain stem, is a collection of nuclei that are loosely connected. The reticular formation receives ascending somatosensory information from the spinal cord, and also descending fibres from the cerebral cortex that terminate bilaterally. There are two descending reticulospinal tracts. The function of the lateral tract, which originates in the medulla, is in positioning and support by the proximal muscles of the limbs during movement. The medial reticulospinal tract, which originates in the pons, is more concerned with the activation of the extensor muscles of the neck and trunk to maintain the upright posture and the balance of the whole body.

Summary

The descending pathways from the brain stem motor centres together form a part of the motor system that regulates activity in the muscles to:

- stabilise the position of the head and the eyes;
- provide proximal support during skilled movement of the hands and feet;
- maintain activity in extensor antigravity muscles to keep the body upright.

Practice note-pad 12B: upper motor neurone lesion

Interruption of upper motor neurones may be due to a stroke, traumatic brain injury or cerebral tumour. The outcome is variable. Lesions can cause increased tendon reflexes and spasticity owing to loss of higher centre control of the stretch reflex. Movement is often most affected in the fine co-ordinated movements of the fingers and hands. Abnormal movement patterns may appear. The upper limb may show flexor synergy, and the lower limb may demonstrate an extensor synergy, so that normal movements are difficult to perform. There is a risk of muscle shortening.

Terminology

The upper motor neurones have been divided into:

- the **pyramidal system** for the direct descending pathway from the cortical motor areas to the lower motor neurones;
- the **extrapyramidal system** for all the other descending pathways from the brain to the lower motor neurones. These routes are largely polysynaptic.

A distinction between the pyramidal and extrapyramidal systems was originally based on the assumption that the pyramidal system, originating in the cortical motor areas, is concerned with voluntary movement; while the extrapyramidal system, originating in the brain stem, is involved in background postural activity during movement. This distinction is not reflected in the presenting features of upper motor neurone lesions and the terms are no longer used in most up-to-date textbooks.

Planning, co-ordination and motor learning

The basal ganglia and the cerebellum regulate movement as it progresses by interaction with the cortical and brain stem motor centres. Their influence on movement is exerted via the descending pathways from these centres. There are no direct descending pathways from the basal ganglia and cerebellum to the spinal level. The basal ganglia form motor control loops with the cortical motor centres of the same side, while the cerebellum interacts with the contralateral cerebral cortex.

Basal ganglia

The individual nuclei of the basal ganglia link together to form a functional unit. Information enters the basal ganglia system from almost all areas of the cerebral cortex, especially from the motor areas and the somatosensory cortex. Output from the basal ganglia projects back to the cortex of the same side via the thalamus. Two control loops are formed in this way: (i) cortex, caudate and putamen (striatum), globus pallidus, thalamus, cortex; and (ii) cortex, caudate and putamen (striatum), substantia nigra, thalamus, cortex (Figure 12.7). These two motor loops act independently and in parallel.

The exact way in which the basal ganglia influence movement remains unclear. There is evidence that the activity in the neurones linking the basal ganglia to the thalamus is inhibitory. This has led to the hypothesis that the basal ganglia act as a braking system for motor control. Variations in the level of this inhibition could affect movement performance in several different ways: unwanted movements are eliminated when inhibition is increased; movements are initiated when the inhibition is removed; and the sequential stages in a complex movement are started and stopped by the alternation of low and high levels of inhibition, respectively. The variation in the level of inhibition in the basal ganglia system could explain some of the features of diseases of the basal ganglia, which range from the presence of involuntary spontaneous movements (hyperkinesia) to a poverty of movement with an inability to initiate voluntary movements (hypokinesia).

The basal ganglia play a role in **motor planning**. Some of the information entering the basal ganglia system originates in the supplementary motor area of the cerebral cortex, which is active before a movements starts. Other sources of input are from the somatosensory area and premotor area, which have links with the sensory system monitoring the current environment. Some movements are initiated by internal decision making. For example, when a person decides to switch on the television, a motor plan is activated that selects the correct motor programme for the execution of this action. This type of movement occurs when a patient is asked to perform a movement to command. Other movements are generated more by sensory input from the environment, for example by the visual input from objects or the sound of a doorbell. In this case, the environmental stimuli facilitate the activation of motor programmes to initiate the movement. Patients with basal ganglia disease have difficulty in initiating movements, particularly those that are internally generated, and they can be assisted by cueing, which provides additional sensory input.

Cerebellum

The cerebellum is not necessary for the generation of movement. However, it plays a major role in the regulation of movement and posture indirectly by adjusting the output of the descending motor systems of the brain. The cerebellum is said to act as a comparator which compensates for

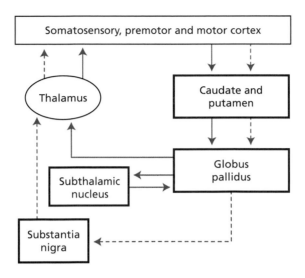

Figure 12.7   Motor control loop between the basal ganglia and motor centres in the cortex.

errors in movement by comparing intention with performance. In more detail, this is accomplished by comparing feedback signals that reflect the intended movement (motor commands) with external feedback signals from the sensory system that reflect the actual movement. In response, the cerebellum modifies descending motor commands accordingly.

The cerebellum acts principally on the descending pathways to proximal muscles that control posture via the muscles of the back, the neck, and the pectoral and pelvic girdles.

Figure 12.8 shows the input of the intended movement from the primary motor cortex, which enters the cerebellum after crossing the midline in the pons. The sensory information from the vestibule of the ear and from the muscle proprioceptors, giving information about current head and body position, enters the ipsilateral side of the cerebellum. The output from the cerebellum returns to the motor cortex via the thalamus or relays in the red nucleus of the brain stem before entering the descending system.

Theories of cerebellar function

Current theories on how the cerebellum modifies movement have been developed from studies in neurophysiology and the observation of patients with cerebellar damage. Three main functions have been proposed:

- co-ordination of the activity in all the muscles involved in multijoint movements;
- timing of muscle activity so that the muscle groups are recruited in the correct order to achieve the goal;
- motor learning.

Most actions involve ongoing changes in the position of several joints moving together to produce a movement synergy. This requires the **co-ordination** of all the active muscles moving the joints. Loss of co-ordination is seen in patients with cerebellar damage when asked to reach

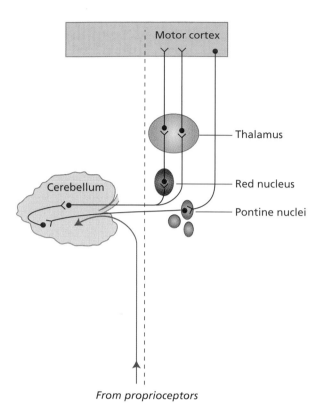

Figure 12.8 Motor control loop between the cerebellum and the contralateral motor cortex.

out to grasp a cup. The movement is decomposed into separate actions at the shoulder, the elbow, and then the wrist and fingers.

In cerebellar damage, patients show disruption of **timing** when asked to perform repetitive movements, for example rapidly pronating and supinating the forearm to turn the hand over and back. Poor timing is also demonstrated by a staggering and wide-based gait. A further problem with timing is seen as poor initiation and termination of movement after cerebellar damage.

The role of the cerebellum in **motor learning** has been studied extensively in studies of animals and the theories developed have been applied to the acquisition of motor skills. An example of motor skill learning experienced by many people is learning to drive a car, when a complex sequence of movements of the upper and lower limbs is executed in relation to the activation of the handbrake, footbrakes, accelerator and clutch. After extended practice of the same sequence, the correct movements can be performed automatically.

In the early stages, the execution of the movements is initiated by motor commands from the cortical motor areas with conscious awareness. It has been suggested that the motor programmes of successful movements are developed and stored in the cerebellum. After many repetitions the motor programmes can be activated without reference to the cortical areas. This means that there is a change over time to a performance without conscious awareness. If there is any alteration in the pattern of input to the cerebellum, for example a driver may change to a new car, then the learning process is repeated and the motor programme updated. After a short period of practice, the movements become automatic again.

This theory of motor learning involving the cerebellum was supported by studies of the cellular structure of the cerebellum.

Cellular structure of the cerebellum

The cerebellar cortex has layers of cells that are distributed in a uniform way over the entire surface of the cerebellum (Figure 12.9), unlike the cerebral cortex where there are variations in the cell layers in different areas. The output from the cerebellum is from a layer of large Purkinje cells, the axons of which end in the deep nuclei of the cerebellum and then relay to the brain stem. Two systems of incoming fibres affect the activity of the Purkinje cells: the climbing fibres, which have direct connections with the Purkinje cells; and the mossy fibres, which interact with cells in other layers before they synapse with the Purkinje cells. The climbing fibre system originates solely in a nucleus in the medulla (the inferior olive), while the mossy fibres have their origin in all other inputs to the cerebellum. The indirect connections of the mossy fibres synapse in the granule cells of the deep cell layer before sending ascending axons to the molecular layer. In this layer each axon divides into two to form the parallel fibres. They traverse the molecular layer of the cortex like telephone wires, and each branches to make contact with a large number of Purkinje cells. The arrangement of the parallel fibres allows for the integration of the activity occurring at several joints simultaneously.

A model of motor learning developed in the 1970s proposed that in the early stages the Purkinje cells are excited by the climbing and the mossy fibres associated with a particular pattern of sensory feedback from the muscles, skin, eyes and ears. It was shown that after many repetitions of the same sequence, the direct excitation by the climbing fibres originating in the inferior olive

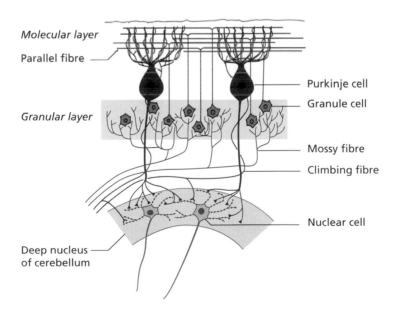

Figure 12.9   Cellular structure of the cerebellar cortex (simplified).

275

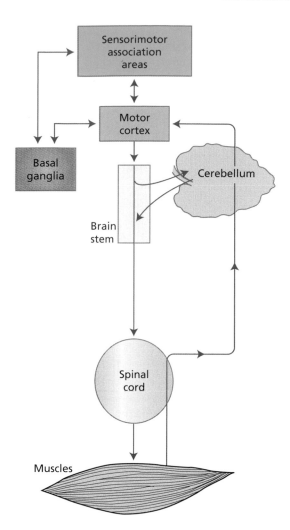

Figure 12.10 Interaction of the basal ganglia and the cerebellum with the cortical areas, the brain stem and the spinal cord.

was no longer required. This change with practice led to the idea that motor programmes for skilled movements are developed with practice and stored in the cerebellum, which became known as a 'skills bank'. More recent studies have demonstrated that both the climbing and mossy fibre systems are active in motor adaptation, and this leads to the co-ordination of complex movements from simple components, as well as providing a basis for motor learning. There is currently a debate about the number of sites in the brain where the memories for motor skills may be stored. Since other components of memory, for example semantic memory, are distributed over more than one brain area, it seems likely that the cerebellum is not the only site for motor memories.

Figure 12.10 shows a summary of the interaction between the cerebral cortical areas, basal ganglia and cerebellum, the motor nuclei in the brain stem and the spinal cord.

Summary

- This chapter has considered how the motor system functions at three levels of control.
- The **spinal** level is the integration of (i) incoming proprioceptor activity from the muscles, tendons and joints; (ii) motor commands from the cortical motor centres via the descending system; and (iii) activity in local networks of interneurones acting as basic pattern generators. The fine tuning of lower motor neurone activity at this level maintains the correct length and tension in synergistic muscles during the execution of the movement.
- The **brain stem** level of control is based on sensory inputs from the eyes, the vestibule of the ear and the muscle proprioceptors via the cerebellum. The output of integration in the brain stem nuclei is to descending pathways of the spinal cord to maintain extensor activity to keep the body upright and provide proximal stability for skilled movements of the hands and feet. Processing of visual and vestibular input stabilises the position of the head and eyes and maintains maximum visual discrimination of the environment ahead.
- The **higher centres** level of control is mediated by the primary motor cortex, interacting with sensory areas in the parietal lobe and with the basal ganglia and the cerebellum. The basal ganglia are particularly concerned with the planning of internally cued movements. In actions that are stimulus driven or externally prompted, the cerebellum compensates for errors by comparing intention with performance. The basal ganglia and the cerebellum exert their control via the primary motor area and the brain stem motor centres, which have direct links to the spinal level.
- The hierarchical organisation of the motor system incorporates the modulation of activity by information entering from the sensory system at each level. In Chapter 13 motor control will be extended to include parallel processing for the integration of input from the cognitive and limbic systems.

Section IV

Human occupation

Occupational performance skills and capacities and occupational performance

- Occupational performance skills and capacities
- Occupational performance

13

Occupational performance skills and capacities

Key terms

Occupational performance skills and capacities, multiple factors in control of occupational performance skills, core positions and patterns of occupational performance skills

Conceptual overview

This chapter will outine the **occupational performance skills** that are used in everyday life as part of an individual's occupational performance. Occupational performance skills that are addressed in this chapter include; lying, rolling and sitting up, sitting, standing and squatting, standing, walking and climbing stairs and reaching and retrieving. This chapter will also consider the **capacities** and other factors necessary for the production and control of these skills. In occupational performances, the body moves through sequences of movements. Each stage in the sequence involves simultaneous movements at several joints and the goal for the task may be reached in a variety of ways.

To interact effectively with the environment, the body utilises a number of core positions. From these positions a range of movement patterns is carried out to move from one position to another, and to orientate the body in a stable functional position for the performance of skills and tasks. An example is answering the doorbell, which involves rising from sitting to standing, walking to the door and reaching for the handle to open it.

Tyldesley & Grieve's Muscles, Nerves and Movement in Human Occupation, Fourth Edition. Ian R. McMillan, Gail Carin-Levy.
© 2012 Ian R. McMillan, Gail Carin-Levy, Barbara Tyldesley and June I. Grieve. Published 2012 by Blackwell Publishing Ltd.

Multiple factors in control of occupational performance skills

The execution of skills is seen in movements which are the outcome of the integration of muscular and neural components of motor control interacting with psychological, social and environmental factors. Consider how a person gets out of bed in the morning. This is not only the result of biomechanical and neurological activity. The quality, speed and precise nature of the movements produced will vary according to circumstances. Hence, if the person has overslept and is late for work, his movements will be hurried and less well controlled. If getting up and not wanting to disturb a sleeping partner, movements may be slow and cautious. In terms of the physical environment, the precise performance of this skill will vary with the qualities of the bed and its relationship to the floor and other objects in the room. A soft, low bed will require different qualities and degrees of movement to get out of, compared with a high, firm bed. Such examples demonstrate the multiple factors that determine the characteristics of this performance and skilled movements.

In the hierarchical model of motor control presented in previous chapters, the motor commands issued at the highest levels of the central nervous system drive the activity in the subcortical, brain stem and spinal motor areas in top-down processing. When psychological and social factors of task performance are included, the motor system needs to be viewed functionally as a series of interconnected centres that work in series and in parallel and feature numerous feedback and feedforward circuits. The focus for control of movement is thought to shift between these centres, depending on the needs and demands of a given performnace, and the environmental conditions experienced at the time. The cognitive system is a major component of the motor control of movement, particularly when decision making and problem solving are involved.

In organising and producing movement, the brain regulates posture to ensure that the body can maintain and restore equilibrium and be safe from the threat of harm. For example, when reaching for an object, if the line of gravity begins to move beyond the base of support, compensatory adjustments are made to maintain equilibrium. If these adjustments are not made, the intended goal is abandoned as righting and saving reactions are initiated. Another priority is the adoption of body positions that allow any given task to be carried out in the most efficient way possible.

Consider the skills of crossing one of the moving walkways found at fairgrounds. The priority in movement is directed to the negotiation of the walkway. The attention is fully engaged in the task of keeping upright while walking. The simultaneous execution of other activities, such as talking or reading signs, becomes impossible, whereas these would pose no difficulties when walking along a clear, level corridor.

To interact effectively with the environment, the body uses a number of basic, or core, positions. From these positions, a sequence of movement patterns is carried out to move from one position to another, and to orientate the body in a stable position for the performance of occupations.

The objectives guiding the selection of these positions are:

- to position the head for optimal visual and auditory monitoring of events;
- to bring the trunk and upper limbs into the most effective and efficient position for the execution of skills;
- to ensure optimal stability and equilibrium;
- to minimise the amount of physical effort required to execute skills and achieve performances;
- to achieve human occupation.

The core positions are lying, sitting, squatting and standing. The choice of the position to be adopted for skill performance depends on the attributes of the skill and the environment. An understanding of the performance demands and the priorities for stability in these positions and movements leads to the identification of abnormalities in movement and the facilitation of effective performance.

Emotional and cognitive factors

Skill performance is orientated towards the achievement of a goal. A person's ability to reach the goal is determined by their mood at the time and by their ability to organise and use stored knowledge about the movements involved and the environment. The ways in which emotional and cognitive factors affect movement will now be considered.

Emotional factors have been shown to have a significant effect on movement performance. Studies of human responses to stress have established that links exist between psychological state and physiological functioning. Neural connections between areas of the brain that apparently serve disparate functions suggest the potential for psychological factors to influence motor behaviour. The reverse, that physical activity can influence psychological state, is well accepted. The ability of physical exercise to stimulate the release of endorphins in the brain (neurotransmitters with some of the properties of opiates) has been established, and physical practices such as relaxation and breathing exercises are used in the treatment of some mental illnesses. Stress, or more specifically distress, is known to be a risk factor in the development of some physical conditions such as high blood pressure, heart disease and stroke. How then do psychological factors influence motor behaviour?

In previous chapters we have seen how sensory inputs are relayed to many areas, cortical and subcortical, and are used to provide knowledge to an individual in relation to the world, and to formulate appropriate actions and behaviours. The prefrontal areas of the frontal lobe interact with cortical areas in which meaning and significance are attached to the information received. These areas are also richly connected to the network of fibres and nuclei that form the limbic system (Figure 13.1). Hence connections exist that permit the attribution of emotional value to experiences, and emotional influences upon behaviour.

The limbic system also projects fibres to the hypothalamus and is influential in determining the relative balance of autonomic activity within the body. Thus there are two ways in which emotion may influence motor activity. One is its contribution at the conscious level, to decision making, motor planning and the execution of voluntary movements. The other is its influence upon skeletal muscle tone through up- or down-regulation of central nervous system activity, depending how stressed or at ease an individual is.

Reflective task

- Think about an occasion when you have seen a friend really angry. On a piece of paper, write a list of all the things you saw that conveyed that mood. Everything in your friend's behaviour will be the result of muscle activity.
- Think about yourself when you are happy and relaxed, and when you are angry. What are the differences in your speech, facial expressions, gestures and body movements between these two states?

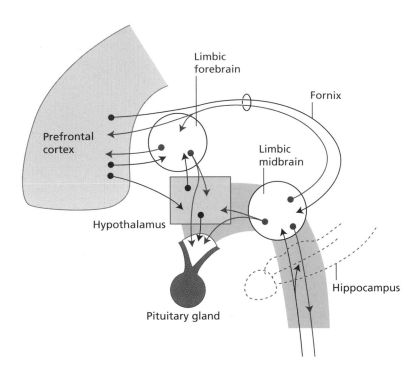

Figure 13.1   Connections between the limbic system, hypothalamus and prefrontal cortex.

Cognition is a complex system of interrelated parts that allows people to organise and use knowledge about themselves and the changing environment to achieve goals. The output of cognitive processing may be action, decision making or storage of information for future use. In the effective performance of all occupations, the sensorimotor system interacts with the cognitive system. There are many components of the cognitive system.

Perception is the component of cognition that makes sense of the environment by integrating all the sensory input to the nervous system for meaning. Visual, auditory and tactile input is processed for the recognition of objects and tools. The perception of the position of all the parts of the body in space, known as body scheme, is based on information from proprioceptors in the muscles and the joints. Body scheme must be integrated with visual and spatial perception of objects to perform the accurate movements of reaching and grasping.

Attention is another component of cognition. In task performance, an object or a tool is grasped, and attention must first be focused on it during perceptual processing for recognition. Selective attention allows any distracting noise in the environment, for example people talking in the same room, to be ignored. Attention must then be sustained long enough until the task has been completed. It is also possible to divide one's attention, for example talk to a friend while doing the task.

Memory is the stored knowledge of objects, faces, environmental landmarks, movements and experiences. When an activity is performed, motor programmes, stored in procedural memory, are activated by the environment or from decision making. Stored motor programmes allow people to plan movements and to execute the correct sequence of actions. Orientation in time is based on prospective memory of when actions must be performed in the future. Everyday routine actions are mostly automatic, but prospective memory is required for non-routine actions that have to be remembered once in a while, for example phoning a friend on her birthday. Autobiographical memory of past experiences gives someone a personal identity and self-esteem. Shared experiences are important parts of interactions with family and friends.

The highest level of cognitive processes is the **executive functions** that allow people to set realistic goals and to modify movements and behaviour when conditions change. Tasks can be initiated and a judgement on the performance made at the end. Executive functions are important when people are confronted with an unfamiliar situation and flexible problem solving is needed to complete a task.

Reflective task

Walk round your local supermarket selecting the items you need from the shelves. Think about examples of all the components of perception and cognition that are basic to shopping: attention; visuospatial perception and body scheme; visual and verbal recognition; memory; executive functions. Evaluate the outcome when you unload your shopping at home.

Many areas of the cerebral cortex are implicated in cognition. The visual processing in the occipital lobe is an important part of visual perception. The parietal lobe processes tactile and spatial perception, body scheme and attention. The brain areas involved in memory include the temporal lobe for recent and spatial memory, the thalamus and hypothalamus for procedural memory; and the frontal lobes for prospective and autobiographical memory.

Figure 13.2 outlines the serial and parallel processing between the sensorimotor, cognitive, limbic and subcortical (basal ganglia and cerebellum) systems for the output to the muscles in motor behaviour.

Practice note-pad 13A: perceptual and cognitive impairments

Perceptual and cognitive deficits, which can significantly restrict movement, occur in many neurological conditions, especially stroke and traumatic brain injury. The problems relate to the component of the cognitive system that is impaired:

- **attention**: inactivity due to poor arousal, distractions interrupt movement; failure to complete a task;
- **visual and spatial perception**: poor object and/or face recognition (agnosia), under- or over-reaching; difficulty in finding the way round rooms and buildings and in the street;
- **memory**: poor orientation in time; loss of self-identity; procedural memory is usually spared;
- **executive functions**: poor motor planning and initiation, movement stops when a new situation arises; unable to judge the effectiveness of movements.

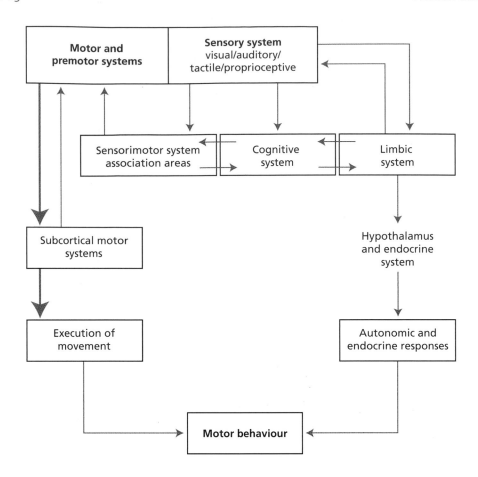

Figure 13.2   Serial and parallel processing in the sensory, motor, limbic and cognitive systems in the control of movement.

Core positions and patterns of occupational performance skills

The core positions and movement patterns that are fundamental to all movements will now be considered in four sections: (i) lying, rolling and sitting up; (ii) sitting; standing and squatting; (iii) walking, and stair ascent and descent; and (iv) reaching and retrieving.

Framework for the analysis of movements

A systematic approach to the analysis of movements enables clear identification of any limitations imposed by musculoskeletal, neurological and cognitive deficits. This can form part of a broader analysis of any task performance. The components of the movement analysis are as follows:

- occupational relevance and context;
- description of the starting position;
- breakdown of the movements into sequential stages;
- description of any postural adjustments within each stage, followed by the movements of the limbs, starting proximally and moving distally. Multijoint movements are identified;
- consideration of the cognitive and emotional factors that relate to the specific movement.

The ability to formulate movement analysis leads to an implicit understanding of a client's movement problems.

Lying, rolling and sitting up

Lying down is the position of rest and sleep. It is a position that renders the person vulnerable, as neither vigilance nor rapid movement is easy when lying down, and is most often adopted in privacy. There are exceptions such as sunbathing, giving blood or receiving a massage, but in such activities the person does not have to be active. Some of the few activities performed in the lying position that have biological and interpersonal significance are those concerning sexual behaviour.

Lying is the most stable body position because the largest possible surface area of the body is in contact with a supporting surface, the bed or the floor. Side lying, which allows free movement of the upper limb and the pectoral girdle on the uppermost side, is the preferred position for reaching movements from lying. Side lying is also the optimum starting position for sitting up from lying, when the hand of the uppermost limb pushes on the bed to lift the trunk to the upright position.

Rolling is a sequence of movements to change from one lying position to another. It can also be a component in the process of moving from lying to sitting and the reverse.

There is considerable variability between individuals in the way in which rolling is performed. This can be seen by observing a group of people rolling over on the floor. In changing from supine to side lying, some initiate from the shoulders, others from the legs. Some raise the arms above the head during the roll. As the body rolls into prone lying, the head must be lifted by extension of the neck to keep the face clear of the ground. In all rolling movements, muscle tone is important to hold the body segments in alignment. The trunk must act as a rigid tube while the limbs are used to generate force for movement and then positioned to stabilise the body. The following exercise demonstrates rolling initiated by the lower limbs.

Reflective task

Working with a partner, one person lies on the floor, the other kneels down level with the pelvis. The person lying down must first keep the body completely relaxed while the kneeling person tries to roll him or her by lifting one side of the pelvis. Now the supine person should flex one hip and knee to bring the foot flat on the floor and at the same time consciously increase muscle tension throughout the body. The kneeling person starts to lift the pelvis again. Note how much more easily the supine body can now be rolled.

The properties of the supporting surface determine the effort needed. A soft, conforming surface offers limited stability and little resistance for the generation of momentum. Bedcovers may need to be considered as heavy layers hinder movement. Some people may need persuading to change from traditional sheets and blankets to a lighter duvet.

287

The movement from **lying to sitting** takes the person from a position of rest to a position preparatory for activity. Without it, a person cannot commence purposeful activity or interact effectively with the environment. This movement sequence, together with moving between sitting and standing, is a prerequisite for independence in basic self-care tasks, mobility and hence all occupations.

To sit up in bed, co-ordinated and simultaneous actions of the head, trunk and all four limbs are required. In moving from lying to sitting on the side of the bed prior to standing, the upper limbs drive the movement and lower limb activity varies according to how the person is lying at the start.

To move from side lying to side sitting the uppermost arm pushes down on the bed to start to lift the head and trunk. With sufficient clearance, the opposite arm can be positioned to take the weight of the trunk and then push down to raise the trunk further by stabilising the pectoral girdle and extending the elbow. The momentum generated, together with lateral flexion of the trunk on the side of the original uppermost arm, brings the head and trunk to the vertical. As the pelvis comes to the vertical the legs fall into a parallel position over the side of the bed with the knees flexed and the feet on the floor (Figure 13.3).

Reflective task

Practise the movement sequence from side lying to sitting on a plinth or a bed several times. Stop at certain points and feel which muscles are working. Refer to pushing movements of the shoulder in Chapter 5 and of lateral flexion of the trunk in Chapter 10. Repeat for the return movement from sitting to lying.

Sitting, standing and squatting

Sitting is a position from which many tasks are carried out. Typically these tasks have one or more of the following features.

- They occur in one location.
- They require sustained attention and finely controlled movements.
- They take long periods of time.
- They allow the line of gravity to remain within only one base area of support.

Sitting is essential to effective task accomplishment within many occupations and for the performance of a range of personal and social roles. Sitting and standing are positions that send social signals; think of religious or civic ceremonies where the use of each position is clearly delineated. Sitting also creates a lap. The thighs can be used for resting and stabilising objects or for holding a young child safely for reading and playing.

By sitting a lower centre of gravity and larger base area of support are achieved, so reducing neurological and muscular activity for maintaining position and equilibrium, and allowing more energy and attention to be directed to the task at hand. Many occupations traditionally carried out in standing can be done sitting, sometimes with some modification to the environment. A compromise between the two can also be achieved by the use of a high stool or perching stool, which confers the height advantage of standing with the energy conservation of sitting.

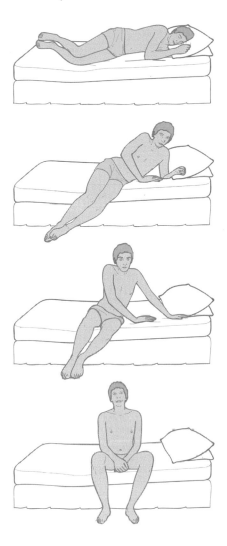

Figure 13.3　A movement strategy for sitting up from lying on the side.

> **Reflective task**
>
> Find three different types of chair, for example a chair for writing at a desk, an easy chair and a stool. Observe a person sitting in each of the chairs. Look at the vertical alignment of the head and trunk, the tilt of the pelvis and the angle of the thigh with the horizontal.

Figure 13.4 shows three different sitting positions.

In everyday life we adopt a whole range of asymmetric and highly variable sitting postures. These are determined by the type of chair, the relationship between the chair and other furniture, the activities we undertake, and even the social situation and the clothes we are wearing. The

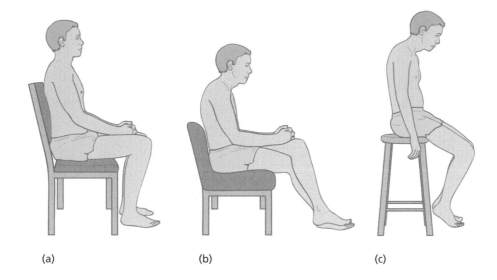

(a)   (b)   (c)

Figure 13.4   Sitting: (a) position; (b) low seat; (c) high stool.

sitting posture also sends non-verbal signals to others about our attitude, mood and degree of co-operation in a given situation or activity.

Why, then, is it necessary to think about a standardised **sitting position**? Because for any occupational performance an effective and stable starting position is needed, from which posture, orientation and movement can be varied with minimal effort and optimum stability. A good sitting position allows sufficient movements of the trunk and the upper limbs for reaching and manipulating, and to bring objects into the visual field. It is important for therapists to appreciate that for many people with limited mobility and movement control, the sitting position may be their only option for engagement in daily activities and occupations, and movement within the seated position may be restricted or severely limited.

The orientation of the pelvis is key to the alignment of the trunk and the head in the sitting position (Figure 13.4a). In turn, the pelvis will be influenced by the angle of the femur imposed by the characteristics of the seat and the position of the feet in contact with the floor. In the sitting position adopted by many for relaxation (Figure 13.4b), or in sitting on a high stool with no back support (Figure 13.4c), the pelvis tilts posteriorly and the lumbar lordosis is obliterated, intervertebral discs are compressed anteriorly, and strain is imposed upon the posterior ligaments and muscles of the vertebral column. This position also compresses the abdominal organs, and respiratory capacity is reduced. However, sitting in an easy chair for relaxation does allow for changes in position.

Moving from **sitting to standing**, and the reverse, are essential to move the body between its two most frequently used positions. Being able to move between the two enables selection of the most effective position for any activity. The inability to stand up restricts activity and participation in a range of environments and social situations, and can have major physical and psychological consequences.

Rising from sitting involves a change from a very stable position, with a large base of support around the legs of the chair and the feet, to a much less stable one, with a relatively small foot

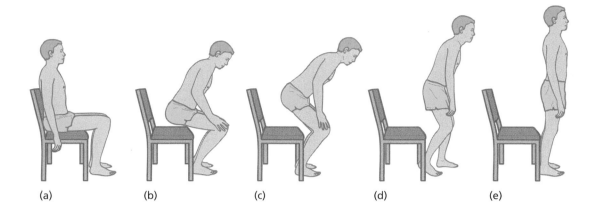

(a)   (b)   (c)   (d)   (e)

Figure 13.5 Rising from sitting to standing: (a) start position; (b) preparation; (c) lift-off; (d) extension; (e) stabilisation in standing.

base. The centre of gravity of the body moves forwards and upwards and the line of gravity must be kept within the changing base of support. Large movements are required at the hip and knee from flexion into extension. Momentum must be generated and then checked to prevent the body from moving forwards. Muscles that oppose the direction of movement are active to operate as a brake.

Reflective task

Observe the movements of a subject sitting on a chair as he or she rises to standing up. The movement can be divided into four phases: (i) preparation: flexion of the trunk and foot placement; (II) lift-off from the seat; (iii) extension; and (iv) stabilisation in upright standing: adjustment of the feet. Describe the movements of the trunk, hip, knee and ankle in each phase.

The sequence of movements shown in Figure 13.5 starts with the sitting position, followed by four phases in rising to standing.

The **preparation** for standing phase involves foot placement and flexion at the hips to bring the trunk and head forwards (Figure 13.5b). The most effective foot placement in terms of stability requires that the feet are drawn back so that they lie close to the front edge of the seat of the chair. The feet may be parallel to each other, but if forward movement is anticipated immediately after rising, one foot may be placed further forward than the other. It is important for a therapist to bear in mind that such anticipatory or preparatory movements, which are normally automatic, may be absent or reduced in people with movement disorders or sensory impairments. In this phase the pelvis tilts forwards, controlled by the hip extensors working eccentrically.

The **lift-off** phase (Figure 13.5c) begins by dorsiflexion of the ankle and extension of the knee. If the line of gravity is not sufficiently forward at this point, lift-off cannot occur, or if attempted will fail. Initiation of lift-off is possibly triggered by tactile sensation conveyed from the plantar surface of the feet and proprioceptors in the lower limb. These inform the brain that the body weight is adequately within the base area of support and that weight-bearing joints and muscles are prepared for optimal generation and control of movement.

In the **extension** phase (Figure 13.5d) simultaneous, forceful concentric contraction of the hip and knee extensors occurs. At the same time the trunk extends, thus maintaining alignment over the pelvis. The plantar flexors of the ankle straighten the leg and move the line of gravity over the foot base.

Rising progresses to the full upright posture (Figure 13.5e), with appropriate adjustment of the feet for stability.

The speed of rising depends on the amount of momentum generated at the beginning of lift-off. People who have difficulty initiating movement, or whose lower limb muscles are weak, compensate by using the upper limbs to provide additional lifting force.

292

> **Reflective task**
>
> Talk through with a partner the action of pushing down on the arms of the chair to assist body to rise. Refer to Chapter 5, Summary of the shoulder and elbow in movements, and Figure 5.14b.

The ability to **sit down from standing** is as essential as being able to stand up, although relatively little is written about it. Sitting down is the movement for rest from standing activities. One might argue that sitting down moves the body from a less stable to a more stable position, and that, as the movement goes with gravity rather than against it, it is less demanding. It also requires the same range of movement at the same joints as standing up. What makes this movement different to most others is that it is done backwards. In what other daily actions do people deliberately execute a backward movement without direct visual monitoring?

When approaching a chair, a person notes its position and dimensions, but in turning to prepare for sitting, the chair is lost to view and they then rely upon short-term visuoperceptual memory to predict contact with the seat. The movement in effect becomes open-loop because a commitment is made to it and it cannot be adjusted once a certain point has been passed. Remember the childish, and dangerous, trick of pulling someone's chair away as he or she sits down. In the moments before expected contact with the seat surface, the individual has committed himself to the movement that shifts the line of gravity backwards and outside the base area of support afforded by the feet, hence it cannot be reversed.

Sitting down can be likened to a form of controlled falling. The movement goes with gravity, and so neither force nor momentum needs to be generated. The extensors of the hip and the knee work eccentrically for the lowering of the body to bring the buttocks and thighs on to the seat. Once seated, the hip extensors pull the pelvis to vertical from its anterior tilt. The trunk is extended and an upright seated position is achieved.

People with weak muscles or limited joint range in the lower limb may develop the habit of sitting down by allowing themselves to fall, especially into a low armchair.

The design and dimensions of the chair affect the demands of moving between sitting and standing. A low seat increases the effort needed to initiate rising, to generate momentum and to carry the body from a lower starting point up to standing. It also increases the time taken to complete the movement, and so decreases stability. A low seat also increases the degree of flexion needed at the hips and knees, and dorsiflexion at the ankle, and so creates difficulties for those with limited joint range.

The movements between sitting and standing are difficult for many elderly people who experience some loss of muscle strength and of the range of joint mobility in the lower limb. In addition, deficits in visual, tactile and proprioceptive perception reduce stability. Movement problems in getting in and out of chairs can have a major impact on mobility, occupations and quality of life.

Squatting is a position that is rarely considered in movement texts, yet it is an important functional position. Young children frequently adopt this position in play activities, and adults may do so when playing with young children, or assisting them with personal care tasks such as dressing or drying themselves. It is also a position that some adults may habitually adopt for specific tasks, for example gardening. In many cultures, elimination functions are performed in squatting. In some situations and circumstances, food preparation and other domestic tasks may be carried out on the floor. Even with modern fitted kitchens, a large social or family occasion may necessitate the use of floor space for food preparation.

Compared with sitting on the floor, squatting is a less stable position and requires more muscle work. However, the advantages of squatting as a position are:

- it confers a height advantage over sitting on the floor;
- it allows more trunk movement and a greater reach within the position;
- it enables an individual to move quickly into standing.

Squatting is an intermediate position that a person may move through between standing and kneeling, or standing and floor sitting. It is also a position adopted temporarily when reaching for low objects or into low cupboards.

In lifting heavy objects from a low position squatting ensures a straight back, and enables the large muscles of the lower limbs to generate the force required for the lift. Using this position minimises strain on the back and helps to avoid serious damage to the spine (see Chapter 10, Figure 10.5).

The achievement of the squat position (Figure 13.6) requires a continuation of the movement pattern needed for sitting down on a chair, but with adjustments to keep the line of gravity forward over the base of support, and maximal flexion at the hips and knees.

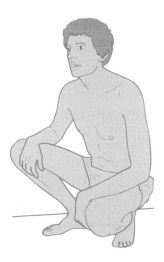

Figure 13.6   Squatting.

As the hips and knees flex to lower the body, the extensors of the hip and knee work eccentri-ally, and the ankles dorsiflex. The trunk remains upright, aligned over the pelvis. The movement then departs from that of sitting down because plantar flexion is not initiated to move the trunk backwards. Instead, the ankle continues to dorsiflex, keeping the trunk centred over the feet as the centre of gravity is lowered. When maximum dorsiflexion is reached, the heels begin to rise off the ground and the trunk is tilted forwards (Figure 13.6).

Some individuals are able to squat with the pelvis very close to the floor and the feet everted. This requires great flexibility of the lower limb muscles and joints. It is most often seen in young children and in particular cultural settings.

Reflective task

- Stand upright with the hands on the anterior thigh palpating the quadriceps muscle. Move slowly into a squat position, feeling the increase in muscle tension as the quad-riceps works eccentrically to lower the body.
- Compare a high squat with a low squat position with hips adducted and abducted. Note the changes in the freedom of the upper limbs to perform activity.

Rising from squatting requires an initial forceful contraction of the hip and knee extensors to produce the upward momentum. The force needed to overcome the effects of gravity is greater than in rising from sitting.

Standing, walking and climbing up and down stairs

Standing is a more effective position for task performance than sitting since the hand can be positioned over a larger area around the body. In the kitchen, where work surfaces are usually designed for the standing position, reaching can be extended further by bending the trunk or standing on the toes. Dressing and washing are easier when upright, especially for the lower half of the body. Standing in a shower may be the only option for washing by those who cannot get in and out of the bath. However, the base of support for the body is smaller in standing than in sitting, therefore the maintenance of standing balance is a crucial factor for all occupations. Many activities that are usually performed standing can be adapted for the sitting position, but this reduces the area available for reaching and retrieving. Some jobs inevitably include long periods of standing, for example teaching or working in large department stores.

Transferring loads from the standing position puts less strain on the low back than sitting (see Chapter 10, Figure 10.5). Child-care activities include transferring a baby or toddler from cot to pram, or into a car seat. These can only be done from the standing position. Standing is the start-ing position for many leisure activities, for example all ball games and darts. In gardening, activities such as digging, mowing the lawn and cutting hedges are usually done in the standing position. On social occasions, standing allows the interaction between a large number of people, or may be the only possibility if the room is small. In social and work situations, an individual adopting a standing position engenders feelings of command and authority.

Refer to Chapter 8, Figure 8.5a to see standing viewed from the side. Trace the line of gravity from the head to the base of support provided by the feet. The shape of the vertebral column (see Chapter 10, upright posture) forms a balanced support for the trunk over the pelvis. In relaxed standing, the weight of the head and the trunk may be aligned over one foot and then the other. The head and the trunk may be habitually aligned over one foot in those who experience chronic pain in the joints of the opposite leg.

The standing position is affected by the features of the floor and the height of the heels of shoes. The slope of the ground alters the position of the feet and in turn the tilting of the pelvis. High heels tip the trunk forwards. This leads to anterior tilting of the pelvis and lumbar lordosis. There is more strain on the quadriceps muscles to keep the knee stable. Standing on rough, slippery or icy ground demands more muscle activity at the ankle to maintain balance. If the floor is moving, for example when standing in a train or bus, more muscle activity is needed to counteract lateral sway of the trunk.

The upper limbs are not involved in maintaining balance in standing, they are therefore free to perform the movements required in tasks. Standing still for long periods increases venous pressure at the ankle, causing local oedema and poor blood flow back to the heart. In a hot environment this may lead to fainting. The energy expenditure in standing activities is higher than similar tasks in the sitting position, therefore fatigue is a factor in long periods of standing activity.

Standing is the final stage in achieving independent mobility. Only when the body can be balanced over the feet in standing can progress be made towards walking.

Walking allows people to be engaged in occupations where they need to move around in a variety of directions. Public areas and transport systems that are not adapted for wheelchairs remain inaccessible for those who are unable to walk. The ability to walk extends the options for work and leisure. Walking as a leisure activity has the added bonus of keeping joints mobile, improving cardiovascular fitness, and experiencing the sights and sounds of the changing seasons.

Changing both speed and direction, adapting to different surfaces and avoiding obstacles are essential features of mobility. A person must be safe and free from tripping by making automatic adjustments, especially when carrying a heavy or a delicate load. The construction worker on a building site has very different demands in walking compared with a secretary in a carpeted office.

Although a large amount of communication between people and organisations can now be done by electronic mail and computer interaction, the inability to walk can lead to social isolation and depression.

Each individual develops a unique habitual way of walking. All the measurable parameters of gait, such as stride length and step frequency, are related to stature. If a person tries to walk in step with someone else, it is always difficult, especially if they are not the same height. Tall people take long strides and make fewer steps per minute compared with short people walking at the same speed. Variations in speed and rhythm occur with changes in mood and the time of day. The way that elderly people walk often reflects poor balance, reduced muscle strength or less sensory processing, as well as cognitive factors, for example inattention and fear of tripping.

> **Reflective task**
>
> Watch people of all ages walking to the shops, to the station and in the park; alone and in groups. Notice the variety of walking speed, length of stride, rate of stepping, position of the head and body, and amount of arm swing.

Walking is the progression of the body forwards by repetitive movements of the lower limbs. There are periods of double support when both feet are in contact with the ground, followed by periods of single support (one foot supporting the body) while the other limb swings forwards to take the next step.

The sequence of movements in walking is known as the **walking cycle**. This is divided into phases punctuated by the events of heel strike and toe-off (Figure 13.7).

For convenience of description it is usual to start the cycle with left heel strike (Figure 13.7a).

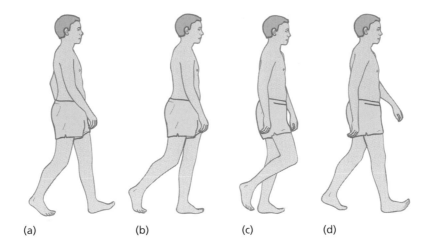

(a)   (b)   (c)   (d)

Figure 13.7   Walking cycle: (a) left heel strike; (b) right toe-off; (c) right swing with foot clearance; (d) right heel strike.

The heel of the leading left leg is lowered to the ground at **heel strike**. This starts the **double support phase**. Next, the whole foot is placed on the ground by the eccentric action of the knee extensors and ankle dorsiflexors (Figure 13.7b). At the same time, plantar flexion of the right ankle transfers the weight on to the left leg. This is known as right **toe-off**.

In the **single support phase**, the left hip and knee extensors convert the limb into a pillar. The pelvis remains level by the action of the hip abductors on the support side (see Chapter 8, Figure 8.6). In this phase the right limb starts the **swing** initiated by the hip flexors and continued by the momentum of the swinging leg. Foot clearance of the ground is achieved by active dorsiflexion of the ankle and some knee flexion (Figure 13.7c).

The swinging right leg rotates the pelvis to the left. Trunk rotation in the opposite direction to the right keeps the head and the eyes facing forwards. This rotation produces the natural arm swing.

At the end of the swing phase in the right limb, the hip extensors halt the thigh, the knee extends and the right heel is placed on the ground to start the next walking cycle (Figure 13.7d).

It can be seen that in walking the lower limb muscles work both concentrically to exert propulsive forces against the ground to move the body forwards and eccentrically to act as a brake to bring the movement of body segments to a halt. For example, just after heel strike, the gluteus maximus in the leading leg is active to control trunk flexion and keep the head and trunk aligned over the supporting limb.

Reflective task

- Observe a partner (preferably wearing shorts) as he or she walks across a large room.
- Identify: heel strike, single support and toe-off in one limb; and the swing phase with toe clearance in the opposite limb. Note the arm movements and trunk rotation.
- Ask your partner to walk across the room at different speeds. Does this make any difference to the time spent in support and swing?

Sensory and perceptual processing increases when walking in a crowd or hurrying across a busy road. This is extended to higher level cognitive processing for topographical orientation, visuospatial memory for landmarks and flexible problem solving trying to find the way in an unfamiliar environment.

Stair ascent and descent: the ability to negotiate stairs allows a person access to transport systems, shops, leisure facilities, friends and neighbours. Many older public buildings and homes still have steps to the front door and to the toilets. These barriers to work and leisure lead to social isolation for those who can walk on level ground but are unsure in stair climbing. The problem is compounded when there is a need to carry loads, for example files and books, shopping or a young child, up and down stairs.

There is a wide variation in the way that people move on stairs. Young adults may run up stairs placing only the forefoot on each step. The elderly with locomotor problems may ascend and descend one step at a time, increasing the time with both feet on one step to gain stability. The most common accident in elderly people at home is falling down the stairs.

In the repeated movement sequence of stair walking, one limb is weight bearing while the opposite limb is being carried through to place the foot on the next step. Differences between walking and stepping lie in the increase in muscle strength and joint mobility required to propel the body upwards in stair ascent, and to perform controlled lowering of the body with respect to the force of gravity in stair descent. Figure 13.8 shows the sequence of movements in walking up one step.

297

Reflective task

Go to a staircase with a partner and ask him or her to walk up stairs slowly and then down stairs. Observe the movements in the joints of the lower limbs and the position of the trunk throughout the sequence of movements View from the front and from the side if possible.

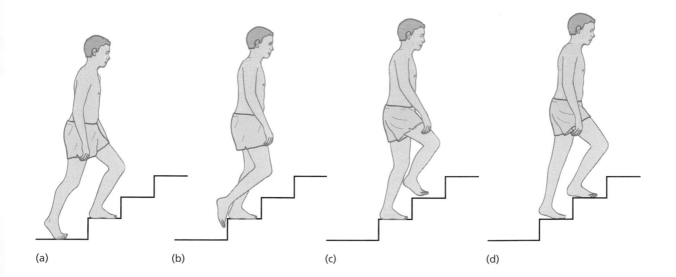

(a)   (b)   (c)   (d)

Figure 13.8 Ascending stairs: (a) right toe-off, left foot placed on step 1; (b) right carry through, left support; (c) right foot clearance; (d) right foot placement on step 2.

Stair ascent will be described starting with the left foot already placed on step 1 (Figure 13.8a). The right limb pushes off from the ground by plantar fexion of the ankle. The trunk flexes to bring the line of gravity forwards, while the body is lifted upwards by the concentric action of the left hip and knee extensors and the ankle dorsiflexors.

As the body moves upwards, the left limb is now in single support and the right limb starts the carry through (swing) phase (Figure 13.8b). The right limb flexes at the hip and knee and dorsiflexes at the ankle. This movement continues until the right foot lies just above step 2 (Figure 13.8c). The foot is lowered on to step 2 by eccentric action of the hip flexors, and the trunk extends to the upright position. The right limb is now prepared for weight bearing and the cycle is repeated.

During carry through of the right limb, the pelvis is lifted by the action of the hip abductors on the supporting left side, and rotated to the left.

Stair descent is described starting from step 2 with the right limb stepping down first. The extended right limb is lowered on to the step below by the eccentric action of the left hip and knee extensors and the plantar flexors of the ankle. The trunk is aligned over the left foot base. This controlled lowering of the body allows the right foot to be placed on step 1 to prepare for weight bearing. At foot placement, the right knee is extended, the hip is slightly flexed and the ankle is plantar flexed. The body weight is now supported by the right limb and the trunk extends into the upright position to prepare for the lowering of the left limb on to the floor.

The environmental factors that influence the movements to ascend and descend stairs are: the rise and depth of steps, the step covering, the type of shoes worn and the lighting. Bifocal lenses can blur vision in stair descent. Visuospatial perception of the height and depth of the steps is crucial in ascent and descent of unfamiliar stairs. A stair rail allows the upper limbs to contribute to stability in ascent and descent.

Reaching and retrieving

Reaching and retrieving movements are key to ocupational performance. The upper limbs play a significant role in supporting, enabling and controlling movements of the body but in reaching and retrieving they are the central players.

This movement demands the adoption of the appropriate posture for the task being undertaken. The degree of involvement of the whole body depends on the duration, direction and speed of movement required and the manipulative goal to be reached. Figure 13.9 shows three reaching movements, each adopting different postures.

Anticipatory movements are part of the motor planning of reaching activities. Such positioning is usually performed automatically. Compensatory movements may be made during the progress of the activity, for example the hand must remain steady when carrying a full cup of tea.

Success in reaching is dependent upon mobility at the shoulder joint. Without freedom of movement of the shoulder, only limited reaching can occur. Once the reach has been accomplished, the shoulder/pectoral girdle complex must be capable of stability and fixation to keep the hand in the desired position and facilitate its functions. Retrieval movements can entail returning the arm and hand to a resting position after performing a task, or bringing an object towards the body, for example bringing food to the mouth or putting on clothing. It is not always a simple reversal of reaching, and it may form an important link between one component movement and another in occupational performance.

Analysis of a reaching and retrieving task

Table 13.1 presents a musculoskeletal analysis of a reaching and retrieving movement. The object characteristics and the environment determine the position and movements of the body segments.

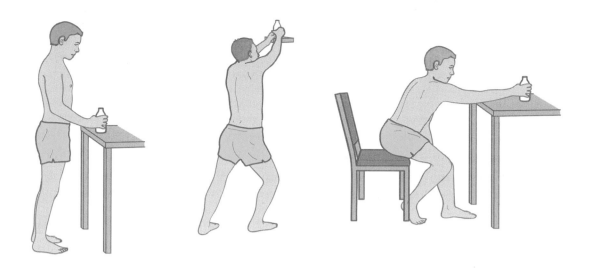

Figure 13.9   Reaching and retrieving, variations in posture.

Table 13.1   Musculoskeletal analysis of reaching and retrieving (occupational performance skills).

Movement	Picking up a cup with one hand to take to the mouth and drink
Environment	Domestic dining room.
Object characteristics	Standard cylindrical 150 ml cup, full of water
Starting position	Seated on an upright dining chair pulled up to the table
Stage of movement	**Performance skill demands**
Reach for the cup	The movement sequence can be performed within the starting base area of support. Postural adjustments are not required In the upright seated position. The arm is relaxed, with the hand resting in the lap. The elbow flexes to lift the hand clear of the table edge. There is simultaneous flexion at the shoulder joint and extension of the elbow to reach forwards. Protraction of the pectoral girdle occurs
Grasp the cup	The humerus is maintained in medial (internal) rotation. The forearm is held in the midprone position. The wrist is extended. The thumb is abducted, the fingers are abducted and extended, with slight flexion of the proximal interphalangeal joints. The cup is grasped in a cylinder grip
Retrieve; bring the cup to the mouth	Increase in muscle tone of all the antigravity muscles of the upper limb to bear the weight of the cup. Forearm, wrist and hand positions are stabilised while elbow flexion and shoulder extension bring the cup to the mouth. The pectoral girdle retracts. As the cup nears the mouth, small adjustments of position occur. Ulnar deviation and slight flexion at the wrist hold the cup level. Slight lateral (external) rotation of the humerus and shoulder flexion bring the cup into contact with the mouth. Pronation of the forearm tips the cup for drinking

(Continued)

Table 13.1   (*Continued*)

Task completion	Returning the cup to the table is accomplished by reversal of the retrieval and cup-to-mouth movements. The cup is released from the grasp by extension and abduction of the fingers and thumb. Muscle tone in antigravity muscles decreases
Cognitive factors	These include visuospatial perception, object recognition, body scheme related to hand-to-mouth movement, praxis associated with an open container of fluid

Summary

- This chapter has brought together knowledge presented in Sections I, II and III to assist occupational therapists' understanding of the performance of movement.
- Motor control is now extended to include the sensorimotor, cognitive and limbic systems, interconnected in series and in parallel. The focus of control shifts between these centres depending on the demands of the task and the environment. The neuropsychological aspects of performance and the occupational relevance (context, goal and environment) to the individual of movement patterns are considered.
- The progression from lying through the core positions and movement patterns to walking and stair climbing has been described. As one moves through the core positions, the demand for muscle strength and the range of movement at the joints increases; new patterns of movement emerge that require a complex interplay between concentric and eccentric muscle work.
- Sitting up from lying requires sufficient muscle tone to keep the body segments aligned, stability in the pectoral and pelvic girdles, and muscle strength in the upper or lower limbs to exert pressure on the floor.
- Moving to standing up requires greater strength and range of movement in the lower limbs; the stability of the trunk and its alignment over the feet become crucial factors.
- Walking and climbing stairs demand the co-ordination of a repeated cycle of movements when the whole body is supported by one lower limb while the other limb swings forwards to take the next step.
- Few problems for balance are found in reaching and retrieving movements in the sitting position with its stable base of support.
- The execution of sequences of precise and skilful movements of the hands and fingers to reach a goal increases the role of perception and cognition.
- The reader should now feel able to apply the framework for description and analysis that has been described and used here to any purposeful movement. This in turn should enable the recognition of movement components and skills, and facilitate identification of component and skill deficits in the context of practice.
- Such ability is central to the diagnosis of occupational dysfunction, and the remediation of identified problems in physical performance.
- In Chapter 14, occupational performance is examined in more detail. The case scenarios that are presented provide opportunities for reflection and application of the content of this chapter.

14

Occupational performance

Key terms

Framework for understanding human occupation: role, performance, skills, capacities and environment; case scenarios

Conceptual overview

The first three sections of this book looked at the structure and functions of the tissues that make up the musculoskeletal and the nervous systems, the mechanics of the joints of the body, the bony architecture and ligamentous support that determines the range and limitation of movement; the organisation and strength of the muscles surrounding the joints, and the way in which areas of the brain harmonise these muscle groups to perform the movements and skills that make up the performances of everyday occupations. This chapter will specifically address the significance of occupational performance in more detail through the presentation of a series of case scenarios.

Tyldesley & Grieve's Muscles, Nerves and Movement in Human Occupation, Fourth Edition. Ian R. McMillan, Gail Carin-Levy.
© 2012 Ian R. McMillan, Gail Carin-Levy, Barbara Tyldesley and June I. Grieve. Published 2012 by Blackwell Publishing Ltd.

Introduction

People are occupational beings. From very early childhood they explore the world around them to discover the ways in which they can learn about, manipulate, utilise and dominate their environment. From first waking up in the morning, getting out of bed, washing and dressing, preparing and eating breakfast, communicating and responding to all surrounding stimuli; these are all occupations. The group of Canadian occupational therapists who developed the Canadian Occupational Performance Measure (Law *et al.*, 2005) devised an exercise to direct colleagues and students towards an understanding of the concepts of everyday occupational performance. This exercise suggests that you sit down with a friend, preferably someone who is not a fellow student. Each of you should take a clean piece of paper and, starting in the bottom, left-hand corner, write down the time as it is at the moment. Above that write down each previous half hour until you have covered 24 hours. Next think back and list all the things you have done in the past 24 hours. Once you have made your list, identify those occupations that you consider to have been carried as a result of habit, and those that you have judiciously or spontaneously decided upon. Now make a summary.

- How many of your occupations were directed towards looking after yourself?
- How many were related to your current work?
- Were some of them part of your leisure?

Go through your list and work out how much time you spend on each category of occupation. Would the result be different if the list was made in term time compared with the weekend or holiday?

Compare your list with that of your friend. How similar are your lists and the categories of occupations? Is your interpretation of work and leisure the same as that of your friend? If you were 10 years younger what differences would there be in your average daily occupations? This exercise highlights the importance of our everyday occupational performance, and how each person may have a different interpretation of their everyday occupations. For example, cooking may feel like work for one person, but pleasurable leisure to another. Whereas a mother may enjoy and look forward to bathing her baby, a carer may consider this aspect of the working day as arduous.

Framework for understanding human occupation

At this point it would be helpful to reflect on a framework to organise your thinking, when interacting with individuals who have occupational performance problems in daily life.

The core values and beliefs about human occupation are located within a paradigm of occupation and these ideas are articulated fully within the study of Occupational Science (Clark & Zemke, 1996) which studies the importance of the relationship between occupation and human beings. The occupational role issues (e.g. mother, worker, friend etc.) that people experience and how to intervene can be located in different models of human occupation, for example the Model of Human Occupation (MOHO) (Kielhofner, 2007), the Canadian Model of Occupational Performance-Enablement (CMOP-E) (Townsend & Polatajko, 2007) and the Kawa Model (Iwama, 2006) to name but a few. These and other models of human occupation share similar concepts in relation to the factors that need to be considered for understanding the occupations of an individual, these are broadly:

- **occupational roles**: identifies the perceived roles held by the individual;
- **occupational performance**: identifies the particular performances, relating them to self-care, work and productivity, and leisure;
- **occupational performance skills**: identifies the motor and process skills required to perform the occupations;
- **occupational performance skill capacities** that underlie the maintenance of performance skills, including sensorimotor, cognitive and pyschosocial aspects;
- **environment**: identifies how the individual interacts with the temporal, physical (architectural), social and cultural environments, and their spiritual response to their present existence.

Occupational role

A person's occupational life is closely linked to the roles that they fulfil in everyday living. An individual may play a number of roles in one day, for example acting as a mother, employee, carer and wife at different times of the day. Another example could be the roles of flatmate, friend, student, teammate and lover. Behaviour and occupational lifestyle can be determined by the roles that an individual is called upon to fulfil, and these will also have an effect on occupational performance. When one is highly motivated performance may be enhanced, for example preparing a meal for a much-loved friend. Conversely, a task that is routine or boring may be performed less effectively, for example in the role of homemaker, doing the ironing may be a tedious task.

Occupational performance

Each human occupation has a level of performance that must be achieved in order to be effective. Problems caused by trauma, disease or arrested development affect performance in many different ways. The changes may present in areas of mobility, manipulation, cognitive function or social interaction. Refer back to the summary of your own daily occupations, of which some were self-care, some work and productivity, and others leisure.

- The daily occupations relating to **self-care** would include dressing, feeding, grooming, toileting, bathing/showering and using transportation.
- **Work and productivity** would include finding and keeping a job, voluntary/unpaid work, education at school or university, instructive play, cleaning the house, doing the ironing, etc.
- **Leisure** occupations include visiting and socialising, reading, sport, travel, hobbies and crafts whether individually or in a group.

A therapist, in conversation with a client, will be able to elicit the client's interpretation of daily occupations, a process that may assist in the understanding of the particular client's motivation and attitude towards aspects of the problems in everyday life.

Occupational performance skills

The level of skill required to perform occupations is different between tasks. A computer operator must achieve a high level of manipulative skill in operating the keyboard and the mouse. As well as manipulation, other important skills in the operation of a computer would be:

303

- **motor skills**, including positioning, stability and alignment; bending, reaching and gripping;
- **process skills**, including the ability to choose, enquire, continue, organise and terminate.

The assessment of motor and process skills (Fisher, 2010) can take place during performance of the client's chosen occupation of daily living, giving the therapist essential information on the impact that the client's condition has had upon their everyday life.

Occupational performance skill capacities

Occupations depend on the basic processing and integration of all the information entering the nervous system from the world around us, which then activates the correct motor performance. Sensorimotor processing is also the basis for cognitive processing which allows people to make decisions, to modify performance, and to recall past experience of successful outcomes. These capacities are:

- sensory awareness, sensory processing and perceptual processing;
- higher cortical functions of cognition and strategic planning;
- psychosocial components related to psychological, social and self-management skills, for example, how people express their values and interests, conduct themselves with others in a social gathering and manage their time during the day.

Environment

The environment has an important effect on occupational performance. An older person who can function reasonably well in their own home may be unable to be independent if he or she has to move to a different environment. The presence of steps, a slippery floor or a gravel path can all interfere with safe and confident walking. A soft chair, a low bed and the absence of adequate heating can impede successful independent living. Adaptation of the environment may be a major factor in assisting an individual to learn to perform effectively. The components of the environment to be considered are as follows:

- **Temporal factors**, including the context of the client's past, present and possibilities for the future, may influence the time it takes to complete an occupation and the capacity of the client to sustain effort for the period involved.
- The **physical architectural environment**, that is the layout of the area and objects within it. This may vary in different situations, which may alter the patterns and strategies needed to perform an occupation.
- The **social environment** can have a marked effect on performance, for example being watched and assessed increases performance stress and may interfere with normal sequencing.
- The **cultural environment** plays a significant role in performance, influencing the way that an occupation may be carried out and the tools and equipment used.

An individual's spiritual response to each of the performance components may have an effect on the sense of the meaning and purpose of occupations. For example, feelings of self-esteem and personal dignity, responsibility and personal courage, and other personal spiritual beliefs may be important.

Case scenarios

Chapter 13 analysed the core positions and movement patterns of an individual that underpin occupational performance skills..

Here, performance skills are extended into occupation, identifying the many interactive factors that may have an influence. These include: the role of the individual within a family and work context, personal motivation, and the motor and process skills required for particular tasks. These are the factors that a therapist can assess and learn to assemble to assist an individual to learn to improve performance, or to take advantage of assistive devices and adaptive methods of performance in their daily lives.

Case scenario exercises

Six case scenario exercises have been devised to encourage the reader to use this book as a source of reference and to apply thought to the way in which a therapist might direct intervention and advice to assist a client. It is suggested that you form a small group with your colleagues and discuss and think through each case scenario and, using the framework given below, put together ideas related to working with each client.

Format for discussion

1. **Referral information**: to be read carefully, making suitable notes.
2. **Therapist's knowledge**: reference guidance for the revision of the topics being studied.
3. **Preparation for the initial interview**: roles and important aspects of the client's issues that will need to be considered.
4. **Therapist's approach**:
   (i) occupational performance: self-care, work and productivity, leisure;
   (ii) environment and possible adaptations;
   (iii) spiritual aspects.
5. **Comments and future management**, for example:
   (i) psychological effects;
   (ii) medical and surgical management;
   (iii) long-term outcomes.

By working in a group, you will have the opportunity to discuss each case scenario and share ideas. Each exercise will provide the referral information from which the important facts can be ascertained. The relevant normal structure and function of the systems involved should be revised from chapters in the book, together with information given in the practice note-pads. A summary of the background information should be prepared in case the client wants more knowledge of the condition and to equip the therapist for in-depth discussion with other members of the multidisciplinary team. Each client will have a personal approach to the problems that may arise as a result of disease, injury or developmental delay, and the members of the discussion group may have a number of differing ideas. A summary of what actually occurred in each case scenario is presented in Part II. It will be interesting for you to compare your thoughts with this summary, it must be remembered that in the 'real world' the client would respond to the therapist during conversation. The conclusions in the summary may be different from those reached by the group. However, the important part of this exercise is the process of working through the case and preparing adequately for early conversations with the client.

Comment

The approaches and conclusions to the case histories that are presented reflect the ideas of the authors and advisors **and do not relate to specific theoretical models of occupational therapy**. You as the reader are encouraged to consult textbooks and articles that describe and comment on the utility of different models of occupational therapy (see Duncan, 2011). The importance of readers' participation in these exercises is to ensure that you undertand the significance of the the biological and biomechanical capacities alongside the psychosocial, intellectual and environmental issues that may influence the healing and/or coping process. The Canadian Occupational Performance Measure (Law *et al.*, 2005) has been used to guide the reader into thinking about the social, domestic and spiritual aspects of clients' responses to incapacity and the way in which the environment can impinge upon these dimensions of living. The Assessment of Motor and Process Skills (Fisher, 2010) has been cited to alert the reader to the complex interplay of factors that determine the way in which occupational performance skills are carried out. We trust you will find these exercises helpful and that they help you to consider the broader influences on clients' health and everyday occupations.

PART I

Part I begins with an example of a case scenario that has been written to demonstrate how to tackle the other six.

Example case scenario

Information

Kathleen is a 64-year-old librarian in full-time employment with the District Council Library Service. Recently, she has been feeling discomfort and aching in the area of the groin and the front of her thighs, which becomes more acute as she climbs stairs. She discussed this with her husband, a retired businessman, who said it was probably due to her age. Her daughter, a pharmacist at the local hospital, thought otherwise and suggested that Kathleen talk to the family doctor. The doctor thought that Kathleen may have osteoarthritis and he arranged for her to have an X-ray at the local hospital. The letter from the radiologist confirmed his suspicions, saying that Kathleen has osteoarithitic changes in both hip joints and some possible changes in the sacroiliac joints. Kathleen expressed distress at this diagnosis as she had planned her retirement, in 18 months time, to include active grandparenting, working to renovate her garden and planning visits to the National Trust houses and gardens. Because he realised her potential problems her doctor referred her to the community occupational therapist for advice and help.

Therapist's knowledge

Osteoarthritis is a process of degeneration due to the wear and tear on specific joints of the body. (Refer to the hip joint in Chapter 8 and Practice note-pad 1B.) The hip joint is the joint that transfers the weight of the trunk, head and upper limbs to the floor by means of the lower limbs. (Refer to Chapter 13, standing and walking.) Those people who stand for most of their working lives are therefore more prone to this problem, for example teachers, shop assistants, waitresses and librarians. The syndrome is characterised by inflammatory incidents around and within the joints, and particularly within the bursae surrounding the joints. Pain is felt in areas not related to the joint location and is often at its worst in the early hours of the morning and particularly following a busy day. Kathleen's interests are noted by the therapist and she expects to mention these quite early in her discussion with Kathleen.

Therapist's preparation for an initial interview

Looking at the referral, the occupational therapist was able to ascertain that Kathleen was married, and from the address realised that she probably lived in a 1930s semidetached house in the suburban part of the town, quite close to shops but a long way from the town centre. As a married woman Kathleen would fulfil the roles of wife, mother, grandmother (according to the referral), gardener, organiser and a member of a work team. She had worked throughout her life and was someone who was familiar with books and resource information. She would know how to co-operate within a team of employees, for example sharing the workload, working conditions, holiday requests and problems relating to sickness leave.

Therapist's approach

The therapist makes an appointment to talk with Kathleen and asks her about her feelings relating to the recent diagnosis. Kathleen expresses anxiety about her condition and how to deal with it, particularly the possible changes in her roles, but wishes to continue working until she reaches retirement age. The therapist asks how much Kathleen knows about osteoarthritis, and offers further information about bursae and their assistance in muscle action around a joint and why they may become inflamed in the course of the disease. The therapist also suggests that Kathleen find a nursing medical book in the reference library to find out for herself about the hip joints and the surrounding muscles. Kathleen has been taking the new anti-inflammatory drugs, prescribed by her doctor, but that she stills wakes up in pain in the early morning.

Self-care

The therapist suggests that she might try taking her medication at night, instead of the morning, and in this way she should gain the maximum benefit throughout the night. A suggestion is that Kathleen keep a working diary for a month so that she develops an awareness of the situations that may increase the discomfort. For example, is her favourite chair suitable for relaxation or should it be higher and firmer, with better back support? Is her bed easy to get in and out of, is it firm enough? What effect do long periods of standing or long periods of sitting have on her levels of discomfort?

Work and leisure

At work there will be tasks that will allow her to sit down for some of the time. Kathleen could discuss her problems with her colleagues and between them they should be able to organise her contribution to the library work, making the most of her capabilities and experience. In what ways could she tackle her gardening work most effectively? The therapist understands that Kathleen will gain a fuller understanding of her own condition than any outsider, and by encouraging Kathleen to monitor her own progress, she may come to recognise factors of cause and effect, and will therefore become more able to cope with the day-to-day management of the disease and any deterioration over time.

Environmental adaptations

Certainly the therapist will be able to offer ideas that have been tried in the past, such as the use of a kneeling stool for gardening (and even for locating all sorts of objects on low shelves throughout the kitchen and house). She may also discuss Kathleen's driving experience and whether she feels able to continue driving her car. An automatic car may be easier for Kathleen to drive and the therapist might suggest that she takes a test drive to ascertain the advantages or otherwise of making this change. The provision of a high stool to obviate the long standing periods when cooking, washing-up, ironing or working in the greenhouse may be of great assistance, and when she is visiting National Trust properties she should monitor how long she can cope with walking and standing before taking a rest.

Future management

The therapist asks Kathleen about her feelings relating to her future and the changes that will, in time, take place. Will she find the psychological resources to cope with the inevitable restrictions on her life and the possibility of asking others to support her on occasions? Relating to the future, the therapist will be able to give her information concerning total hip replacement and its outcomes, which may be needed if the pain becomes more intense and intolerable.

Further case scenarios

The next six case histories are designed for group discussion (Figure 14.1). The referral information about the case and an indication of the relevant knowledge related to the client's condition are given. Part II presents what actually occurred, so that the outcome of the discussions can be compared.

Case scenario 1: Mabel; the ageing process

Information

Mabel aged 75, is a widow of some years. She has a caring and supportive family of 10 children, all married and living nearby, who see her regularly, bring in hot meals and helping out with her heavier household tasks such as changing the bedding, vacuum cleaning and cleaning windows. Mabel has some hearing impairment but is otherwise a bright, assertive, independent person. She lives in a four-bedroomed terraced house, but has recently put her name down to be rehoused in a bungalow. She was admitted to hospital with fracture dislocation of both malleoli of the right ankle and torn ligaments of the left ankle. It seems that she thought that she had heard the front doorbell, then it rang again and she jumped up quickly and fell. After 3 weeks' postoperative hospitalisation she was discharged to her daughter's home, where a bed was put downstairs for her. At this stage Mabel was partially weight-bearing and using a Zimmer walking frame. At the follow-up clinic 3 weeks later Mabel was referred to the community physiotherapist, and after 2 weeks of physiotherapy treatment Mabel was gaining in confidence and started to work on going up stairs with a view to having a bath. At this time she expressed the wish to return home but her daughter was anxious and doubtful about her ability to manage on her own. The community occupational therapist was asked to carry out an assessment of bathing and kitchen tasks in preparation for her return to her own home.

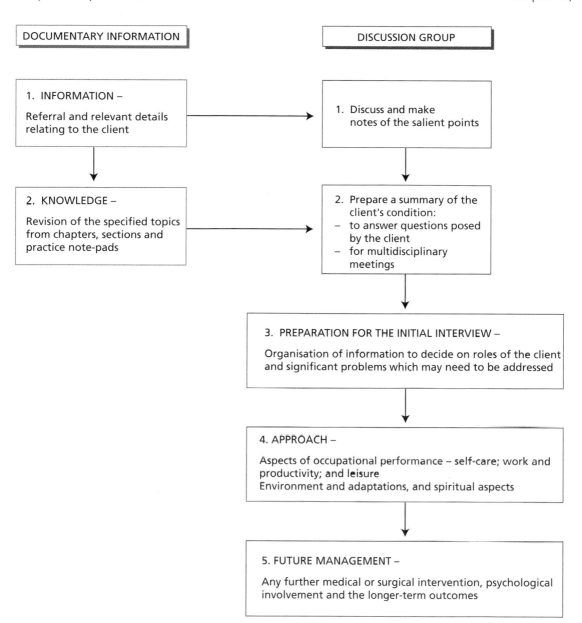

Figure 14.1   Plan for case scenario discussion.

Therapist's knowledge

Refer to Chapter 8, the ankle joint, muscles that move it and the foot. Also refer to Chapter 13, reaching and retrieving, sitting to standing, walking, and going up and down stairs.

Case scenario 2: Mary; Parkinson's disease

Information

Mary is a 72-year-old retired dentist who has lived above the practice in a second-floor flat for 35 years. She retired at the age of 60 and maintained contacts with colleagues until 12 months ago. She went to see her doctor 2 years ago, as she felt stiffness in her right arm and leg and had noticed that her handwriting was becoming smaller. Following referral to a neurologist a diagnosis of Parkinson's disease was confirmed. At this stage a dopamine agonist was prescribed and she coped well on this, remaining independent until 3 months ago when her muscle stiffness increased and she was aware of slurring of her speech. A fall at home precipitated her admission to hospital. Mary was then sent to the local neurological centre, where she was confirmed as being medically stable and was transferred to the elderly medical rehabilitation ward, with the aim being to review her medical management and rehabilitation assessment relating to her ability in independent living.

Therapist's knowledge

Refer to Chapters 3 and 12, the basal ganglia, and Practice note-pad 3G.

Case scenario 3: John; traumatic brain injury

Information

John aged 20 was recently involved in a road traffic accident and sustained a traumatic brain injury (TBI). John spent a few days in intensive care and then 4 weeks in an acute medical unit. He is now beginning his rehabilitation with the multidisciplinary team. Before this accident, John was independent in all aspects of his occupational lifestyle. John appears to have multiple problems at this stage, including physical, cognitive, psychological and social.

The occupational therapist decides to establish contact with John's mother to gain more information. John's mother explains that he currently lives at home with his parents in a bungalow along with his younger brother. John has a girlfriend and they were thinking about becoming engaged and renting a flat in the immediate future. John works as a van driver delivering goods to shops around the city where he lives, and enjoys his job because he likes driving and is interested in cars. He also participates in sports and socialising with his friends.

Therapist's knowledge

Refer to Chapter 3, central nervous system, the brain and spinal cord, practice note-pads 3B–F, and Chapter 13, patterns of movement in functional positions.

TBI is usually seen as damage to brain tissue caused by mechanical forces. This damage may occur both at the primary site of impact (when he struck his head) and as the result of secondary complications, for example, contusions, lacerations and the effects of shearing and rotational forces through the brain tissue causing diffuse axonal damage. This can result in a complex picture where the individual will display multiple problems.

The nature of these multiple problems in TBI may be observed in John's occupational performance and this can be traced back to the underlying performance components. John may have some or all of the performance component problems identified in Practice note-pad 3F.

Case scenario 4: Patrick; hand injury

Information

Patrick, aged 47, has been referred to the occupational therapist following an operation to correct Dupuytren's contracture to the left little and ring fingers. He has bilateral contractures and is right hand dominant, but the left hand was more severely affected. At present, Patrick's little and ring fingers of the right hand are flexed to 120 degrees at the metacarpophalangeal joints and the proximal interphalangeal joints, which does not interfere with his ability to obtain a power grip, but is a nuisance when he is washing and dressing. Patrick's left hand was first operated upon 8 years ago, when he gained good extension of the ring finger but very limited extension in the three joints of the little finger. During the period since his first operation contracture of the left-hand little finger has increased to such an extent that a second operation has been necessary. Patrick works for the Water Board and in his first years was employed as a labourer using pneumatic drills and other vibrating tools. At this time he sometimes developed 'white finger' if he used the equipment for a long period and, because of this, he asked to be transferred to lighter work. At present he works in the sewage branch, tending valves, hosing down areas and monitoring the machinery. Patrick wishes to return to work. His wife has a part-time clerical job and his children are at school, one in the lower sixth form and the other is approaching examinations. Patrick is a keen snooker player; in the past he played for his club in the local league but in recent years he has been coaching younger members. He hopes that this second release of his left little finger will permit him to play once more for his club team.

Therapist's knowledge

Refer to Chapter 6, manipulative movements of the hand, Practice note-pad 6B, and Chapter 13, reaching and retrieving.

Case scenario 5: Christopher; spinal cord injury

Information

Christopher aged 40 has a 15-year history of spinal cord injury. Christopher originally injured his neck in a competitive sporting accident. He spent a few days in intensive care, where it became obvious to Christopher that he had 'broken his neck'. He then spent 8 months at a specialist unit for individuals with spinal cord injury. During his time at the rehabilitation unit he worked every day with various members of the multidisciplinary team including the occupational therapist to maximise his physical capacity, adjust psychologically and rebuild his life from an occupational point of view. Before his accident, Christopher was independent in all aspects of his occupational lifestyle.

Christopher is attending his annual check-up appointment at the spinal rehabilitation unit, where he will see the occupational therapist as part of this routine contact so that his occupational needs can be assessed and any intervention and management carried out.

The occupational therapist has been in the post for several years, and has met Christopher before, and is aware that Christopher sustained a fracture of his sixth cervical vertebra during his accident and this has caused damage to the spinal segment C6/7 of his spinal cord. The therapist also knows that the majority of individuals who sustain this damage are young males who are frequently involved in accidents on the road, at work or, as in Christopher's case, occasionally playing sport. The damage sustained at the level of C6/7 implies that Christopher is functionally tetraplegic, although a large amount of variation can be perceived in different people with the same level of injury. Through reading his notes the therapist remembers that Christopher has a partner, lives in a ground-floor flat, works part time and drives a car.

Therapist's knowledge

Refer to Chapter 3, control systems: the brain and spinal cord, Practice note-pads 4C and 11A, and Chapter 13, lying, rolling and sitting.

Case scenario 6: Susan; chronic pain

Information

Susan is a 28-year-old secretary who injured her back some 10 years ago when out jogging with a friend. At that time, she was recommended to rest, take painkillers prescribed by her doctor and stay off work for 3 months.

Over the past 10 years increasing levels of pain have impinged on her occupations and motor skills in terms of bending, walking and lifting heavy objects. Her pain originally started in the lumbar region of her back but now appears to have spread up to her neck and sometimes involves her upper and lower limbs to some extent. Her current levels of pain affect all of her occupational performances with respect to self-care on occasions. She has had frequent sick leave from work and especially from leisure activities, which has meant that she has withdrawn from various social pursuits. During this 10-year period she has consulted her doctor and hospital specialists regarding the condition of her lumbar spine. She has been prescribed various drugs, been given advice about posture, taken regular exercise, worn numerous surgical corsets and received physiotherapy on many occasions. These treatments have worked to some extent but have never been fully effective and she still reports the perception of pain to her doctor.

Susan has been married for 7 years and she and her husband would like to start a family, however she is fearful that her back condition may deteriorate and she doubts her potential ability to cope with a baby. In summary, Susan feels anxious about her future, guilty about withdrawing from various occupations and concerned that her life may be completely dominated by pain.

Therapist's knowledge

Refer to Chapter 11, interpretation of pain, Practice note-pad 11B and Chapter 13, posture in sitting.

The nervous system in some individuals appears to change over time in response to the initial injury and produce a 'maladaptive state'. This is the result of structural neuroplastic changes taking place in the nervous system created by chronic disease, in this case low back damage. The persistence of chronic pain originates in changes in the sensitivity of peripheral nociceptors in the low back and the transmission neurones of the adjacent area of the spinal cord, together with altered processing in the cerebral cortex. These changes in the neural pathways may outlast the original condition, which seems to be the problem in Susan's case. Susan's chronic pain can still be perceived even when the tissues have healed. The peripheral and central neuroplastic changes have created negative perceptions and led to Susan's occupational disengagement.

PART II

This section presents what actually occurred in the six case histories given in Part I.

Case scenario 1: Mabel; the ageing process

313

Refer to Part I for referral information and therapist's knowledge.

Therapist's preparation for the initial interview

Mabel, who had been an independent person before her admission and brought up 10 children in the house in which she now lives, is not finding it easy to be dependent on her daughter. There are her daughter's husband and two grandchildren who also live in the house and she feels that she is a burden, and that she would like to be back in her own home where she would be familiar with everything once more. The therapist realises that Mabel's roles are those of housewife, mother and mother-in-law, grandmother and friend.

Therapist's approach

Self-care

Mabel can dress and carry out her own personal care on a daily basis but she cannot bathe without assistance.

Work and productivity

Initially, Mabel was not keen to try a kitchen assessment in her daughter's home but the occupational therapist discussed a treatment plan for a written contract of achievement to be reviewed weekly with Mabel and her daughter, so that Mabel could build up confidence and strength over a suitable period. In this way her daughter would be assured of her capabilities and Mabel would have proved to herself that she could cope. The treatment contract would be progressive and would include all the aspects of Mabel's life that she enjoys:

- carrying out everyday kitchen tasks;
- using kitchen trolley in place of the Zimmer walking frame when working in the kitchen and carrying things into the living room;
- weight-bearing going up and down stairs;

- using the bath board and seat to assist both Mabel and her daughter in bathing. This equipment would, in time, be transferred to Mabel's home;
- practising reaching up to high and down to low cupboards to retrieve objects and put them away safely;
- visiting her home once a week with her daughter and carrying out the specified tasks, first practised in her daughter's home, and using the trolley and bath equipment in her own surroundings.

Leisure

Mabel enjoys going out in the car for shopping, to a place of entertainment or to see a friend.

For the first try-out of each aspect of the programme the therapist would be present, then the daughter would monitor and assist if necessary, and finally Mabel would achieve things on her own. The programme progressed quickly and well, with Mabel regaining her confidence and the daughter feeling reassured that her mother would be able live on her own once more. Recognising the cause of Mabel's accident the occupational therapist contacted the Deaf Society before recommending a trial stay at home for a weekend. An adapted telephone and doorbell with flashing lights were fitted, and a television amplifier. Mabel was offered a Piper Life Line Personal Alarm but she refused. She said that she had such regular visits from her family that this type of alarm was not necessary.

Future management

The trial went successfully and Mabel moved back into her own home. Mabel had already applied for rehousing in a bungalow, but bungalows as social housing are scarce, and once someone is rehoused in this type of accommodation they usually cope very well, therefore vacant ones are only infrequently available. It is hoped that Mabel will eventually move into accommodation that is on one level and easier to manage.

Case scenario 2: Mary; Parkinson's disease

Therapist's preparation for the initial interview

The occupational therapist realises that Mary will experience difficulty in initiating and adjusting movement, for example problems relating to moving across visual barriers, such as thresholds to doorways and painted lines on the roadways. As a professional person Mary will probably be able to understand her symptoms and this may cause an increase in apprehension as to her ability to overcome them. Mary is a single, independent person, with a few close friends. The slurring of speech has a detrimental effect socially, and the reduction in her ability to react with appropriate facial expression will compound this problem and her confidence. Mary is likely to experience increased fatigue and anxiety which will impede her ability to socialise as she had done in the past. Other aspects of Mary's illness that should be considered are potential disturbance in perceptual and cognitive function leading to slowness in thought processes, inattention, and impaired motor planning and spatial negotiation.

314

Therapist's approach

Mary is a determined person who has read carefully about her condition and its medical management and wishes to use every opportunity to increase her functional ability. She appreciates the way in which the therapist discusses matters with her, identifies specific aspects of her problems and offers solutions, and as a result she is both frank and honest about her difficulties. She reports that she can use the stairs to her flat without too much difficulty and can walk quite well with her Zimmer frame. Her main problem is negotiating doorways. To overcome this the therapist suggests that she practise walking on the spot and counting out loud before stepping forward, which will assist in allowing her to progress through a visual barrier.

Self-care

Following assessment in washing and dressing Mary was found to have some problems with standing tolerance, reduced fine finger control, limited ability to initiate movement and, as a result of this, an increased level of anxiety. The therapist helps her to overcome her anxiety, and therefore the extent of the tremor, by adopting a more relaxed position for dressing, for example sitting, choosing clothing that is easy for her to manage and by practising breathing exercises and self-pacing. This ensures that getting dressed is tackled in a more relaxed frame of mind, so giving a greater likelihood of success, the aim being to enhance her abilities and reduce tension. Similar techniques are adopted to assist her with eating, drinking, swallowing and speaking. Mary has also been referred to the speech and language therapist for specific treatment for these aspects of her condition.

Work and leisure

Mary is very keen to continue cooking, writing and using her computer, all of which have been interrupted by increased tremor. After a kitchen assessment Mary is advised to break her activities into shorter stages to avoid unnecessary fatigue. The use of a high stool in the kitchen is suggested, as well as a trolley for moving items. However, negotiating the trolley around the kitchen and other furniture proved to be more of a hindrance than an asset and was abandoned. Advice relating to positioning for writing, and adapted pen grips has assisted with writing and the use of a key guard and wrist support has meant that Mary can use her computer more effectively.

Cognitive and psychosocial aspects

Mary reports that she is having difficulty in recalling verbal information. She indicates that she finds that she cannot always concentrate and it was thought that this may be a result of apprehension and anxiety. The therapist suggests that she could compensate for this problem by the use of word association and imagery.

Mary has always been a very independent person and so becomes easily frustrated and often needs encouragement to focus on her positive achievements. On an intellectual basis she was able to accept the effect of anxiety and low mood on her performance, and is finding ways of thinking in a more constructive manner to help her to cope more effectively, and thus build up her self-confidence.

Medical management

Mary's drug regimen has been monitored. Changes were made to the dosage in medication by monitoring her own responses, and Mary has gained an awareness of the relationship between taking medication and the optimal time for most efficient mobility and functioning. This understanding has also assisted in recognition of the periods of reduced rigidity, increased movement initiation and swallowing.

Future management

Environmental factors

Mary had a home assessment before discharge from the rehabilitation ward. She feels that she has gained an improved level of mobility and greater control over the symptoms that occur in Parkinson's disease. She has been referred to the community therapy team for regular monitoring and has been given an appointment to see the neurologist in 6 months' time for review.

Case scenario 3: John; traumatic brain injury

Therapist's preparation for the initial interview

On receipt of the referral the occupational therapist remembers that a majority of individuals who sustain a TBI are young males in road traffic accidents and this is consistent with John's profile. The therapist is also aware that a young man like John will probably have multiple problems in relation to his injury and this will have some effect on his occupational performance for some time.

Following the important conversation with his mother it can be seen that John occupies the roles of son, brother, worker, partner and friend.

Therapist's approach

The occupational therapist decides to make contact with John in the rehabilitation unit, where initially she finds communication with John difficult, as he appears slightly confused about the time, his location, his interests and occupational performance up to the point of his accident. At times he seems agitated and frustrated, and unable to concentrate long enough to sustain a conversation. His speech sounds slurred, especially when he reports being tired. John is beginning to appreciate that he has been in a serious accident and that he may require rehabilitation for some time. The therapist is aware that these problems will have implications for John's occupational performance and his relationship with his girlfriend and family.

Self-care

John is beginning to wash and dress with assistance and take some interest in his appearance, although he lacks motivation regarding shaving and brushing his teeth and requires prompting to do so. He is managing to control his limbs and is also beginning to express a desire to choose certain clothes rather than being passive about the process. Through conversation with the therapist, John has expressed an interest in living independently with his girlfriend. This will need close and detailed work with John's girlfriend so that she understands John's problems (especially cognitive and behavioural problems), so that realistic, informed and shared progress can be made. The therapist would educate both of them together through John's occupations so that issues about motivation, understanding and concentration would be discussed. A collaborative plan of occupations that John could complete independently would be necessary, for example helping his girl-friend to prepare meals, washing the dishes afterwards and being involved in planning more social interaction with friends. Other problems that may interfere with John's everyday life are issues such as poor sleep patterns, staying up at night and wanting to sleep during the day, frequent headaches and the possibility John may suffer a single or frequent seizures. Seizure activity may undermine John's confidence in his abilities and requires compliance with medication that can have serious side-effects, especially if mixed with alcohol.

Work and leisure

John has also informed the occupational therapist that he wishes to return to his job as a van driver in the city. This may be problematic, since John is legally unfit to drive at present. The Driver and Vehicle Licence Authority regulations state that John would not be able to drive for at least 6 months to 1 year, depending on the severity of his TBI. The therapist knows that a driving centre is available at the local brain injury unit and that, when appropriate, John could be tested formally for competence. If driving was ultimately ruled out the occupational therapist could liaise with John's employer to assess whether John could return to work undertaking a different role in dis-patching goods in the company stores. Another possibility would be to suggest that John return to some form of education or training course so that he can learn new skills.

Leisure pursuits may also require some management, since John may not be motivated to resume his interests or interact with friends, or he may display inappropriate behaviour, for example becoming uncharacteristically angry in public.

Environment

John may not require any devices within his home environment to assist mobility and other aspects of his life, but he may have difficulties maintaining his environment because of lack of motivation and apathy. In order to engage meaningfully in his occupations he may need help from the therapist and his girlfriend and family to structure his day.

Future management

John will require contact with the occupational therapist for some time, especially when he goes home and thinks about his future. Ultimately, John's initial physical impairments may resolve and the major issues for future management might be centred on cognitive, behavioural and long-term relationship issues.

Case scenario 4: Patrick; hand injury

Therapist's preparation for the initial interview

The left hand is the support hand in a right-handed person, but with the little finger in a flexed position this hand is unable to open out sufficiently to employ a power grip. If Patrick is to return to work he must be able to use both his hands to operate the pressure hose and to turn the wheels that open and close the valves. The therapist will carry out a functional assessment of his upper limb and a sensory test to the ulnar side of the hand, as this area of the hand can be vulnerable to burns and other forms of injury. Work will be targeted at maintaining and increasing extension at the metacarpophalangeal (MCP), and distal and proximal interphalangeal (DIP and PIP) joints of the little finger, and discouraging the formation of scar nodules in the area of the hypothenar eminence.

Therapist's approach

During the interview the occupational therapist asks Patrick to take off his coat and his shoes and put them back on again. This allows the therapist to assess the function of the upper limb and the extent to which the flexed fingers of both hands interfere with normal dressing tasks. This exercise may be repeated at each visit to reassess normal function. The therapist also asks him about other coping strategies that he employs when carrying out everyday activities and may advise him of ways in which mobility of the left little finger could be encouraged. Patrick will be very much involved in the initial treatment of his left hand, massaging the scar area, trying to achieve active extension and assisting the process with passive extension exercises to improve occupational function of the little and ring fingers. The therapist assesses the sensation on the medial border of the hand and discovers that he does not have two-point discrimination, is unable to detect hot and cold, but can feel deep pressure and, as this has occurred since the surgery, it may remain or improve. The therapist supplies him with a night resting splint to overcome undue flexion during sleep and a three-point active extension orthosis to maintain and/or increase little finger extension, while allowing active flexion. (Note. It will be important for the therapist to emphasise that gentle stretching is the way to achieve success and that the apparatus should not be used too vigorously and thereby cause tearing of the soft tissue. Tearing causes scar tissue to form, which in turn will be prone to contract.) The night resting splint may be remoulded at each visit to the occupational therapy department to ensure that the increase in extension is maintained. Once the scar has stabilised, which should take 6 weeks, Patrick could return to work. He must be careful in his observation and work practice to protect the ulnar side of the hand, and not to carry heavy bags or equipment in the left hand to avoid shearing damage to the skin on the medial border. Furthermore, it would be sensible for him to continue to wear the night resting splint and practise extension of the finger for 3–6 months until scar maturation is established. In relation to snooker, the left hand gives the bridge support and regular play should reinforce a pattern of extension in the DIP and PIP joints of the left little finger.

Case scenario 5: Christopher; spinal cord injury

Therapist's preparation for the initial interview

Recovery of function at the level of C6/7 is variable and observations of Christopher's occupational performance will give a clear picture of his present status. The therapist is aware that the roles that Christopher occupies are those of partner, worker, brother and friend.

Therapist's approach

The occupational therapist makes contact with Christopher in the rehabilitation unit. He is a very positive outgoing individual who has worked hard to overcome the majority of his occupational performance problems by various means. Christopher is sitting in his wheelchair, which he can self-propel along flat surfaces and to some extent up small gradients without assistance. He uses 'palm mitts' to protect the skin on his hands when propelling his chair. His sitting balance in his chair is very competent and he does not require thoracic supports. He can operate the brakes independently, and he has learned how to remove the chair armrests independently, since this is required to fit his chair under a desk.

Self-care

Christopher's day starts when he wakes up in his special bed, which has an air mattress and is capable of turning him without assistance, so helping to prevent the risk of pressure sores. Christopher can move in bed to some extent by hooking his elbow into flexion through the handle of a monkey pole mounted above the bed. He is mostly dependent on his partner for his dressing needs, however he can wash and shave his face independently. Christopher spends a lot of the day in his wheelchair, which is very important to him and is fitted with a special gel cushion. While sitting in his chair, Christopher manages to lift himself sufficiently to relieve pressure from his bottom every so often, reducing the development of pressure sores. In terms of self-care, the occupational therapist reinforces that prevention of skin abrasions or potential sores is of the utmost priority. Christopher is relatively independent in feeding and drinking. Although he finds exerting pressure when cutting food difficult, he can manage everything else. Insulated mugs prevent him from sustaining burn damage to his hands when drinking coffee or tea.

319

Work and leisure

Christopher had worked for the same insurance company for many years before his accident, and his employer, with assistance from the occupational therapist, was keen to facilitate his return to work. Christopher now works part time so that he does not become unduly fatigued over the space of a week. The therapist reinforces the technique of pacing and energy conservation whenever possible. Christopher's current work duties include using a computer, answering the phone and talking directly to the public in the office. He uses a standard computer, keyboard and monitor. He has learned how to use the equipment without recourse to any special adaptations, by using a pen to tap the keys. He does not want any specialised devices or orthoses for his hands. When sitting behind a desk, people cannot see his wheelchair and this is important to Christopher, since he does not want to be treated any differently from other staff by the public. As the office is all on the level and the entrance to the front door only has a slight inclination, Christopher can move freely about his work space. He uses his own car to travel to work, which has been especially adapted with hand controls for accelerating and braking, and has a wrist support and handle mounted on the steering wheel to facilitate turning. The car also has an automatic gearbox and power steering. He has a hands-free mobile phone for emergencies. Christopher uses a sliding board to transfer from his wheelchair to car and vice versa. Although he is independent when driving, he requires assistance in terms of another person folding and loading his chair into the boot of his car. His partner fulfils this role at his home when he leaves for the office. In the parking area attached to his office one of his colleagues unloads and positions his wheelchair for him to transfer independently. The occupational therapist, in discussion with Christopher, mentions that a work site visit could be made to assess his place of work, and that this, together with liaison with his employer, could identify any further environmental adaptations that would increase his independence. Application to the local Disability Service Team, based at Job Centre Plus, could facilitate improvements by recommending government funding for the necessary work or equipment.

Christopher does not have any problems related to his leisure pursuits; occasionally he will research the possibility of cinemas and restaurants being wheelchair accessible.

Environment

Following his discharge Christopher moved into a new flat and therefore, before moving in, he had an opportunity to modify the environment with help and advice from the occupational therapist and the builder. Christopher and his partner live on the ground floor. A small ramp was fitted at the front entrance to facilitate access. All of the internal doors were widened slightly to facilitate his wheelchair comfortably. All of the electrical sockets were moved up from the floor to a reasonable height so that Christopher could use them sitting in his wheelchair. The bathroom has a special lifting device to facilitate transfers in and out of the bath, and Christopher's partner uses a small mobile hoist to lift Christopher onto and off the toilet in order to empty his bowel. A special inflatable rubber ring is fitted over the toilet seat to prevent pressure sores. Christopher's bladder management involves the use of a sheath and leg bag to collect urine, which is then emptied during the day.

Parking at home has not been a problem up until very recently, and the therapist suggests that Christopher might want to consider applying to the local council for permission to have a designated disabled space nearer his flat.

One aspect that has recently revolutionised Christopher's life was the purchase, assisted by the occupational therapist, of a home computer with a grant from a charitable sporting organisation. This new computer is connected to the Internet and this helps Christopher to exert more control over various aspects of his life. Internet shopping is particularly helpful, especially for food from the local supermarket, which is delivered from the store to his kitchen. He can now pay all of his bills via the Internet and set up other banking facilities. He has also started to look for holiday accommodation in Britain that could cater for his special needs. Other uses of the Internet are to research information about rights for the disabled, products from special disability companies and the details of the Disability Discrimination Act.

Future management

Christopher believes that life is going well, however from a practical and spiritual point of view he recognises that skin problems, bladder or other infections could have a serious effect on his current and future level of independence. The therapist encourages him to continue to monitor his skin condition, especially on his bottom, and reminds him that he should request assistance for help with the maintenance or replacement of any assistive devices or adaptations when necessary. Christopher is aware that he should pay attention to these aspects of everyday life and rejoice in the independence he has so far achieved.

Christopher's partner works part time from home and she is the principal carer who also requires support. Although Christopher is very independently minded, he needs to be aware that his partner may need assistance to manage the situation, for example some form of home help or care assistants to carry out more of the regular duties associated with keeping Christopher independent in the future.

Case scenario 6: Susan; chronic pain

Therapist's preparation for the initial interview

The occupational therapist is aware that Susan now experiences chronic pain, as it is 10 years since the initial tissue damage took place. The therapist also remembers that pain is ultimately a perception and although Susan started with low back pain, it now affects her whole life, her personality and the manner in which she copes. It is important for the therapist to gain an impression of Susan's past and present occupations and to gauge the degree of disengagement from her occupations over the past 10 years. The therapist also realises that Susan will never be cured of her pain in the medical sense of the term and that she will need to learn to manage the effects of her pain on her occupational lifestyle. Susan's roles are those of wife, daughter, worker and friend.

Therapist's approach

The occupational therapist quickly senses that Susan is somewhat disillusioned with the healthcare system with regard to past attempts at 'curing' her pain. The therapist affirms the belief that Susan continues to have chronic pain despite no tissue damage being demonstrated on medical testing, this being entirely consistent with a thorough knowledge of the neural mechanisms of pain. The therapist explains the neural mechanisms of pain and chronic pain to Susan, so that she can appreciate what has happened and what will happen to her nervous system in the future. The principal therapeutic aim is to alter Susan's cognition and behaviour, through engagement in more occupations, to create neuroplastic changes and positive changes in Susan's perceptions. Susan tells the occupational therapist that she is fearful of further injury to her back and that she 'holds' herself in awkward postures to prevent people banging into her and causing further damage. The therapist reassures Susan that pain is not necessarily a sign of further damage or degeneration of her back and that holding certain postures may make the pain worse, because of increased muscle tension. From a spiritual perspective Susan admits being afraid of the future and does not see much chance of getting rid of the pain or even starting a family. This is a difficult belief to confront. From a professional perspective, it is unlikely that Susan will ever be cured. However, if she can learn to manage the effects of her pain in her life, she will regain more control and increased confidence. Susan will be encouraged to re-engage in her occupations through the use of various techniques advocated by the Pain Society, for example self-pacing, goal setting, education about pain, learning to relax, becoming more aware of her body mechanics, posture and physical reconditioning. Susan acknowledges that she has reduced her occupational engagement over the years and feels very physically and mentally unfit. The therapist will encourage Susan to engage in previous and new occupations that will help her to recondition her muscles and improve her endurance and self-esteem. The therapist knows that when Susan feels more in control, change will occur in her perceptions, and she may then be more able to think about starting a family.

Self-care

Susan does not have major self-care problems in terms of undertaking performances such as dressing, feeding and putting on make-up, however she does report fatigue and exacerbation of pain at times during these occupations, which means that at times she cannot be bothered to do them. On other days, she feels much better and attempts to do a lot to compensate fearing that she may not be able to complete things the next day. In this way she is demonstrating the typical error of the overactivity/rest cycle, doing too much on good days and nothing on bad days. The therapist explains about pacing performance during occupations, doing less than she is capable of achieving in her chosen occupations over a specified period, irrespective of how she feels. This will mean that Susan will begin to engage in her self-care occupations every day, rather than only on some days as before. This technique, energised by her occupations, should improve her self-esteem and perceived success, and increase her perception of control. Education on good and poor body mechanics when carrying out occupations such as ironing, loading the washing machine and making the bed will assist in reducing muscle tension and fatigue. Similarly, Susan also has to learn to pace herself when she experiences feelings of stress in anticipation of cleaning the house, and she can learn to conserve energy by pacing her own involvement and by delegating certain household tasks to her husband.

Work

This is a difficult area for Susan since she has a long record of absence from work because of her pain. She feels guilty about letting people down and, because of this patchy record, being perceived by her work colleagues as not accepting responsibilities for projects at work. The occupational therapist carries out a work site evaluation to assesses Susan's computer work station. Various changes regarding her chair, the height of her monitor and other small modifications that ought to prevent her back pain becoming worse are recommended. The therapist also advises her to pace herself at work, by regularly changing her posture, standing up occasionally and learning to implement her newly acquired relaxation techniques.

Leisure

Susan feels that she no longer has anything in common with her social circle of friends. She now gains very little enjoyment from her leisure and has gradually given up running, playing tennis and horse-riding, since all of these tend to make her pain worse. The occupational therapist could teach Susan relaxation techniques so that during leisure activities, she could decrease muscle tension and increase perceptions of the feelings associated with comfort. She could also use mental imagery to divert her cognitive processes from pain. Susan could be encouraged to apply her new problem-solving skills by setting small, manageable goals, so applying self-pacing techniques with the aim of returning to one of her leisure pursuits.

Environment

This is a contentious area for the therapist. Susan has been using various devices to assist her occupations in the past, becoming more dependent on devices and adaptations over time. The belief is that overreliance on these devices reinforces negative perceptions of pain and encourages the maladaptive behaviours associated with pain. As Susan learns to manage the effects of her pain more efficiently, she should be encouraged to give up using devices.

Future management

To reinforce the approach of the occupational therapist it may be beneficial for Susan to attend a specifically structured programme along with other individuals with chronic pain. This would help Susan to appreciate that chronic pain is relatively common in the population, and that individuals who have chronic pain tend to have similar thought processes and exhibit maladaptive behaviours regarding pain. Staff who work on pain management units hold common sets of beliefs and messages about pain to help people to manage their pain. Susan would also see other people improving in terms of performing more occupations, and this would reinforce the perception of efficacy of pain management.

Conclusion

This concludes the case scenario exercises. The authors hope that you have found them interesting and challenging and that you feel you have learned how to use the information in this book to guide you in your preparation for work with future clients by undertanding occupational performance skills and capacities in more detail.

References

Clark, F. and Zemke, R. (1996) *Occupational Science: The Evolving Discipline*, F.A. Davis, Philadelphia.

Duncan, E.A.S. (2011) *Foundations for Practice in Occupational Therapy*, 5th edn, Elsevier Churchill Livingstone, Edinburgh.

Fisher, A.G. (2010) *Assessment of Motor and Process Skills*, 7th edn, Three Star Press, Fort Collins.

Iwama, M.K. (2006) *The Kawa Model: Culturally Relevant Occupational Therapy*, Churchill Livingstone Elsevier, Edinburgh.

Kielhofner, G. (2007) *A Model of Human Occupation: Theory and Application*, 4th edn, Lippincott Williams & Wilkins, Baltimore.

Law, M., Baptiste, S., Carswell, A., McColl, M., Polatajko, H. and Pollock, N. (2005) *Canadian Occupational Performance Measure*, 4th edn, Canadian Association of Occupational Therapists, Ottowa.

Townsend, E.A. and Polatajko, H.J. (2007) *Enabling Occupation II: Advancing an Occupational Therapy Vision for Health, Well Being & Justice through Occupation*, Canadian Association of Occupational Therapists, Ottawa.

Further reading

Abrahams, P.H., Boon, J.M. and Spratt, J.D. (2008) *McMinn's Clinical Atlas of Human Anatomy*, 6th edn, Mosby Elsevier, St. Louis.

Agur, A. and Daley, A.F. (2009) *Grant's Atlas of Anatomy*, 12th edn, Lippincott, Williams & Wilkins, Philadelphia.

Andrew, W.A.A.A., Garden, J.O., Bradbury, A.W., Forsythe, J.L.R. and Parks, R.W. (2007) *Principles and Practice of Surgery*, 5th edn, Churchill Livingstone, Edinburgh.

Atchison, B. and Dirette, D.K. (2007) *Conditions in Occupational Therapy: Effect on Occupational Performance*, 3rd edn, Lippincott, Williams & Wilkins, Philadelphia.

Bray, J.J., Cragg, J.A., MacKnight, A.D.C., Mills, R.G. and Taylor, D. (1999) *Lecture Notes on Human Physiology*, 4th edn, Blackwell, Oxford.

Bundy, C., Lane, S.J. and Murray, E. (2002) *Sensory Integration: Theory and Practice*, 2nd edn, F.A. Davis, Philadelphia.

Caillet, R. (1994) *Hand Pain and Impairment*, 4th edn, F.A. Davis, Philadelphia.

Carr, J. and Shepherd, R. (2010) *Neurological Rehabilitation: Optimising Motor Performance*, 2nd edn, Churchill Livingstone, Edinburgh.

Clancy, J. and McVicar, A. (2009) *Physiology and Anatomy for Nurses and Healthcare Practitioners a Homeostatic Approach*, Hodder Arnold, London.

Clark, F. and Zemke, R. (1996) *Occupational Science: The Evolving Discipline*, F.A. Davis, Philadelphia.

Cohen, H. (1999) *Neuroscience for Rehabilitation*, 2nd edn, Lippincott, Williams & Wilkins, Philadelphia.

Colledge, N.R., Walker, B.R. and Ralston, S.H. (2010) *Davidsons Principles and Practice of Medicine*, 21st edn, Churchill Livingstone, Edinburgh.

Duncan, E.A.S. (2011) *Foundations for Practice in Occupational Therapy*, 5th edn, Elsevier Churchill Livingstone, Edinburgh.

Durward, B.R., Baer, G.D. and Rowe, P.J. (1999) *Functional Human Movement: Measurement and Analysis*, Butterworth Heinemann, Oxford.

Ekman-Lundy, L. (2002) *Neuroscience: Fundamentals for Rehabilitation*, 2nd edn, Lippincott, Williams & Wilkins, Philadelphia.

Everett, T. and Kell, C. (2010) *Human Movement: an Introductory Text*, 6th edn, Churchill Livingstone, Edinburgh.

Fisher, A.G. (2010) *Assessment of Motor and Process Skills*, 7th edn, Three Star Press, Fort Collins.

Floyd, R.T and Thompson, C. (2004) *Manual of Structural Kinesiology*, 15th edn, McGraw-Hill, London.

Grieve, J. and Gnanasekaran, L. (2007) *Neuropsychology for Occupational Therapists: Cognition in Occupational Performance*, 3rd edn, Blackwell, Oxford.

Hall, S.J. (2006) *Basic Biomechanics*, 5th edn, McGraw-Hill, Singapore.

Iwama, M.K. (2006) *The Kawa Model: Culturally Relevant Occupational Therapy*, Churchill Livingstone Elsevier, Edinburgh.

Kielhofner, G. (2007) *A Model of Human Occupation: Theory and Application*, 4th edn, Lippincott Williams & Wilkins, Baltimore.

Kiernan, J.A. (2005) *Barr's The Human Nervous System*, 8th edn, Lippincott, Williams & Wilkins, Philadelphia.

Kingsley, R.E. (1999) *Concise Text of Neuroscience*, 2nd edn, Lippincott, Williams & Wilkins, Baltimore.

Kingston, B. (2005) *Understanding Muscles: a Practical Guide to Muscle Function*, 2nd edn, Nelson Thornes, Cheltenham.

Law, M., Baptiste, S., Carswell, A., McColl, M., Polatajko, H. and Pollock, N. (2005) *Canadian Occupational Performance Measure*, 4th edn, Canadian Association of Occupational Therapists, Ottowa.

Lehmkulh, L.D., Smith, L.K. and Weiss, E.L. (1995) *Brunnstrom's Clinical Kinesiology*, 5th edn, F.A. Davis, Philadelphia.

Lovallo, W. (2004) *Stress and Health – Biological and Psychological Interactions*, 2nd edn, Sage, Beverly Hills.

Main, C.J. and Spanswick, C.C. (2000) *Pain Management – an Interdisciplinary Approach*, Churchill Livingstone, Edinburgh.

Melzack, R. and Wall, P.D. (1985) *The Challenge of Pain*, Basic Books, New York.

Nair, M. and Peate, I. (2009) *Fundamentals of Applied Pathophysiology: an Essential Guide for Nursing Students*, Wiley-Blackwell, Chichester.

Neirynck, J. and Garey, L. (2009) *Your Brain and Your Self: What You Need to Know*, Springer, Berlin.

Netter, F.H. (2003) *Atlas of Human Anatomy*, 3rd edn, Teterboro, New Jersey.

Orrison, W.W. (2009) *An Atlas of Brain Function*, Thieme, New York.

Palastanga, N., Field, D. and Soames, R. (2006) *Anatomy and Human Movement*, 5th edn, Butterworth Heinemann, Oxford.

Robinson, S.E. and Fisher, A.G. (1996) A study to examine the relationship of the Assessment of Motor and Process Skills (AMPS) to other tests of cognition and function. *British Journal of Occupational Therapy*, 59(6), 260–263.

Rothwell, R. (1994) *Control of Voluntary Movement*, 2nd edn, Chapman & Hall, London.

Seeley, R., Stephens, T. and Tate, P. (2004) *Essentials of Anatomy and Physiology*, 5th edn, McGraw-Hill, New York.

Shumway-Cook, A. and Woollacott, M.J. (2011) *Motor Control: Translating Research into Clinical Practice*, 4th edn, Lippincott, Williams & Wilkins, Philadelphia.

Solomon, L., Warwick, D. and Nayagam, S. (2005) *Apley's Concise System of Orthopaedics and Fractures*, 3rd edn, Arnold, London.

Stirling, J. and Elliot, R. (2008) *Introducing Neuropsychology*, 2nd edn, Psychology Press, Hove.

Stone, R. and Stone, J. (2002) *Atlas of Skeletal Muscles*, 4th edn, McGraw-Hill Publishing, New York.

Strong, J., Unrah, A.M., Wright, A. and Wall, P.D. (2002) *Pain: A Textbook for Therapists*. Churchill Livingstone, Edinburgh.

Tortora, G. and Derrickson, B. (2010) *Essentials of Anatomy and Physiology*, 8th edn, Wiley-Blackwell, Chichester.

Tortora, G.J. (2011) *Principles of Anatomy and Physiology*, 13th edn, John Wiley & Sons, Inc., Hoboken.

Townsend, E.A. and Polatajko, H.J. (2007) *Enabling Occupation II: Advancing an Occupational Therapy Vision for Health, Well Being & Justice through Occupation*, Canadian Association of Occupational Therapists, Ottawa.

Watkins, J. (2009) *Functional Anatomy*, Churchill Livingstone Elsevier, Edinburgh.

Wirhed, R. (1997) *Athletic Ability and the Anatomy of Human Motion*, 2nd edn, Mosby, St Louis.

Appendix I
Bones

Right clavicle – superior aspect

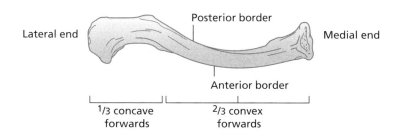

Lateral end

Posterior border

Medial end

Anterior border

1/3 concave forwards

2/3 convex forwards

Right scapula – anterior aspect

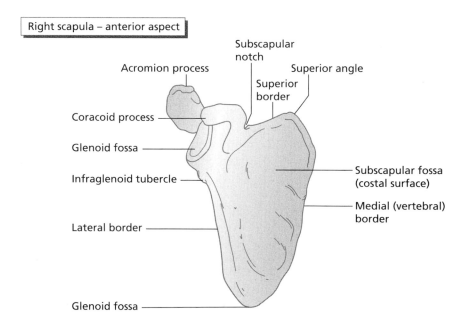

Acromion process

Subscapular notch

Superior angle

Superior border

Coracoid process

Glenoid fossa

Infraglenoid tubercle

Subscapular fossa (costal surface)

Medial (vertebral) border

Lateral border

Glenoid fossa

Tyldesley & Grieve's Muscles, Nerves and Movement in Human Occupation, Fourth Edition. Ian R. McMillan, Gail Carin-Levy.
© 2012 Ian R. McMillan, Gail Carin-Levy, Barbara Tyldesley and June I. Grieve. Published 2012 by Blackwell Publishing Ltd.

Right clavicle – inferior aspect

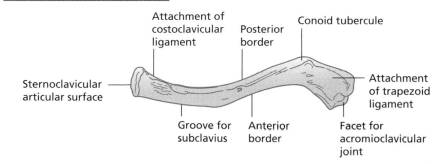

Attachment of
costoclavicular
ligament

Posterior
border

Conoid tubercule

Sternoclavicular
articular surface

Attachment
of trapezoid
ligament

Groove for
subclavius

Anterior
border

Facet for
acromioclavicular
joint

Right scapula – posterior aspect

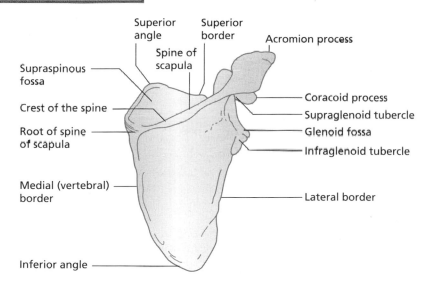

Superior
angle

Superior
border

Acromion process

Spine of
scapula

Supraspinous
fossa

Coracoid process

Crest of the spine

Supraglenoid tubercle

Root of spine
of scapula

Glenoid fossa

Infraglenoid tubercle

Medial (vertebral)
border

Lateral border

Inferior angle

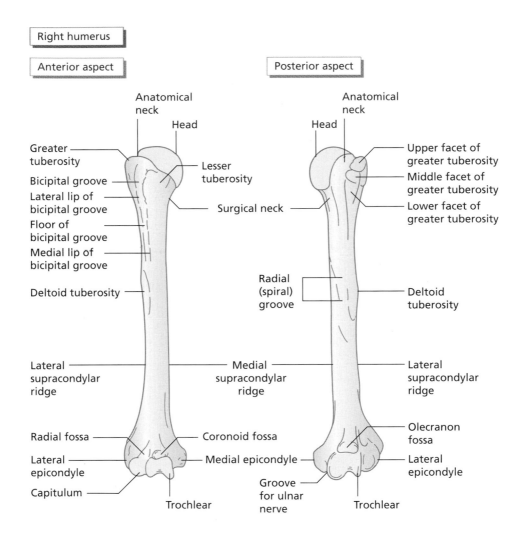

Right humerus

Anterior aspect

Posterior aspect

Anatomical neck

Head

Anatomical neck

Head

Greater tuberosity

Bicipital groove

Lateral lip of bicipital groove

Floor of bicipital groove

Medial lip of bicipital groove

Deltoid tuberosity

Lesser tuberosity

Surgical neck

Upper facet of greater tuberosity

Middle facet of greater tuberosity

Lower facet of greater tuberosity

Radial (spiral) groove

Deltoid tuberosity

Lateral supracondylar ridge

Medial supracondylar ridge

Lateral supracondylar ridge

Radial fossa

Lateral epicondyle

Capitulum

Coronoid fossa

Medial epicondyle

Trochlear

Olecranon fossa

Lateral epicondyle

Groove for ulnar nerve

Trochlear

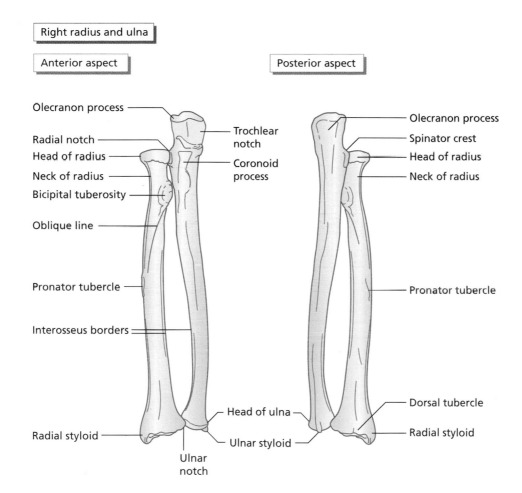

Right radius and ulna

Anterior aspect   Posterior aspect

Olecranon process ——————   —————— Olecranon process
                                —— Trochlear   —————— Spinator crest
Radial notch ——————————   notch   —————— Head of radius
Head of radius ——————————   —————— Neck of radius
                                —— Coronoid
Neck of radius ——————————   process
Bicipital tuberosity ——————

Oblique line ——————————

Pronator tubercle ——————   —————— Pronator tubercle

Interosseus borders ——————

                                                    —————— Dorsal tubercle
                                —— Head of ulna   —————— Radial styloid
Radial styloid ——————————   —— Ulnar styloid
                        Ulnar
                        notch

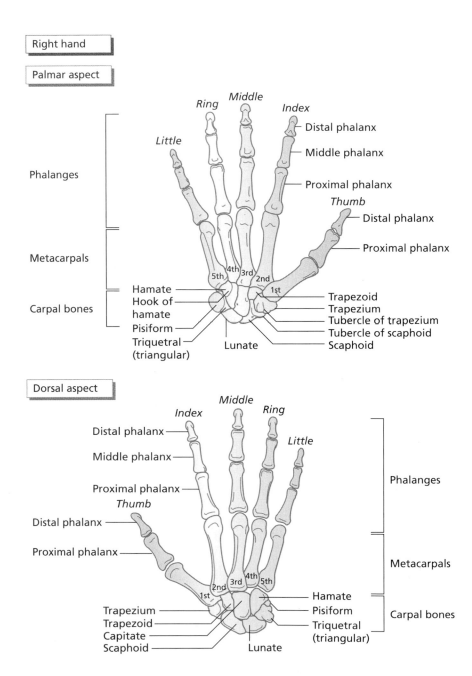

Right hand

Palmar aspect

Ring   Middle
Little   Index

Phalanges

Distal phalanx
Middle phalanx
Proximal phalanx
Thumb
Distal phalanx
Proximal phalanx

Metacarpals

5th 4th 3rd 2nd
1st

Carpal bones

Hamate
Hook of hamate
Pisiform
Triquetral (triangular)
Lunate

Trapezoid
Trapezium
Tubercle of trapezium
Tubercle of scaphoid
Scaphoid

Dorsal aspect

Index   Middle   Ring
Little

Distal phalanx
Middle phalanx
Proximal phalanx
Thumb
Distal phalanx
Proximal phalanx

Phalanges

1st 2nd 3rd 4th 5th

Metacarpals

Trapezium
Trapezoid
Capitate
Scaphoid
Lunate

Hamate
Pisiform
Triquetral (triangular)

Carpal bones

Pelvis

Anterior aspect

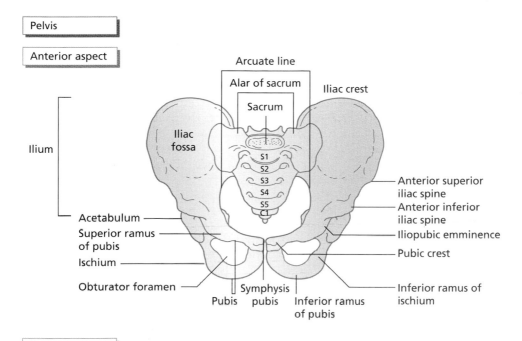

Arcuate line

Alar of sacrum

Iliac crest

Sacrum

Iliac fossa

Ilium

S1
S2
S3
S4
S5
C1

Anterior superior iliac spine

Anterior inferior iliac spine

Acetabulum

Superior ramus of pubis

Ischium

Obturator foramen

Iliopubic emminence

Pubic crest

Inferior ramus of ischium

Pubis

Symphysis pubis

Inferior ramus of pubis

Posterior aspect

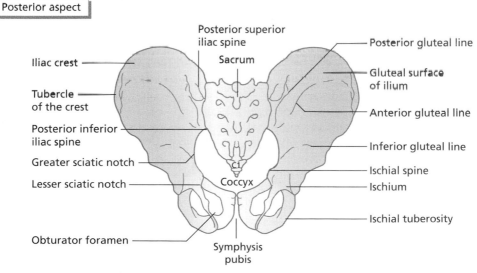

Posterior superior iliac spine

Sacrum

Posterior gluteal line

Iliac crest

Tubercle of the crest

Posterior inferior iliac spine

Greater sciatic notch

Lesser sciatic notch

Obturator foramen

Gluteal surface of ilium

Anterior gluteal line

Inferior gluteal line

Ischial spine

Ischium

Ischial tuberosity

C1

Coccyx

Symphysis pubis

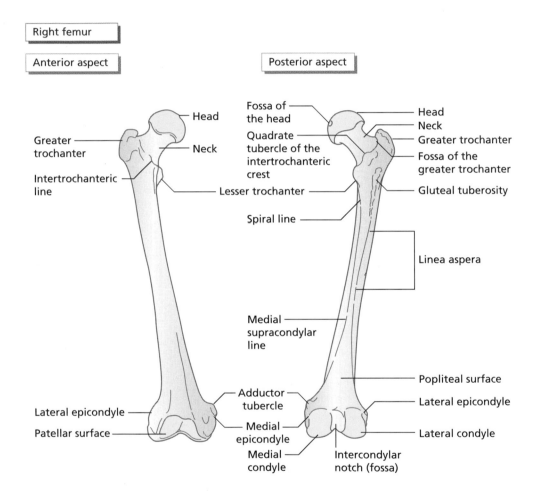

Right femur

Anterior aspect

Posterior aspect

Head

Greater
trochanter

Neck

Intertrochanteric
line

Fossa of
the head

Quadrate
tubercle of the
intertrochanteric
crest

Lesser trochanter

Spiral line

Head
Neck
Greater trochanter
Fossa of the
greater trochanter

Gluteal tuberosity

Linea aspera

Medial
supracondylar
line

Popliteal surface

Adductor
tubercle

Medial
epicondyle

Medial
condyle

Lateral epicondyle

Lateral condyle

Intercondylar
notch (fossa)

Lateral epicondyle

Patellar surface

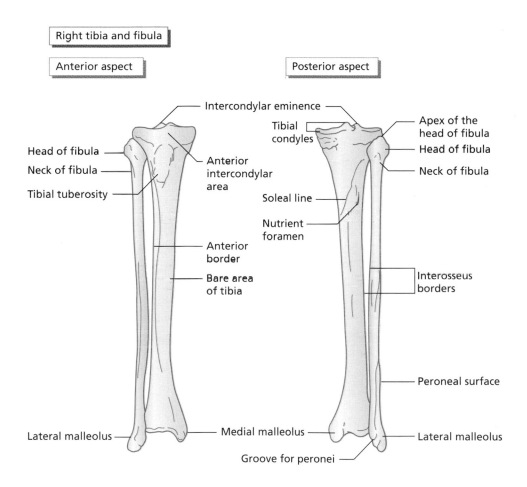

Right tibia and fibula

Anterior aspect

Posterior aspect

Intercondylar eminence

Head of fibula

Neck of fibula

Tibial tuberosity

Anterior intercondylar area

Anterior border

Bare area of tibia

Lateral malleolus

Medial malleolus

Groove for peronei

Tibial condyles

Apex of the head of fibula

Head of fibula

Neck of fibula

Soleal line

Nutrient foramen

Interosseus borders

Peroneal surface

Lateral malleolus

Right foot

Lateral aspect

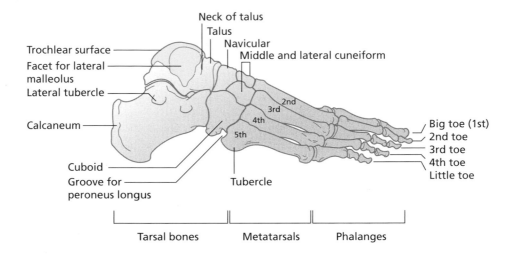

Neck of talus
Talus
Navicular
Middle and lateral cuneiform
Trochlear surface
Facet for lateral
malleolus
Lateral tubercle
Calcaneum
2nd
3rd
4th
5th
Big toe (1st)
2nd toe
3rd toe
4th toe
Little toe
Cuboid
Groove for
peroneus longus
Tubercle

Tarsal bones   Metatarsals   Phalanges

Medial aspect

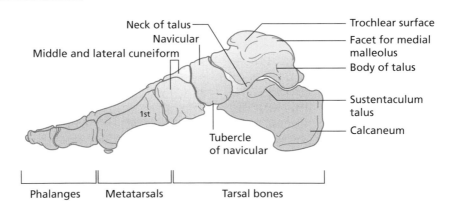

Neck of talus
Navicular
Middle and lateral cuneiform
Trochlear surface
Facet for medial
malleolus
Body of talus
1st
Sustentaculum
talus
Calcaneum
Tubercle
of navicular

Phalanges   Metatarsals   Tarsal bones

A typical (thoracic) vertebra

Superior aspect

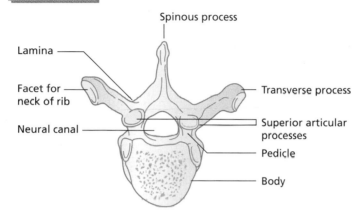

Spinous process

Lamina

Facet for
neck of rib

Neural canal

Transverse process

Superior articular
processes

Pedicle

Body

Lateral aspect

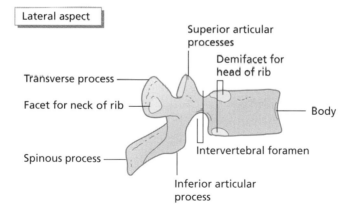

Superior articular
processes

Demifacet for
head of rib

Transverse process

Facet for neck of rib

Body

Spinous process

Intervertebral foramen

Inferior articular
process

Appendix II

Segmental nerve supply of muscles

Table A2.1 Cranial nerves.

I	Olfactory	Sensory from roof of the nose. Smell
II	Optic	Sensory from retina of the eye. Vision
III	Oculomotor	Motor to four of the muscles of the eye (superior, inferior and medial rectus, inferior oblique), motor to the sphincter muscle of the iris and the ciliary muscle of the lens
IV	Trochlear	Motor to the superior oblique eye muscle
V	Trigeminal	Sensory to the skin of the face and anterior tongue
		Motor to salivary glands and muscles of mastication (temporalis and masseter)
VI	Abducens	Motor to the lateral rectus eye muscle
VII	Facial	Sensory to anterior tongue. Taste Motor to muscles of the face and salivary glands
VIII	Vestibulocochlear	Sensory from vestibule. Balance
		Sensory from coclea of ear. Sound
IX	Glossopharyngeal	Sensory from posterior tongue. Taste
X	Vagus	Sensory and motor to pharynx, larynx, thoracic and abdominal organs
XI	Spinal assessory	
	Cranial root	Motor to the muscles of the pharynx and larynx
	Spinal root (C1–C5)	Motor to sternomastoid and trapezius
XII	Hypoglossal	Motor to muscles of the tongue

Note: Cranial nerves supplying muscles contain sensory proprioceptor fibres, except the facial nerve. Proprioception from facial muscles is carried in the trigeminal nerve

Tyldesley & Grieve's Muscles, Nerves and Movement in Human Occupation, Fourth Edition. Ian R. McMillan, Gail Carin-Levy.
© 2012 Ian R. McMillan, Gail Carin-Levy, Barbara Tyldesley and June I. Grieve. Published 2012 by Blackwell Publishing Ltd.

Table A2.2   Spinal nerves. Segmental origin in the spinal cord of the nerves supplying the muscle groups moving the limbs.

C5, C6	Shoulder	Abductors and lateral rotators
C5, C6, C7, C8		Flexors, extensors, adductors and medial rotators
C5, C6	Elbow	Flexors
C7, C8		Extensors
C5, C6	Forearm	Supinators
C6, C7, C8		Pronators
C6, C7, C8	Wrist	Flexors, extensors and deviators
C7, C8, T1	Digits	Long flexors and extensors
C8, T1	Hand	Intrinsic muscles
L2, L3	Hip	Flexors
L2, L3, L4		Abductors
L4, L5, S1		Extensors, medial and lateral rotators and abductors
L2, L3, L4	Knee	Extensors
L4, L5, S1, S2	Flexors	
L4, L5, S1	Ankle	Dorsiflexors
L4, L5, S1, S2		Plantarflexors
L4, L5, S1	Foot	Invertors
L5, S1		Evertors
L5, S1, S2		Intrinsic muscles

Table A2.3 Segmental innervation of the muscles of the upper limb [after Basmajian, J. (ed.) (1980) *Grant's Method of Anatomy*, 10th edn, published by Williams & Wilkins].

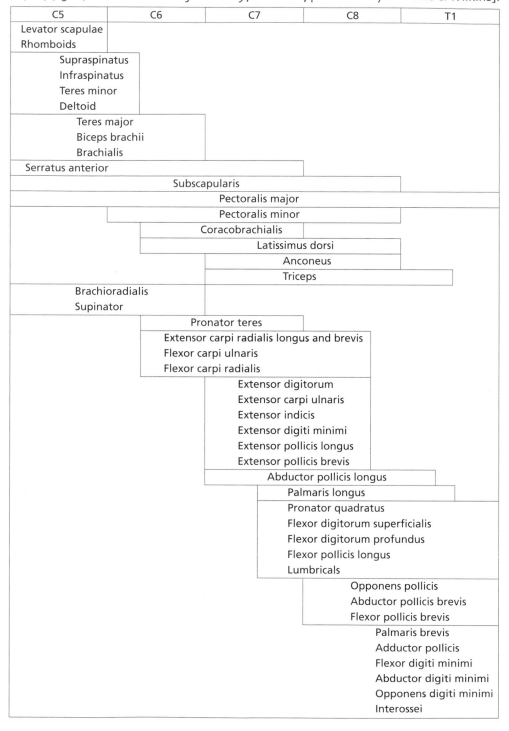

Muscle	C5	C6	C7	C8	T1
Levator scapulae	X				
Rhomboids	X				
Supraspinatus	X	X			
Infraspinatus	X	X			
Teres minor	X	X			
Deltoid	X	X			
Teres major	X	X	X		
Biceps brachii	X	X	X		
Brachialis	X	X	X		
Serratus anterior	X	X	X		
Subscapularis	X	X	X	X	
Pectoralis major	X	X	X	X	X
Pectoralis minor		X	X	X	
Coracobrachialis		X	X		
Latissimus dorsi		X	X	X	
Anconeus			X	X	
Triceps			X	X	X
Brachioradialis	X	X	X		
Supinator	X	X	X		
Pronator teres		X	X		
Extensor carpi radialis longus and brevis		X	X	X	
Flexor carpi ulnaris		X	X	X	
Flexor carpi radialis		X	X	X	
Extensor digitorum			X	X	
Extensor carpi ulnaris			X	X	
Extensor indicis			X	X	
Extensor digiti minimi			X	X	
Extensor pollicis longus			X	X	
Extensor pollicis brevis			X	X	
Abductor pollicis longus			X	X	
Palmaris longus			X	X	X
Pronator quadratus				X	X
Flexor digitorum superficialis				X	X
Flexor digitorum profundus				X	X
Flexor pollicis longus				X	X
Lumbricals				X	X
Opponens pollicis				X	X
Abductor pollicis brevis				X	X
Flexor pollicis brevis				X	X
Palmaris brevis					X
Adductor pollicis					X
Flexor digiti minimi					X
Abductor digiti minimi					X
Opponens digiti minimi					X
Interossei					X

Table A2.4   Segmental innervation of the muscles of the lower limb [after Basmajian, J. (ed.) (1980) *Grant's Method of Anatomy*, 10th edn, published by Williams & Wilkins].

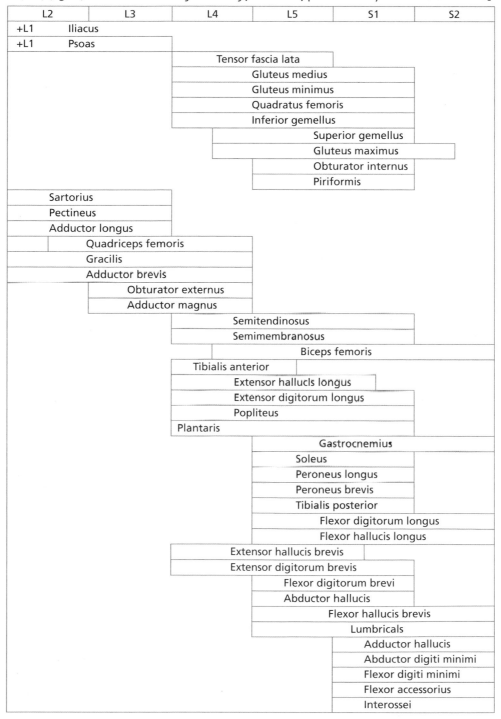

Muscle	L2	L3	L4	L5	S1	S2
Iliacus (+L1)	■	■				
Psoas (+L1)	■	■				
Tensor fascia lata			■	■		
Gluteus medius			■	■	■	
Gluteus minimus			■	■	■	
Quadratus femoris			■	■	■	
Inferior gemellus			■	■	■	
Superior gemellus				■	■	
Gluteus maximus				■	■	■
Obturator internus				■	■	
Piriformis				■	■	
Sartorius	■	■				
Pectineus	■	■				
Adductor longus	■	■				
Quadriceps femoris	■	■	■			
Gracilis	■	■	■			
Adductor brevis	■	■	■			
Obturator externus		■	■			
Adductor magnus		■	■			
Semitendinosus			■	■	■	
Semimembranosus			■	■	■	
Biceps femoris				■	■	■
Tibialis anterior			■	■		
Extensor hallucis longus			■	■	■	
Extensor digitorum longus			■	■	■	
Popliteus			■	■	■	
Plantaris			■	■	■	
Gastrocnemius				■	■	■
Soleus				■	■	
Peroneus longus				■	■	
Peroneus brevis				■	■	
Tibialis posterior				■	■	
Flexor digitorum longus				■	■	■
Flexor hallucis longus				■	■	■
Extensor hallucis brevis			■	■	■	
Extensor digitorum brevis			■	■	■	
Flexor digitorum brevi				■	■	
Abductor hallucis				■	■	
Flexor hallucis brevis				■	■	■
Lumbricals				■	■	■
Adductor hallucis					■	■
Abductor digiti minimi					■	■
Flexor digiti minimi					■	■
Flexor accessorius					■	■
Interossei					■	■

Glossary

abduction　　movement of a body segment that takes it away from the midline of the body in the coronal (frontal) plane.

action potential　　reversal of the membrane potential in a localised area of a neurone or muscle fibre due to the movement of charged particles (ions) across the membrane.

adduction　　movement of a body segment towards the midline of the body in the coronal (frontal) plane.

aerobic metabolism　　chemical reactions in the mitochondria of a cell that replenish ATP using oxygen and glucose.

afferent　　'towards', e.g. afferent (sensory) neurones carry impulses towards the central nervous system.

agonist　　the muscle primarily responsible for the intiation of a specific movement, also known as the prime mover.

allodynia　　the experience of pain from a stimulus that would not normally be harmful.

ampulla　　a specialised receptor area in one of the semicircular canals of the inner ear.

antagonist　　a muscle that opposes the action of the agonist (prime mover).

aponeurosis　　a broad sheet of dense fibrous tissue that: (i) attaches muscles to each other, e.g. abdominal muscles; (ii) forms the attachment of a muscle to bone, e.g. tensor fascia lata; or (iii) forms a protective layer for tendons, e.g. plantar aponeurosis.

arthroplasty　　replacement of a joint by an artificial one.

astereognosis　　inability to identify an object by manipulation in the hand without vision.

ataxia　　movement errors that include the inability to place a body part accurately, or to perform smooth, co-ordinated movement of the limbs.

Tyldesley & Grieve's Muscles, Nerves and Movement in Human Occupation, Fourth Edition. Ian R. McMillan, Gail Carin-Levy.
© 2012 Ian R. McMillan, Gail Carin-Levy, Barbara Tyldesley and June I. Grieve. Published 2012 by Blackwell Publishing Ltd.

ATP   (adenosine triphosphate) the major energy-storing molecule in the cells of the body.

autonomic nervous system   part of the peripheral nervous system that innervates cardiac and smooth muscle, and glands.

axon   main process of the neurone that conducts impulses away from the cell body to another neurone or an effector.

basal ganglia   subcortical motor nuclei that modulate the activity in the descending motor system.

body scheme   the perception of the position of parts of the body in space and their relationship to each other.

bouton   enlarged bulbous end of a terminal branch of an axon or dendrite.

brachial   related to the upper limb.

brain stem   a long cylindrical structure at the base of the brain leading to the spinal cord. There are three parts: midbrain, pons and medulla.

bursa   a closed sac of fibrous tissue, containing synovial fluid associated with the large joints. Bursitis is inflammation of a bursa.

capsule   the sleeve of dense fibrous tissue surrounding and uniting the ends of the bones in a synovial joint.

carpal   one of eight bones of the wrist, which link the radius and the ulna of the forearm with the metacarpals in the hand.

carpal tunnel   anatomical space on the palmar surface of the wrist for the long tendons passing from the forearm into the hand.

CAT scan   (computed axial tomography) A thin, fan-shaped X-ray beam views a 'slice' of the brain. The X-ray tube revolves round the patient so that the brain is viewed from all angles. A computer combines all the views, and the changes in soft tissue at the lesion site are revealed in a single image.

cauda equina   the lower spinal nerves that lie in the spinal canal below the level of the first lumbar vertebra.

central nervous system   division of the nervous system containing the brain and spinal cord.

centre of gravity	the point around which the body's weight and mass are equally balanced in all directions.
cerebral vascular accident	(CVA) a stroke: the term used to describe rapidly developing focal brain damage resulting from a reduction in blood flow (ischaemia) or a haemorrhage in the brain.
cerebrospinal fluid	circulates in the cavities of the brain, the central canal of the spinal cord and the subarachnoid space of the meninges.
circumduction	circular (conical) movement made by a body segment (not to be confused with rotation movement at a joint).
closed loop	motor control that uses feedback to make corrections during the progress of a movement.
cognition	the ability to organise and use knowledge about oneself and the environment to function effectively.
cognitive system	a complex system of interrelated parts that processes visual and spatial perception, attention, body scheme, memory and the executive functions.
collagen	fibrous protein found in connective tissue that has tensile strength.
concentric muscle work	active muscles shorten to produce a movement.
conduction velocity	the speed at which a neurone conducts impulses.
contracture	the permanent shortening of a muscle or tendon producing a deformity and limiting movement.
contralateral	the opposite side of the body.
corpus callosum	a thick band of axons connecting the right and left hemispheres in the forebrain.
corpus striatum	collective term used for the caudate, putamen and globus pallidus, which form the main components of the basal ganglia.
cortex	outer layer of an organ, e.g. surface grey matter of cerebral hemispheres or cerebellum.
cranial nerve	one of 12 pairs of nerves leaving the brain, which are sensory, motor or mixed.

depolarisation a change in the electrical potential across the membrane of a neurone, produced by the movement of charged particles (ions).

dermatome sensory innervation of one spinal nerve.

diaphysis the shaft of a long bone.

diencephalon part of the forebrain found buried deep in the cerebral hemispheres that includes the thalamus and hypothalamus.

dorsiflexion movement of the foot at the ankle joint that lifts the toes up towards the leg.

dysmetria inability to make active placement of a body part, e.g. touching the nose.

eccentric muscle work active muscles lengthening to control the effect of an external force, such as gravity.

efferent away from, e.g. efferent (motor) neurones carry impulses away from the central nervous system (motor).

epiphyseal plate cartilaginous layer between the epiphysis and diaphysis of long bone during growth in length.

epiphysis the end of a long bone that develops from a secondary centre of ossification.

equilibrium reaction a reflex response to a disturbance of balance, e.g. when the line of gravity of the body moves outside the base of support.

eversion movement in the joints of the foot that turns the sole of the foot outwards or laterally.

excitation changes in the membrane of a neurone that allows impulses to be propagated.

executive functions the mental operations involved in goal setting, organising, monitoring and completing action and behaviour.

extension return movement from flexion in the sagittal plane back to the anatomical position. Extensor muscles increase the joint angle or straighten a limb when they contract.

extrafusal fibres form the bulk of a skeletal muscle.

extrapyramidal system polysynaptic descending pathways from cortical and subcortical brain areas involved in motor control, balance and posture.

fascia lata	*see* **iliotibial tract**
fasciculus	bundle of muscle fibres or axons surrounded by fibrous connective tissue.
fast muscle fibres	(glycolytic, type II) generate energy from glycogen without oxygen. Specialised for short bursts of high-level muscle activity.
feedback control	the modification of action as it progresses based on changes in the environment.
feedforward control	the modification of the motor command for action before the movement is executed.
first-order neurone	the initial neurone in a sensory system that carries information from the receptors to the central nervous system.
flaccidity	state of hypotonia in muscles that is characteristic of lower motor neurone lesions.
flexion	movement in the sagittal plane that moves body segments towards each other.
force	(muscle) is generated by the tension in a muscle acting at its point of attachment to a bone.
forearm	body segment between the elbow and the wrist containing the radius and the ulna.
fusimotor neurone	innervates the intrafusal muscle fibres found inside a muscle spindle.
ganglion	a collection of the cell bodies of neurones located in the peripheral nervous system.
girdle	the bones that attach the limbs to the body; the pectoral girdle for the upper limb, and the pelvic girdle for the lower limb.
grey matter	collections of the cell bodies of neurones, their dendrites and the neuroglia cells that support them within the central nervous system.
gyrus	a raised area of cortex seen on the surface of the cerebral hemisphere or cerebellum.
hemianopia	'blindness' in part of the visual field of one or both eyes, originating in a lesion in the occipital lobe of the cerebral hemisphere.

hierarchy	the organisation of levels of neural processing in a ranked order in relation to one another.
hippocampus	a curved gyrus that lies deep in the medial temporal lobe, adjacent to the temporal part of the lateral ventricle, forming part of the limbic system.
homunculus	a representation of the parts of the body in the brain, usually drawn as a distorted image of a person.
hypertonia	muscle tone that is higher than normal which is felt as increased resistance to passive stretch of a limb.
hypothenar	muscles in the palm of the hand at the base of the little finger.
hypotonia	muscle tone that is lower than normal which is felt as decreased resistance to passive stretch of a limb.
iliotibial tract	(fascia lata) a band of dense fibrous tissue on the lateral side of the thigh, extending from the iliac crest to below the posterior aspect of the lateral tibial condyle.
impulse	(nerve) a localised change in the membrane potential in a neurone, which is self-propagating and travels down the axon in one direction only.
inhibition	a decrease in the excitability of a neurone so that no impulses can be propagated. The source of inhibition may be from presynaptic interneurones or the release of inhibitory neurotransmitter substances.
innervation	the nerve supply to a muscle or to an end organ or gland.
insertion	the distal or lateral attachment of a muscle to a bone that usually moves when the muscle contracts.
interneurone	a neurone in the central nervous system that has no branches in a peripheral nerve.
intrafusal muscle fibres	lie in a muscle spindle innervated by annulospiral (sensory) and fusimotor nerve endings.
inversion	movement in the joints of the foot that turns the sole of the foot inwards or medially.
ipsilateral	the same side of the body.
isometric (static) muscle work	active muscles that remain the same length to hold a position.

kyphosis   an increase in the primary thoracic curve of the spine, which may appear as rounded shoulders.

labyrinth (bony)   a system of tunnels within part of the temporal bone containing the utricle, saccule and semicircular canals of the inner ear.

lentiform nucleus   the putamen and globus pallidus of the basal ganglia.

lesion   focal damage of brain tissue, vascular in origin.

lever   a rigid bar (or bone) that moves about a pivot (fulcrum).

ligament   dense fibrous tissue that joins bone to bone around a joint in the form of a cord or band. The fibrous capsule that surrounds synovial joints is also known as a capsular ligament.

limbic system   a complex system of interconnected structures in the cerebral hemispheres and the diencephalon, including the cingulate gyrus of the medial cerebral cortex, and the hippocampus of the temporal lobe. The limbic system attributes emotional value to movement and behaviour.

lobe   discrete rounded part of an organ, e.g. the brain.

lordosis   an increase in the secondary lumbar curve of the spine, often referred to as hollow back.

lower motor neurone   originates in the anterior horn of the spinal grey matter and its axon supplies skeletal muscle fibres (also used to describe the neurones of cranial motor nerves).

lower motor neurone lesion   interruption of nerve impulses at any point in a lower motor neurone. The result is loss of muscle tone and of tendon reflexes.

macula lutea (fovea)   area of the retina of the eye opposite the lens where visual acuity is greatest.

mechanoreceptor   a receptor found in the skin that responds to touch and pressure stimuli. Those in the palm of the hand and the sole of the foot are important in the manipulation of objects, and for the balance of the body in standing, respectively.

membrane potential   the electrical potential due to the distribution of ions across a cell membrane.

meninges	the membranes that surround and protect the brain and spinal cord.
metacarpal	one of five bones found in the palm of the hand and the base of the thumb. The metacarpals join the distal row of carpals to the proximal phalanges of the fingers and the thumb.
metatarsal	one of five bones in the forefoot that link the distal row of tarsals with the proximal phalanges of the toes.
mitochondrion	a sausage-shaped structure with a double membrane, found in the cytoplasm of cells, forming the site of production of ATP.
mixed nerve	contains both sensory and motor axons.
modality	a system of receptors that respond to specific type of stimulus, e.g. tactile, visual, auditory.
modulation	the process by which the level of excitability of a group of neurones is changed. The base level of response may be raised or lowered in the short term or the long term.
moment of force	the product of the magnitude of a force and its distance from the fulcrum (centre of the joint).
momentum	of a moving body part, generated by muscle action, depends on the product of its mass and its speed of movement.
motor neurone	*see* **efferent**
motor programme	a plan for action that includes force, timing and sequence of muscle activity.
motor unit	one motor neurone in the spinal cord and all the muscle fibres supplied by it.
MRI	(magnetic resonance imaging) a strong magnetic field is produced by electromagnets distributed around the head. A radio pulse excites the hydrogen atoms in the water in the brain tissue. A computer translates the signals from the movement of the hydrogen atoms into an image, which identifies where lesions have occurred.
muscle fibre	multinucleated unit of structure of skeletal muscle.
muscle spindle	a complex receptor lying in parallel with skeletal muscle fibres that is stimulated by changes in muscle length.

muscle tone   the tension in a muscle resulting from background neural activity in the muscle stretch reflex. Clinically, muscle tone is felt as the resistance that is felt when passively manipulating the limb of a patient.

myelin sheath   a fatty layer surrounding the axon of some neurones that acts as an insulator and increases the rate of conduction of impulses.

myofibril   strand of protein along the whole length of a muscle fibre. There are several hundred myofibrils in each muscle fibre.

myofilaments   strands of actin and myosin, arranged in a particular way in a sarcomere.

myotome   all the muscles supplied by one spinal segment and its pair of spinal nerves.

nerve tract   bundle of parallel axons in the central nervous system carrying information towards (ascending) or away from (descending) centres in the brain.

neuroglia   support cells in the nervous system, other than neurones, which are not primarily involved in the propagation of nerve impulses.

neuromuscular junction   a specialised synapse between a motor neurone and a muscle fibre.

neuropathy   a pathology that affects the peripheral nervous system.

neuroplasticity   structural and biochemical changes in neurones that may establish new learning or restore function in the brain.

neurotransmitter   a specific chemical released by a presynaptic neurone that crosses the synaptic cleft and stimulates or inhibits the postsynaptic neurone.

nociceptor   a receptor responding to harmful stimuli that lead to the perception of pain.

nucleus pulposus   semi-fluid central portion of the intervertebral disc.

nystagmus   movement of the eyes from side to side with alternate slow and fast phases.

opposition   movement of the thumb that turns the pad or the tip of the thumb towards one or more fingers.

osteoblast   a bone-forming cell.

osteoclast   a cell that absorbs bone in remodelling during growth or repair.

pennate muscle   fasciculi of muscle fibres arranged diagonally along a common tendon like a feather.

perception   the integration of all the sensory information entering the brain to make a meaningful whole.

peripheral nervous system   the division of the nervous system that conducts information towards and away from the brain and spinal cord.

PET scan   (positron emission tomography) reveals the level of activity in the different areas of the brain over time. A solution containing a radioactive isotope is injected intravenously and accumulates in the brain in amounts proportional to the local blood flow. The positrons emitted by the isotope are detected by sensors placed around the head.

phalanx   a bone of a finger or toe (plural = phalanges).

pia mater   innermost layer of the meninges covering the brain and spinal cord.

plane of movement   an imaginary line of reference passing through the body in a particular direction used to describe movement.

  sagittal plane   passes through the body from front to back, dividing it into right and left halves. Flexion and extension movements occur in this plane.

  coronal (frontal) plane   passes through the body from top to bottom, dividing it into anterior and posterior halves. Abduction and adduction movements occur in this plane.

  transverse (horizontal) plane   passes through the body horizontally, dividing it into upper and lower parts. Rotation movements occur in this plane.

plantar flexion   movement of the foot at the ankle joint that points the toes downwards, or in standing, lifts the body on to the toes.

plaque   an area of demyelination in the central nervous system.

plexus   network of nerves or blood vessels branching and joining, e.g. brachial plexus.

popliteal fossa   posterior region of the knee.

power grip   all the fingers are flexed and the thumb is curled in the opposite direction around a handle or an object.

power (muscle) the product of force times speed of movement. A high level of muscle power is required for fast dynamic movement such as jumping and throwing.

precision grip the hand holds an object between the pads or the tips of the thumb and one, two or three fingers.

prime mover *see* **agonist**

processing a series of operations in the nervous system directed to some end. The output of the activity in a processing centre or neural network is relayed to other centres.

  serial processing occurs in centres that are arranged in serial order.

  parallel processing occurs simultaneously in different centres and the outputs are integrated in another centre.

pronation movement of the radius over the ulna in the forearm that turns the palm of the hand downwards or backwards.

proprioceptors the receptors lying in skeletal muscle, tendon and joints, which collectively respond to changes in the length and tension in muscle and the angulation of joints.

pyramidal system the monosynaptic descending pathway from the primary motor area to the lower motor neurones.

receptor a specialised area of membrane at the distal end of a sensory neurone, which responds to a specific stimulus.

reciprocal innervation the integration of spinal motor neurones to excite one muscle group and inhibit the opposing group.

red nucleus an area of grey matter in the midbrain receiving fibres from the cerebellum and projecting fibres into the rubrospinal tract for activation of the proximal muscles of the limbs in positioning movements.

reticular formation a diffuse network of neurones in the brain stem concerned with levels of arousal.

retinaculum a band of dense fibrous tissue that binds the tendons of muscles and prevents bowstring.

rigidity the resistance to passive movement over the whole range of movement at a joint, due to the presence of abnormal muscle tone.

sarcomere	the unit of the myofibril between adjacent Z-lines.
scoliosis	lateral curvature of the spine.
semicircular canals	thin tubes found in the inner ear with receptors responding to movements of the head in three planes.
sensory neurone	*see* **afferent**
sesamoid bone	found within a tendon, e.g. patella.
skeletomotor neurone	innervates skeletal muscle fibres.
slow muscle fibres	(aerobic, type I) generate energy from ATP in the presence of oxygen. Specialised for long periods of muscle activity without fatigue.
somatic	referring to the skin and the muscles.
somatosensory	the part of the nervous system concerned with information from the body, including the skin, muscles and joints.
spasticity	a pathological state of hypertonia.
spinal nerve	one of 31 pairs of nerves leaving the spinal cord. Each nerve is formed by the joining of an anterior and a posterior root from the spinal cord.
spinal segment	portion of the spinal cord that gives origin to one pair of spinal nerves.
stereognosis	the ability to identify an object by manipulation and without vision.
striate cortex	the area of the cerebral cortex on the medial aspect of the occipital lobe where processing of visual information occurs.
subarachnoid space	the space, filled with cerebrospinal fluid, between the arachnoid mater and the pia mater of the meninges.
substantia gelatinosa	a band of grey matter in the spinal cord round the apex of the posterior horn. The neurones form a spinal control mechanism in the transmission of nociception to the brain.
sulcus	(also known as a **fissure**) a groove or furrow between adjacent gyri on the surface of the brain.
supination	movement of the radius around the ulna that turns the palm of the hand to face upwards or forwards.

suture	a fibrous joint between the bones of the skull.
symphysis	a secondary cartilaginous joint where the bones are joined by fibrocartilage.
synapse	a junction between a neurone with another neurone, a muscle fibre or a cell of a gland, where the transmission of nerve impulses occurs.
synaptic cleft	the microscopic space between the membranes of the presynaptic and postsynaptic neurones at a synapse.
syndesmosis	the type of fibrous joint where the bones are a distance apart and they are connected by a sheet or band of fibrous tissue, e.g. middle radioulnar joint.
synergist	a muscle, other than the agonist or antagonist, whose activity assists in a movement.
synergy	co-ordinated activity in muscle groups acting over several joints to perform commonly occurring movements of a limb.
synovial fluid	viscous fluid secreted by the synovial membrane into the cavity of a joint or a tendon sheath.
synovial joint	the articulation of the ends of two bones that are separated by a joint cavity and surrounded by a fibrous capsule lined with a synovial membrane.
tarsal	one of seven bones that link the tibia and fibula of the leg with the bones of the forefoot (metatarsals and phalanges).
tectum	the roof of the midbrain.
tendon	a cord or band of dense fibrous tissue that unites muscle to bone.
tension	(muscle) force generated by an active muscle to produce movement, or to resist movement.
thalamus	the large oval mass of grey matter in the diencephalon on either side of the slit-like third ventricle.
thenar	muscles in the palm of the hand at the base of the thumb.
tremor	involuntary rhythmic contractions of agonist and antagonist muscles, commonly in the distal segments of the limbs. May occur at rest, or on initiation of a movement (intention tremor).
tubercle	a lump on a bone, created by muscle traction.

upper motor neurone	originates in a motor area of the brain that regulates the activity in lower motor neurones via descending pathways in the spinal cord.
upper motor neurone lesion	an interruption of conduction of nerve impulses at any point in upper motor neurones. The outcome is an exaggeration of reflexes, abnormal movement patterns and changes in muscle tone.
ventricle	a cavity inside the brain filled with cerebrospinal fluid.
vestibule	the part of the inner ear with receptors responding to the position of the head with respect to gravity.
vestibulo-ocular reflex	the reflex movement of the eyes in the opposite direction to the movement of the head that maintains a constant image on the retina.
visceral	referring to internal organs.
visual field	the area of the visual world that is visible out of the eye in a given position.
white matter	the parts of the central nevous system that are mainly composed of collections of axons whose myelin sheaths glve a white appearance.
Z-line	the dark line seen by the electron microscope that marks the separation of adjacent sarcomeres in a myofibril.

Index

Tyldesley & Grieve's Muscles, Nerves and Movement in Human Occupation, Fourth Edition. Ian R. McMillan, Gail Carin-Levy.
© 2012 Ian R. McMillan, Gail Carin-Levy, Barbara Tyldesley and June I. Grieve. Published 2012 by Blackwell Publishing Ltd.

Practice note-pad list

Tyldesley & Grieve's Muscles, Nerves and Movement in Human Occupation, Fourth Edition. Ian R. McMillan, Gail Carin-Levy.
© 2012 Ian R. McMillan, Gail Carin-Levy, Barbara Tyldesley and June I. Grieve. Published 2012 by Blackwell Publishing Ltd.